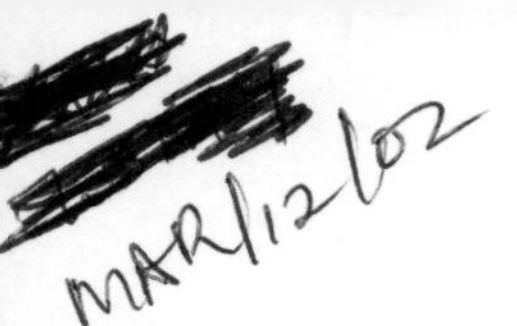

# Toxicology and Clinical Pharmacology of Herbal Products

# FORENSIC SCIENCE AND MEDICINE

***Steven B. Karch,*** *MD,* SERIES EDITOR

TOXICOLOGY AND CLINICAL PHARMACOLOGY OF HERBAL PRODUCTS,
edited by ***Melanie Johns Cupp,*** *2000*

CRIMINAL POISONING: *INVESTIGATIONAL GUIDE FOR LAW ENFORCEMENT, TOXICOLOGISTS, FORENSIC SCIENTISTS, AND ATTORNEYS,*
by ***John H. Trestrail, III,*** *2000*

A PHYSICIAN'S GUIDE TO CLINICAL FORENSIC MEDICINE,
edited by ***Margaret M. Stark,*** *2000*

# TOXICOLOGY and CLINICAL PHARMACOLOGY of HERBAL PRODUCTS

Edited by

**Melanie Johns Cupp,** PharmD, BCPS

*West Virginia University*
*Morgantown, WV*

**Humana Press** 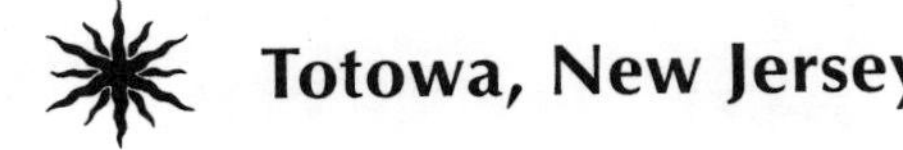 **Totowa, New Jersey**

999 Riverview Drive, Suite 208
Totowa, New Jersey 07512



This publication is printed on acid-free paper. ∞
ANSI Z39.48-1984 (American Standards Institute) Permanence of Paper for Printed Library Materials.

Cover design by Patricia F. Cleary.

For additional copies, pricing for bulk purchases, and/or information about other Humana titles, contact Humana at the above address or at any of the following numbers: Tel: 973-256-1699; Fax: 973-256-8341; E-mail: humana@humanapr.com, or visit our Website at www.humanapress.com


Printed in the United States of America. 10 9 8 7 6 5 4 3 2
Library of Congress Cataloging in Publication Data
Toxicology and clinical pharmacology of herbal products / edited by Melanie Johns Cupp.
p. ; cm. -- (Forensic science and medicine)
Includes bibliographical references and index.
ISBN 0-89603-791-6 (alk. paper)
1. Herbs--Toxicology. 2. Materia medica, Vegetable--Toxicology. I. Title:Herbal products. II. Cupp, Melanie Johns. III. Series.
[DNLM: 1. Herbs--adverse effects. 2. Plants, Medicinal--adverse effects. 3. Pharmacology. QV 767 T755 2000]
RA1250 .T68 2000
615.9'52--dc21

99-046505

# Foreword

The herbal medicine industry is growing at an astounding rate. Trade group estimates suggest that total sales exceeded $4 billion dollars in 1999. Herbal remedies are for sale not just in health food stores, but in supermarkets, drug stores, and even discount warehouses. Along with the proliferation in sales has come a proliferation of information sources. Not all of the sources are equally reliable, or even intelligible. Traditional herbalists classify thistle and mugwort as "cholagogues," substances used to make the gallbladder contract and release bile. Medical school graduates are unlikely to have ever heard the term, or even accept the notion that most right-sided abdominal pain is a result of diminished bile flow.

Heroin and cocaine may not be the only drugs to come from plants, but a practicing physician or toxicologist might be forgiven for thinking so. In 1998, 1264 papers were published about cocaine and only 17 about kava kava, an abused herb that is not without toxic side effects. Unfortunately, the majority of the papers about kava kava were published in journals not found in ordinary hospital libraries. In recognition of this fact, and of the obvious need for a reliable reference work on herbal toxicology, *The Toxicology and Clinical Pharmacology of Herbal Products* was an early addition to our new series in *Forensic Science and Medicine*. It is very badly needed.

The reason that herbalists and physicians use different terminology, and the reason that most herbal medicine books are of little use to the physician confronted with a desperately ill patient, is that herbalists and traditional physicians think about diseases (and the medicines used to treat them) differently. Of course many of the drugs first used in modern medicine are extracted from plants. But herbalists use whole plants and traditional physicians use purified ingredients derived from plants. Traditional physicians and scientists generally believe that, if a plant has any medicinal value at all, it is because it contains one "active" ingredient that must be isolated and purified. Herbalist believe results are better when the whole herb is used, because different components of the plant act synergistically.

There are risks and benefits to both approaches. If an "active" ingredient is isolated, then it can be given in a more concentrated form. This means that the effects, both therapeutic and toxic, will be exaggerated. On the other hand, if the whole plant (or leaves, or roots, depending on the plant) is used, the concentration of the active ingredient may or may not be sufficient to produce the desired therapeutic result, but the chances for toxicity are decreased. The low concentration of active ingredients may explain why, given the enormous numbers of people taking herbal products, relatively few toxic reactions have been reported. Coca leaf is a good example. Indians who chew the leaves never achieve blood cocaine concentrations high enough to produce serious toxicity. But the results of recent studies suggest that coca leaf chewers do absorb other ingredients from the leaves that prevent high-altitude sickness.

Herbalists also believe that combining herbs improves efficacy and reduces adverse effects. When compounded by knowledgeable practitioners, some of the remedies do make sense. The combination of Devil's claw, white willow, and tumeric, all agents with antiinflammatory effects, is rational, and quite probably effective. But combining St. John's Wort, which contains a selective serotonin reuptake inhibitor, with *Ephedra*, which causes increased catecholamine release, is both dangerous and ill advised.

Whether a particular combination of herbs produces good or bad results depends on who is doing the compounding. Under current US laws, anyone is free to market any combination of ingredients, no matter how misguided the underlying science. Herbalists are not the only ones who combine agents. So do patients. And they often forget to tell their physicians about it. Occassionally, this leads to dire results. Terpenoids contained in *Gingko biloba* interact with platelet-activating factor. Fatal brain hemorrhages have occurred in anticoagulated patients who self-medicated with gingko. Traditional physicians generally avoid drugs in combination, because combinations often turn out to be counterproductive or, as in the case of gingko, outright dangerous. For example, tetracycline and penicillin would never be given at the same time, because the former slows bacterial growth, while the later exerts its bactericidal effects only in growing bacteria.

Even without isolating the active principle, some herbal products are very toxic. Comfrey may be an effective treatment for bruises and sprains, but it also contains pyrrazolidine alkaloids which can cause severe liver damage. The alkaloid content is higher in comfrey's roots than in its leaves and higher in plants grown in Europe than in the United States. Yet neither the alkaloid content, the country of origin, nor the portion of the plant used is likely to be indicated on the product label.

Dr. Cupp and her coauthors are to be congratulated for having done an excellent job in combing the scientific literature for reliable, peer-reviewed, information about the most widely used herbal products. They have also done a very good job in presenting that information in such a way that it is easily accessible to practicing physicians and laboratory scientists, not to mention consumers who would be well advised to read about any remedy, whether it is prescribed by their physician or their herbalist. The 28 subsections of this book deal with the herbs that are most often encountered. Hundreds of other herbs exist, but reliable information about them is difficult to acquire. As more is learned, it will be incorporated into future editions.

***Steven B. Karch,*** *MD*
*Berkeley, CA*

# *Preface*

Sales of herbal products have increased dramatically over the past five years. Unfortunately, the knowledge base devoted to the adverse effects of these products has not grown in proportion to their increased usage. Data of questionable accuracy, often designed to sell products rather than to provide objective information, can be found in the print and electronic media, most notably on the Internet. Even in medical journals, misleading information about the beneficial and adverse effects of herbs can be found.

*Toxicology and Clinical Pharmacology of Herbal Products* is designed to provide medical examiners, toxicologists, and health care providers with an objective review of the available information on the pharmacology and toxicology of commonly used herbs. Clinical and pathological findings from case reports of herbal adverse effects are described in detail. Sections on the relevant pharmacokinetics, chemical analysis, and analysis of biofluids are unique to this volume, and will be of use to pathologists and forensic scientists, as well as to clinicians. Animal, human, and in vitro data are presented on the known pharmacologic and toxicologic effects of each herb, arranged by organ, organ system, or therapeutic/toxicologic effect. A good deal of pharmacology and therapeutics information is included in this section, not only because toxicology is an extension of pharmacology, but also to make the book useful for a wide variety of applications by professionals with various interests. Adverse effects noted in clinical trials are noted in this section as well. At the end of the book, a summary table lists herbal toxicities by affected organ, provides a list of herbs involved in drug interactions, and indicates the type of data supporting the reported toxicities.

Each herbal monograph begins with a discussion of the herb's uses, products, and the dosage forms available. This information, in conjuction with color photographs[1] of some of the most popular products, can be of assistance in those situations where the identity of an herbal product is in question.

A chapter on the legal aspects of herbal products provides an overview of the regulation of herbal products in the US and abroad. In addition, each herbal monograph reviews the herb's status internationally, including approved uses.

The incidence of adverse effects associated with the use of herbal products is unknown, and may be underreported. Without a foundation of knowledge upon which to inquire whether an herbal product might be the cause of a given finding, further exploration of the possibility of an herb-induced toxicity might not be undertaken. Even if an herbal product is suspected of causing an adverse outcome, without information about similar cases, toxicological analysis of biofluids, or the pharmacologic or toxicologic effects of the herb, further investigation might prove difficult or impossible. *Toxicology and Clinical Pharmacology of Herbal Products* is designed to provide the necessary knowledge base upon which such investigations may efficaciously proceed.

***Melanie Johns Cupp***

[1]I want to acknowledge Mark Branciaroli of Elkins, WV for producing the photographs of the herbal products.

# Contents

# *Contributors*

JAMES ALLMAN • West Virginia University School of Pharmacy, Morgantown, WV
JENNIFER ANNON • West Virginia University School of Pharmacy, Morgantown, WV
MELISSA DAWN BOSTIC • West Virginia University School of Pharmacy, Morgantown, WV
DAVID BURCH • West Virginia University School of Pharmacy, Morgantown, WV
MELANIE JOHNS CUPP • WV Drug Information Center, Robert C. Byrd Health Sciences, West Virginia University School of Pharmacy, Morgantown, WV
AMANDA DAILEY • West Virginia University School of Pharmacy, Morgantown, WV
TARA DALTON • West Virginia University School of Pharmacy, Morgantown, WV
JULIE DAVIS • Beckley Appalachian Regional Hospital, Beckley, WV
RAYNA DE ROSA • West Virginia University School of Pharmacy, Morgantown, WV
MARLEA GIVENS • West Virginia University School of Pharmacy, Morgantown, WV
DAVID HUTSON • West Virginia University School of Pharmacy, Morgantown, WV
STEVEN B. KARCH • Assistant Medical Examiner, City and County of San Francisco, CA
A. HEATHER KNIGHT-TRENT • West Virginia University School of Pharmacy, Morgantown, WV
ANGELA J. LAWSON • West Virginia University School of Pharmacy, Morgantown, WV
FOROUZANDEH MAHDAVI • West Virginia University School of Pharmacy, Morgantown, WV

**Amy Meadows** • West Virginia University School of Pharmacy, Morgantown, WV

**Kim Melgarejo** • West Virginia University School of Pharmacy, Morgantown, WV

**Charity Metz** • West Virginia University School of Pharmacy, Morgantown, WV

**Angela Morgan** • West Virginia University School of Pharmacy, Morgantown, WV

**Michael Newton** • Department of Pharmaceutical Services, West Virginia University Hospital, Morgantown, WV

**Shawn Reeder** • West Virginia University School of Pharmacy, Morgantown, WV

**Amy Renner** • Mylan Pharmaceuticals, Morgantown, WV

**Brian Schuller** •West Virginia University School of Pharmacy, Morgantown, WV

**Jennifer Schumacher** • West Virginia University School of Pharmacy, Morgantown, WV

**John T. Schwarz** • West Virginia University School of Pharmacy, Morgantown, WV

# Part I

# Legal/Regulatory Aspects of Herbal Products

# Chapter 1

# Legal/Regulatory Aspects of Herbal Products

Melanie Johns Cupp

The US Food, Drug, and Cosmetic Act mandates that drugs be proven safe and effective for their labeled use before marketing. This requirement does not apply to herbs, because herbal products do not fall under the definition of a drug as long as they are not marketed for the prevention, diagnosis, cure, treatment, or mitigation of a disease. Thus, herbal products do not have to be proven safe or effective before marketing (Kurtzweil, 1999).

Herbal products are classified as "dietary supplements" and are marketed pursuant to the Dietary Supplement Health and Education Act of 1994 (DSHEA). The passage of this act was a response to the Food and Drug Administration's (FDA's) intent to remove some herbal products from the market in the early 1990s. Congress reportedly received more mail in 1993 protesting the FDA's restriction of supplement availability than relating to any other issue since the Vietnam war. Obviously, the American public is very interested in self-medication using herbal products (Vance, 1997).

The DSHEA can be regarded as a compromise between patient autonomy and paternalistic oversight by the FDA. Because the cost of drug development may be more than $200 million per drug and usually takes longer than 10 yr, pharmaceutical manufacturers are unlikely to make the financial commitment necessary to amass safety and efficacy data for an herb that cannot be patented (Vance, 1997). Thus, the DSHEA allows consumers access to herbal products, but without the consumer protection provided by the FDA drug approval process. It has been suggested that the dollar value provided by the pharmaceutical manufacturers regarding the expense of developing a

From Forensic Science: *Toxicology and Clinical Pharmacology of Herbal Products*
Edited by: M. J. Cupp © Humana Press Inc., Totowa, New Jersey

new drug are inflated, and that one or two properly designed clinical trials involving large numbers of patients could be quickly and inexpensively performed and would answer safety and efficacy questions about herbal products (Marwick, 1995).

Despite the controversy over whether these products should be held to the same safety and efficacy standards as "conventional medicines," the DSHEA currently allows herbal labeling to carry claims about the product's ability to affect the structure or function of the human body or to promote general well-being (Kurtzweil, 1999). For example, a St. John's wort label may state, "Helps enhance general mental well-being," but it cannot state, "Cures depression." Likewise, a claim such as, "Improves memory and concentration" would be allowed on a ginkgo biloba product, but "Cures Alzheimer's disease" would not be allowed. For consumers, some structure/function claims may be difficult to distinguish from claims of disease treatment/prevention. For example, would most consumers understand that "Supports cardiovascular health" is not synonymous with "Prevents coronary artery disease"? More study is needed in this area.

The FDA uses the "significant scientific agreement" standard to evaluate herbal product claims. However, a federal appeals court ruled in January, 1999 that this standard must be more clearly defined. They also concluded that the FDA's decision to deny four specific dietary supplement health claims was a violation of the First Amendment (Anonymous, 1999c). Even if a claim is allowed by the FDA, at present, herbal product labels must bear the disclaimer: "This statement has not been evaluated by the Food and Drug Administration. This product is not intended to diagnose, treat, cure, or prevent any disease." It has been argued that the use of this disclaimer may serve as a source of confusion for consumers, rather than helping them make a decision regarding use of the product (Anonymous, 1999d). In the future, more federal court rulings may lead to changes in the type of information seen on herbal labels.

One recent labeling change was the result of a rule that went into effect on March 23, 1999. The FDA now requires an information panel titled "Supplement Facts" to appear on the label of dietary supplements. It is similar to the "Nutrition Facts" panel required on foods and includes the herb's common or usual name, or in certain cases its botanical name; the part of the plant used to make the product (e.g., root, stem, leaf); manufacturer's suggested serving size; and amount per serving. If the product contains nutrients (e.g., iron, calcium, vitamins), these must appear on the panel just as they would on a "Nutrition Facts" label on a food, with the percentage of the recommended daily value listed. For "proprietary blends," the total weight of the blend must be listed, but the weights of the individual ingredients do not have to be listed; however, each component of the blend must be listed in order of predominance by weight. Products labeled prior to March 23, 1999 may remain on shelves until stocks are depleted (Anonymous, 1999b).

In addition to the FDA, the United States Pharmacopoeial Convention is also interested in the purity and potency of dietary supplements. The United States Pharmacopeia (USP) was first published in 1820, and has always included standards for botanicals; however, with the advent of modern medicinal chemistry, many of the botanical drugs were replaced by monographs for synthetic chemicals. With the passage of the DSHEA, setting standards for herbal products has become important once again. Herbs are complex because they are not uniform by nature and contain many different chemicals that can vary depending on soil, climate, season, and part of the plant used. Confusing the issue is that for many herbs, the specific active ingredient is unknown, and the effects of an herb might manifest via a combined effect of several different ingredients. In the absence of better data, "marker compounds" are designated that are used to standardize the product. Marker compounds are chemicals most likely to be responsible for the therapeutic effect. The USP has played an important role in designating marker compounds for various herbs (Anonymous, 1999a).

The USP publishes both "USP" and "NF" monographs. The USP and NF are designated as *the* official compendia by the Food, Drug, and Cosmetic Act as well as by state pharmacy practice acts (Valentino, 1983). The difference between a USP (United States Pharmacopeia) and an NF (National Formulary) monograph is that USP monographs include only items with FDA-approved or USP-accepted uses; otherwise, the item is included in the NF. The USP and NF are now published in the same book. The current USP edition is the 24th, and the current NF edition is the 19th, so the book is referred to as the "USP24–NF19." The USP published nine *National Formulary* botanical monographs in the Ninth Supplement to the USP23–NF18, including feverfew, powdered feverfew, ginger, ginkgo, oriental ginseng, powdered oriental ginseng, St. John's wort, powdered St. John's wort, and saw palmetto. These monographs include specifications for identity, purity, packaging, and labeling. In developing the botanical monographs, US and international information is evaluated, including chemical information, historical literature, expert opinion, anecdotal writings, case reports, and clinical trials. The resulting monographs must be supported by good science, so the level of evidence is considered. The USP Committee of Revision and its advisory panels make the final decision on the information included in each monograph (Anonymous, 1999a). When reading an herbal product label, one must be aware that the use of the word "standardized" does not mean that the product meets USP–NF standards. "Standardized" simply means that the manufacturer is claiming that a certain concentration of one or more ingredients is consistent among batches. However, use of "NF" on the label means that the product meets the NF standard for purity, strength of marker compound, and labeling. It does *not* mean that the product meets a safety or efficacy standard (Anonymous, 1999e).

Another function provided by the USP is the Drug Product Problem Reporting Program (DPPR), which reports health care providers' observations of poor product quality, unclear labeling, defective packaging, therapeutic ineffectiveness, suspected counterfeiting, and product tampering to manufacturers, labelers, the FDA, and the USP Committee of Revision. Problems with herbal products, other dietary supplements, or drugs can be reported to this free service by calling 1-800-638–6725. More than 50 reports regarding herbal products, including efficacy concerns and serious adverse effects, have been reported to the DPPR (Anonymous, 1999a). Health care professionals may also contact the FDA's MedWatch program at 1-800-FDA-1088 with reports of serious adverse effects involving herbal products, other dietary supplements, or drugs.

The National Institutes of Health Office of Alternative Medicine has provided funds to the Cochrane Collaboration to produce, maintain, and disseminate a systematic review of complementary medicine. Several reviews pertaining to herbal medicine have been completed, including St. John's wort for depression, garlic for lower-limb atherosclerosis, and cabbage leaves to reduce breast engorgement in nursing mothers. Included in the analysis are randomized controlled trials indexed on Medline as well as trials published in journals not indexed on Medline. Unpublished data existing in manufacturers' and researchers' files are also being collected to evaluate better the volume of data available and to clarify the value of including unpublished data. Publication bias, including whether "complementary medicine" journals tend to publish studies favoring the safety and efficacy of "complementary medicine" while "conventional medicine" journals tend to do the converse; whether non-English language studies are of the same quality as those published in English; whether the publication language influences publication of favorable vs unfavorable results; and whether "complementary medicine" trials are published most often in non-English language journals is being investigated (Ezzo et al., 1998).

Herbal products are regulated differently in countries other than the United States. For example, in the United Kingdom, any substance not granted a license as a medicinal product by the Medicines Control Agency is treated as a food, and cannot carry a health claim or medical advice on the label, although many do (Marwick, 1995). Canada is moving toward a system resembling that in the U.S. (Allen, 1999). Similarly, botanicals are sold as dietary supplements in the Netherlands. In Germany, herbal monographs called the German Commission E monographs are prepared by an interdisciplinary committee using historical information; chemical data; experimental, pharmacological, clinical, and toxicological studies; epidemiological data; case reports; and unpublished manufacturers' data. If an herb has an approved monograph, it can be marketed. References are not published in the monographs. Unlike the USP–NF, Commission E monographs do not include potency and purity standards. In other Western European countries, herbal products are treated as drugs, and are generally sold in pharmacies as licensed prescription and nonprescription drugs, with registrations based on quality, safety, and efficacy. The European Scientific Cooperative on Phytotherapy (ESCP) has produced 50 monographs since 1997. Like the German Commission E monographs, the ESCP monographs address therapeutics, and do not set product quality standards. Both German Commission E monographs and the ESCP monographs include information such as indications, dosage, side effects, contraindications, and recommended duration of use (Blumenthal, 1998).

The German monograph system is not without precedent in the United States. Nonprescription drugs that were on the market prior to 1962 (e.g., pseudoephedrine, acetaminophen, aspirin) are marketed despite not having endured the FDA approval process as it exists today. Such products can be marketed if they meet the standards set forth in monographs developed by FDA advisory committees in the 1970s and 1980s. These monographs delineate which ingredients may be used in nonprescription products; which combinations of active ingredients may be used together; labeling requirements; and quality testing procedures. A general section applies to all nonprescription drugs, and sets forth acceptable inactive ingredients, manufacturing processes, drug registration, container specifications, and labeling requirements for all nonprescription drugs (e.g., "Keep this and all drugs out of reach of children") (Gilbertson, 1986). Drugs that were judged safe and effective, and thus for which monographs are available, are called category I drugs. Drugs deemed unsafe or ineffective are called category II drugs, and category III drugs are those for which data are insufficient to make a determination. This system has been criticized because it relies on data supplied by manufacturers; thus, potentially safe and effective drugs may be placed in category III simply because no manufacturer felt it worthwhile financially to compile and submit the necessary data (Tyler, 1994). Clearly, there are drawbacks to such a monograph system.

As with older nonprescription drugs, perhaps herbal products will one day be marketed in the United States pursuant to monographs prepared by FDA advisory committees, and formulated to meet USP–NF standards. Properly designed clinical trials using adequate numbers of patients and sound statistical methods, funded by government or the private sector, would add to the knowledge base being compiled by the Cochrane Collaboration. Until then, patients and health care professionals must use caution in the "wild west" world of herbal products.

## *References*


Allen D. Canadian perspectives. Natural Pharm 1999;3(10):1.26.

Anonymous. Botanicals: the dilemmas involved in developing standards for natural products. USP quality review 1999a; April (65).

Anonymous. Dietary supplements now labeled with more information. HHS News. March 23, 1999. Available from: URL: http://www.fda.gov/bbs/topics/NEWS/NEW00678.html. Accessed 1999b March 30.

Anonymous. FDA clarification of health claims "scientific agreement" standard ordered. F-D-C Reports. "The Tan Sheet" 1999c;7:3–4.

Anonymous. Health claims with disclaimers may convey "incompatible" message-attorney. F-D-C Reports. "The Tan Sheet" 1999d;7:4–5.

Anonymous. [No title]. Pharmacist's letter 1999e;15.13.

Blumenthal M. The complete German Commission E monographs. Therapeutic guide to herbal medicines. Austin, TX: American Botanical Council, 1998.

Ezzo J, Berman BM, Vickers AJ, Linde K. Complementary medicine and the Cochrane Collboration. JAMA 1998;280:1628–30.

Gilbertson WE. The FDA's OTC drug review. Handbook of nonprescription drugs, 8th edition. Washington, DC: American Pharmaceutical Association, 1986, pp. 1–8.

Kurtzweil P. FDA Consumer: an FDA guide to dietary supplements. U.S. Food and Drug Administration Publication No. (FDA) 99–2323. Available from: URL:http://vm.cfsan.fda.gov/~dms/fdsupp.html. Accessed 1999 April 6.

Marwick C. Growing use of medicinal botanicals forces assessment by drug regulators. JAMA 1995;273:607–9.

Tyler VE. Herbs of choice. Binghamton, NY: Pharmaceutical Products Press, 1994.

Valentino JG. USP—the cornerstone of pharmacy practice. Presentation to the National Council of State Pharmaceutical Association Executives. New Orleans, LA, April 1983.

Vance DA. An ancient heritage beckons pharmacists. Int J Pharmaceut Compound 1997;1(1):22–4.

# PART II

# Monographs

# Chapter 1

# *Ma Huang and the* Ephedra *Alkaloids*

*Steven B. Karch*, MD

## 1.1 Sources

*Ephedra* (*ephérdre du valais* in French and *Walliser meerträubchen* in German) is a small perennial shrub with thin stems. It rarely grows to more than a foot in height, and at first glance, the plant looks very much like a small broom. Different, closely related, species are found in western Europe, southeastern Europe, Asia, and even the New World. Some of the better known species include *Ephedra sinica* and *E. equisentina* (collectively known as *ma haung*) from China, as well as *E. geriardiana*, *E. intermedia*, and *E. major* which grow in India and Pakistan, and countless other members of the family Ephedraceae that grow in Europe and the United States (*E. distachya*, *E. vulgaris*). The various species are collectively known as *ma huang*, even though that name should really be confined to the species grown in China (Namba et al., 1976).

Different ephedra species vary widely in their ephedrine content. One of the most common Chinese cultivars, known as "China 3," contains 1.39% ephedrine, 0.361% pseudoephedrine, and 0.069% methylephedrine (Sagara et al., 1983). This mix is fairly typical for commercially grown ephedra plants. Noncommercial varieties of ephedra may contain no ephedrine at all (Zhang et al., 1989).

## 1.2 History and Traditional Uses

Ephedra, and other plants thought to have medicinal value, have been identified at European Neanderthal burial sites dating from 60,000 BC (Lietava, 1992). Many thousands of years later, Pliny accurately described the medicinal

From Forensic Science: *Toxicology and Clinical Pharmacology of Herbal Products*
Edited by: M. J. Cupp © Humana Press Inc., Totowa, New Jersey

uses of ephedra, but traditional Chinese healers used ephedra extracts thousands of years before the Romans ever contemplated the idea. Fifteenth-century Chinese texts recommended ephedra as an antipyretic and antitussive. In Russia, at about the same time, extracts of ephedra were used to treat joint pain, and recent laboratory studies confirm that ephedra might just be useful for that purpose (Ling et al., 1995). In the 1600s, Indians and Spaniards in the American Southwest used ephedra as a treatment for venereal disease (Grinspoon and Hedblom, 1995). That idea might also have had some merit, as the latest studies show that ephedra contains a novel antibiotic called transtorine (Al-Khalil et al., 1998). Settlers in the American West brewed ephedra teas, referred to by a variety of names including teamsters' tea, Mormon tea, and chaparral tea (Max, 1991).

In 1885 Nagayoshi Nagi, a German-trained, Japanese-born chemist, isolated and synthesized ephedrine. Forty years later, Nagi's original observations were confirmed by Merck chemists (Holmstedt, 1991). Merck's attempts at commercializing ephedrine were initially unsuccessful, at least until 1930, when Chen and Schmidt published a monograph recommending ephedrine as the treatment of choice for asthma (Chen and Schmidt, 1930). During the 1920s and 1930s, epinephrine was the only effective oral agent for treating asthma. Epinephrine, which had been available since the early 1900s was (and still is) an effective bronchodilator, but it has to be given by injection. Ephedrine was nearly as effective, and it could be taken orally. As a result, ephedrine became the first-line drug against asthma.

Unlike the other alkaloids contained in ephedra, ephedrine is also a potent central nervous system (CNS) stimulant (Martin et al., 1971). Injections of ephedrine, called *philopon* (which means "love of work") were given to Japanese *kamikaze* pilots during World War II. A major epidemic of ephedrine abuse occurred in postwar Japan, when stockpiles of ephedrine accumulated for use by the Army were dumped on the black market. Abusers in Tokyo, and other large Japanese cities, injected themselves with ephedrine (then referred to as *hirapon),* in much the same way that methamphetamine is injected today (Deverall, 1954; Suwanwela and Poshyachinda, 1986). In the Philippines, a mixture of ephedrine and caffeine called *shabu* was traditionally smoked for its stimulating effect. In the late 1980s, *shabu* smoking gave way to the practice of smoking methamphetamine ("ice"). In what is perhaps a tribute to the past, some "ice" is sold under the *philopon* name.

## 1.3 Current Promoted Uses

Physicians routinely use intravenous ephedrine for the prophylaxis and treatment of hypotension caused by spinal anesthesia (Yap et al., 1998), particularly during caesarean section. Although it has been largely replaced by other, more selective, synthetic β2 bronchodilators, ephedrine (as the hydrochloride salt, sulfate, or tannate) is still included as a component of prescription asthma and cough medications. (The current PDR lists Quadrinal™, Broncholate™, Mudrane™, Marax,™ and Rynatuss™.) It can also be found in over-the-counter (OTC) cold remedies. Recent studies continue to confirm the effectiveness of ephedra formulations when they are used in the short term as nasal decongestants (Jawad and Eccles, 1998). In the past, ephedrine was used to treat Stokes–Adams attacks (complete heart block), and was also recommended as a treatment for narcolepsy. Over the years ephedrine has been replaced by other, more effective agents (Pomerantz and O'Rourke, 1969), and the advent of highly selective β-agonists has mostly eliminated the need to use ephedrine in treating asthma.

European medical researchers have, for some time, used ephedrine to help promote weight loss, at least in the morbidly obese (Astrup and Lundsgaard, 1998; Ramsey et al., 1998). Ephedra is found in many "food supplements," especially the type used by bodybuilders. Generally, it is compounded with other ingredients such as vitamins, minerals, and amino acids in products designed to increase muscle mass and enhance endurance (Clarkson and Thompson, 1997). The degree of performance improvement associated with ephedrine ingestion has never been established in a controlled clinical trial (Sidney and Lefcoe, 1977; Smith and Perry, 1992; Gruber and Pope, 1998), but the use of ephedrine has nonetheless been prohibited by the International Olympic Committee, and a number of analytic methods have been developed for detecting ephedrine (Chicharro et al., 1993; Hurlbut et al., 1998; Sweeney et al., 1998), and its principal metabolite norephedrine, in the urine.

Ephedra is also sold in combination with other herbs, such as St. John's wort and/or caffeine, as herbal supplement products designed to help build muscle. Other, more obscure combinations, are said to be indicated for a variety of vaguely defined indications. Except in the case of weight loss (Liu et al., 1995; Astrup and Lundsgaard, 1998), in which controlled clinical trials have found some evidence of effectiveness, none of these other combinations has ever been validated. After several well-publicized accidental deaths, products clearly intended for abuse, such as "*herbal ecstasy*," and other "look-alike drugs" (products usually containing ephedrine or phenylpropanolamine designed to look like illicit methamphetamine) have recently been withdrawn from the market.

## 1.4 Available Products

No one government agency is tasked with tracking production of ephedrine-containing products. Nor does it appear that these products are indexed by any industry or trade organization. Ephedrine-containing products are mostly purchased at health food stores or over the Internet. Claims made by some of the Internet vendors are quite outrageous and totally unsupported by any scientific research. The large supplement makers, of course, have Web pages, many of which contain, or have links to, the most recent peer review studies, but in addition to the established names, hundreds of other smaller manufacturers also advertise and sell over the Internet. Whether the smaller companies will still be in business when it comes time to reorder is anyone's guess.

A partial alphabetical listing of companies found in a cursory web search disclosed numerous sites providing ephedra (or ephedrine) on the Web, many of which are located outside of the United States, but clearly are attempting to reach a U.S. market. Some of the companies are: Altered States Herbs (www.alterstatesherbs.com), Bennett International Products (www.dietnutrition.com), DandE Healthcare Products (www.d-n-e.com), Gold Leaf Herbal Products (Canadian) Metabomax (www.pw2.netcom.com), The Herb and Vitamin Shop (www.herbandvitaminshopl.com), Main Labs Inc (www.mmainlablinc.com), Natures Pantry (www.natures-pantry.com), Planetary Herbal Products (www.Global@PlanetaryHerbs.com), Smartbomb (www.smartbomb.com), Stimline (www.stimline.com), Super Power Trim™, Tambu Passionstore ThermoGenics™, Qingthai Medicines and Health Products (with a mailing address in mainland China),Vitamin Research (www.vrp.com), and World Infinity Network (www.roncaskey.com).

In addition to selling their own proprietary mixture, many of these same Web sites also carry the same popular products sold in herbal and general retail outlets such as Twin Labs bestseller "Ripped Fuel," which contain ephedrine in the form of ma huang, combined with guarana, *l*-carnitine, and chromium picolinate. Metabolife 356™ contains guarana (40 mg caffeine), 12 mg ephedrine as ma huang, chromium picolinate 75 mg, and several other ingredients (*See* www.metabolife.com). Another popular product, sold in stores, and at a discount by many of the Web sites, is AST Research's "EPH 833," which is composed mainly of ephedrine-derived from ma huang. Pep Products are similarly compounded. Ever since ephedrine became the precursor of choice for making methamphetamine, federal regulators have severely restricted bulk sales of ephedrine, but these restrictions can be bypassed by illegally ordering from a foreign Web site.

The ephedrine content of these products can range anywhere from 12 to 80 mg per serving, with the majority of products falling into the lower range. Unless the product has been fortified, the expected ephedrine content of ma huang capsules is generally <10%. Thus a capsule said to contain 1000 g of ephedra would probably contain no more than 80 mg of ephedrine. Absent any laws controlling production or sale of these food supplements, the ephedrine content (and the content of other added ingredients) may vary from batch to batch, and month to month. New labeling regulations, which went into effect only in March of 1999, may put an end to some of these problems.

## 1.5 Pharmacology

### 1.5.1 Introduction

All ephedra plants contain phenylalanine-derived alkaloids. These include (–)-ephedrine, (+)-pseudoephedrine, (–)-norephedrine, (+)-norpseudoephedrine (also called cathine because it is a major alkaloid of *Catha edulis* or khat, a plant used as a stimulant in North Africa), (–)-*N*-methylephedrine and (+)-*N*-methylpseudoephedrine, (+)-pseudoephedrine, and (+/–)-norephedrine (phenylpropanolamine). Significant enantioselective differences with regard to both pharmacokinetic and pharmacodynamic effects of these agents are possible. All of these alkaloids have important effects on the cardiovascular and respiratory systems, but not to the same degree.

Ephedrine, the predominant alkaloid in ephedra, is both an α and a β stimulant, but physiologic doses (50 mg or less) do not cause predictable increases in blood pressure, although modest increases in pulse rate can be expected (Wilkinson and Beckett, 1968; White et al., 1997; Waluga et al., 1998; Rosene et al., 1999).

The pharmacokinetic and toxicokinetic behavior of any isomer cannot be used to predict that of any other ephedrine isomer. Methamphetamine is a prime example. The *d*-isomer is a potent, and quite dangerous, central nervous system (CNS) stimulant. The *l*-isomer is merely a decongestant. There is a tendency in the literature, particularly in government monographs, to lump together all "ephedrine alkaloids." Doing so is both foolish and misleading, as it implies that the toxicity of all the enantiomers is equivalent, which is clearly not the case.

Excessive doses of the isomer commonly referred to as phenylpropanolamine, for example, are associated with cardiovascular toxicity (Johnson et al., 1983; Garriott et al., 1985; Jackson et al., 1985; Glick et al., 1987; Forman et al., 1989; Strand et al., 1991; Chung et al., 1998) while no cases of documented ephedrine cardiotoxicity have ever been reported in individuals taking recommended doses (<50 mg two or three times a day). The amount of phenylpropanolamine contained in ma haung is negligible, and not a cause for concern unless very large amounts of the plant are consumed. Similar considerations apply to pseudoephedrine which, unless it is consumed in massive quantities, generally induces only modest blood pressure increases (Mariani, 1986; Waluga et al., 1998; Rosene et al., 1999).

### 1.5.2 Pharmacologic Effects

Because ephedra is both an α- and a β-adrenergic agonist (mainly by virtue of causing the release of norepinephrine from nerve endings), ingestion of quantities much in excess of 50 mg leads to a predictable rise in blood pressure, heart rate, and cardiac output along with variable increases in peripheral resistance. It is for just those reasons that ephedrine is so widely used as a treatment for the type of hypotensive episodes that often occur during caesarean section under spinal anesthesia (Webb and Shipton, 1998). Ephedrine can cause urinary retention via α stimulation of the smooth muscle found in the base of the bladder, and in the past it has been used to promote urinary continence. Ephedrine is a potent CNS stimulant. Cathine is also a CNS stimulant, but not nearly so powerful as cathinone, a related molecule, that gives the khat plant its psychoactivity (Kalix, 1991).

### 1.5.3 Metabolism and Elimination

Phenylpropanolamine is readily and completely absorbed, but pseudoephedrine, with a bioavailability of only approx 38%, is subject to gut wall metabolism, and absorption may be erratic (Kanfer et al., 1993). Pure ephedrine is well absorbed from the stomach, but absorption is much slower when it is given as a component of ma huang, rather than in its pure form (White et al., 1997). Ephedrine ingested in the form of ma huang has a $t_{max}$ of nearly 4 h, compared to only 2 h when pure ephedrine is given. Like its enantiomers, ephedrine is eliminated in the urine largely as unchanged drug, with a half-life of about 3–6 h.

Peak concentrations for the other enantiomers, specifically phenylpropanolamine and pseudoephedrine, occur earlier (0.5 and 2 h, respectively) than for ephedrine, but all three drugs are extensively distributed into extravascular sites (apparent volume of distribution between 2.6 and 5.0 L/kg). No protein-binding data in humans are available. Peak ephedrine levels after ingestion of 400 mg of ma huang, containing 20 mg of ephedrine, resulted in blood concentrations of 81 ng/mL—essentially no different than the peak ephedrine levels observed after giving an equivalent amount of pure ephedrine (White et al., 1997). In another study, 50 mg of ephedrine given orally to six healthy, 21-yr-old women produced mean peak plasma concentrations of 168 ng/mL, 127 min after ingestion, with a half-life of slightly more than 9 h (Vanakoski and Seppala, 1998). The results are comparable to those obtained in studies done nearly 30 yr earlier (Wilkinson and Beckett, 1968).

Very high levels of methylepehdrine have been observed in Japanese polydrug abusers taking a cough medication called BRON. Concentrations of methylephedrine <0.3 mg/L, the range generally observed in individuals taking BRON for therapeutic, rather than recreational purposes (Kunsman et al.,

1998), appear to be nontoxic and devoid of measurable effects. Methylephedrine is a minor component of most ephedra plants, but in Japan (where, unlike in the United States, methylephedrine is legally sold) it is produced synthetically, and is used in cough and cold remedies, especially BRON (Tokunaga et al., 1989; Ishigooka et al., 1991; Levine et al., 1993; Nakahara and Kikura, 1997). In terms of catecholamine stimulation, methylephedrine appears comparable to ephedrine; however, it does not react with most standard urine screening tests for ephedrine (Kunsman et al., 1998). This can be a cause of some forensic confusion, because 10–15% of a given dose of methylephedrine is converted to ephedrine (Kunsman et al., 1998)

Elimination of ephedrine, pseudoephedrine, and phenylpropanolamine is predominantly renal. Urinary excretion of all three enantiomers is pH dependent. Excretion patterns may be much more rapid in children, and a greater dosage may be required to achieve therapeutic effects. Patients with renal impairment are at special risk for toxicity.

### *1.5.4 Workplace and Sports Drug Testing*

The ephedrine content of most commercially available cold remedies is well in excess of the amount necessary to cause users to exceed current International Olympic Committee cutoffs. Healthy volunteers, given realistic doses of ephedrine-containing nasal spray (roughly 14 mg), were found to have urine levels ranging from 0.09 to 1.65 mg/mL (Lefebvre et al., 1992). In addition, depending on which screening test is used, the presence of ephedrine, or one of its enantiomers, could prove to be a problem for individuals subject to workplace drug testing as well. Initial screening tests use antibodies to detect the presence of prohibited drugs, and some of the antibodies may cross-react with ephedrine or pseudoephedrine, giving false-positive readings for amphetamine (Takayasu et al., 1997; ElSohly and Jones, 1995; Taylor et al., 1999). Of course, the true nature of the drug would be revealed by confirmatory testing with gas chromatography and mass spectrometry, but such tests will occur only in programs where confirmatory testing is in fact done.

## *1.6 Drug Interactions*

Phenylpropanolamine also increases caffeine plasma levels. Whether there is also an effect on theophylline distribution kinetics is a matter of some debate (Lake et al., 1990; Upton, 1991). Even if such an effect does exist, however, it is not known whether such an effect would be of any clinical significance in the case of ma huang, which contains only very small amounts of pure phenylpropanolamine. Reduced metabolism of pseudoephedrine is seen with concurrent administration of monoamine oxidase inhibitors (MAO) (Dawson et al., 1995). In extreme cases, combinations of ephedrine with MAO inhibitors can mimic symptoms of pheochromocytoma. Clinical doses of β-agonists such as ephedrine, or ritodrine, can induce hypersecretion of salivary-type amylase, but usually only in pregnant women, and then not in all of them. Whether this effect has any clinical significance is not known (Takahashi, 1997). In some clinical trials, the coadministration of ephedrine with morphine has been shown to increase analgesia (Tekol, 1994). Such an interaction might explain the increasingly common practice of "speedballing"—injecting cocaine or amphetamine along with heroin (Karch et al., 1995; Karch, 1999). Although such synergy has not been demonstrated with cocaine and methamphetamine, there are enough similarities between these molecules to strongly suggest such a possibility.

## 1.7 Toxicology

### 1.7.1 Neurologic Disorders

Reports of ephedra-related stroke on file with the FDA have not yet been published in the peer reviewed literature. In some of the FDA cases, massive doses of ephedrine were consumed (as with products intended for abuse, such as "herbal ecstasy," now withdrawn from the market). In other cases, toxicology testing was not performed, and it is not known with any certainty whether ephedrine was even taken. In still other cases, the drug identified was not ephedrine! Many adverse events attributed to ephedrine have actually been due to ephedrine enantiomers, pseudoephedrine (Loizou et al., 1982; Stoessl et al., 1985) and phenylpropanolamine (Johnson et al., 1983; Glick et al., 1987; Lake et al., 1990; Thomas et al., 1991; Ryu and Lin, 1995; Tapia, 1996; Chung et al., 1998), and even methylephedrine (Ishigooka et al., 1991).

In the only large study ever done to assess risk factors for stroke in young people (age 20–49) over a 1-yr period (in Poland, a country where ephedra-based products are widely used), nearly half the stroke cases were associated with preexisting hypertension, another 15% had hyperlipidemia, and 6% were diabetic (Jovanovic, 1996). None of the individuals were ephedrine users.

Sometimes, especially in Japan and the Philippines, ephedrine is taken specifically as a psychostimulant. In Japan, BRON, the OTC cough medication containing methylephedrine, dihydrocodeine, caffeine, and chlorpheniramine is very widely abused and transient psychosis is not an uncommon result (Tokunaga et al., 1989; Ishigooka et al., 1991; Levine et al., 1993).

Psychosis (Herridge and Brook, 1968; Roxanas and Spalding, 1977; Whitehouse and Duncan, 1987; Kalix, 1991; Shufman et al., 1994; Doyle and

Kargin, 1996) and stroke (Stoessl et al., 1985; Yin, 1990; Bruno et al., 1993; Anonymous, 1996a,b; Waluga et al., 1998) are fairly common complications of ephedrine abuse, although rarely, if ever, are these seen when the drug is taken in recommended doses.

More often than not, psychosis occurs in individuals taking ephedrine-based products for asthma and other respiratory conditions. Ephedrine's usefulness as a bronchodilator is somewhat limited by the fact that chronic use leads to a predictable, and fairly rapid, down regulation of β-receptors and decreased bronchial responsiveness (Neve and Molinoff, 1986). As the medication becomes less and less effective, patients tend to increase the dose. If they take enough, psychosis can occur. Of course, ephedrine, and products containing ephedrine enantiomers, can also be taken specifically with the intent of becoming intoxicated.

One of the studies cited by the FDA in its 1997 proposed "rule making" (21 CFR Part 111, *Federal Register*; 1997:30678-30724) described 44 Japanese polysubstance abusers taking BRON™, which contains 2 mg/mL of racemic methylephedrine, 1 mg/mL of dihydrocodeine, 2.4 mg/mL of caffeine, and 0.4 mg/mL of chlorpheniramine maleate. Half of the group were also smoking marijuana and/or abusing organic solvents. On average, each of the 44 drug abusers was consuming 1060 mg/d of methylephedrine, along with 1392 mg/d of caffeine, and 580 mg of codeine, along with 232 mg of chlorpheniramine. The FDA did not specify just why psychotic behavior in this group of individuals should be attributed to massive ingestion of methylephedrine, rather than massive ingestion of caffeine, chlorpheniramine, or codeine (Ishigooka et al., 1991). Why the FDA assumes that ephedrine in standard clinical doses will produce the same toxicity as methylephedrine in particularly massive doses is anyone's guess.

Ephedrine psychosis closely resembles psychosis induced by amphetamines: paranoia with delusions of persecution and auditory and visual hallucinations, even though consciousness remains unclouded. Typically, patients with ephedrine psychosis will have ingested more than 1000 mg/d. Recovery is rapid after the drug is withdrawn (Shufman et al., 1994). The ephedrine content per serving of most food supplements is on the order of 10–20 mg, making it extremely unlikely that, in recommended doses, use of any of the products would lead to neurologic symptoms.

### *1.7.2 Renal Disorders*

Reports, particularly in the European literature, have described the occurrence of renal calculi in chronic ephedrine users (Bories, 1976; Schweisheimer, 1976; Blau, 1998; Powell et al., 1998). A review of cases from a large commercial laboratory that analyzes kidney stones found that 200 out of 166,466, or 0.064% of stones analyzed by that laboratory, contained either ephedrine or pseudoephedrine. Unfortunately, the analytic technique used could not distinguish ephedrine from pseudoephedrine, and because pseudoephedrine is used so much more widely than ephedrine, it seems that the risk of renal calculus associated with ephedrine use must be quite small.

Direct toxicity, with altered renal function and/or demonstrable kidney lesions, has never been demonstrated. Urinary retention, occurring as a consequence of drug overdose, has rarely been reported (Glidden and DiBona, 1977; Lindberg, 1988). The FDA and Commission E both have warned against the possibility of urinary retention in patients with prostatic enlargement, but the theoretical basis for this concern is unclear, and, in any case, retention in patients with prostate disease has not been reported.

Ephedrine and most of its enantiomers are excreted unchanged in the urine (although small amounts are oxidized in the liver to norephedrine and norpseudoephedrine, both CNS stimulants). In patients with diminished renal function, these drugs may accumulate and cause serious toxicity. None of the enantiomers are easily removed by dialysis, and treatment remains supportive, using pharmacologic antagonists to counter the α- and β-adrenergic effects of these drugs (Lyon and Turney, 1996). Because excretion is pH dependent, patients with renal tubular acidosis are also at risk (Brater et al., 1980).

The FDA reports having received a number of accounts of hematuria after use of ephedra-based products. No such cases have appeared in the peer reviewed literature, and review of the reports published by the FDA shows that all of the affected individuals were taking multiple remedies. There is no question that some herbal medicines cause interstitial nephritis, as well as other renal pathologies. For example, a cluster of more than 100 cases of interstitial nephritis was reported from Belgium in 1992. All of the cases involved young women who had been prescribed an herbal remedy for weight loss. Renal biopsies from these women disclosed acellular, interstitial fibrosis, often with precancerous transformation of the urinary tract epithelia. Many of these same women were also found to have aortic valve disease. Epidemiologic investigation disclosed that the renal injury was a result of the inadvertent substitution of *Stephnania tetrandra* with *Aristolochia fangji*, an herb known to contain aristilochic acid, a potent carcinogen. The valvular damage may have been a consequence of the fenfluramine and diethylpropion that had also been added to the mixture. It seems extremely unlikely that ephedrine was in any way associated with the hematuria reported in the FDA ADRs.

### *1.7.3 Cardiovascular Diseases*

Ephedrine and pseudoephedrine share properties with cocaine and with the amphetamines because they: (1) stimulate β-receptors directly and (2) also cause the increased release of norepinephrine. Chronic exposure to abnormally high levels of circulating catecholamines can damage the heart. This is certainly the case with cocaine and methamphetamine (Karch et al., 1995; Karch, 1999), but ephedrine-related cardiomyopathy is an extremely rare occurrence, occurring only in individuals who take massive amounts of drug for prolonged periods of time.

The literature contains three case reports describing heart failure in ephedrine users; one was a 35-yr-old asthmatic taking 4000 mg of ephedrine per day and "liberal doses of prednisolone" for 14 yr. Another involved a woman who had been abusing ephedrine (300–600 mg/d) for 10 yr, and a third case, involving a 28-yr-old, cigarette smoking, 321-pound woman taking 2000 mg of ephedrine every day for 8 yr (To et al., 1980; Gaultieri, 1996; Schafers et al., 1998). The difficulty in interpreting these reports is that histologic findings were not described and angiography was not performed, making the diagnosis of cardiomyopathy impossible to prove.

Similar considerations apply to the relationship (if any) between myocardial infarction and ephedrine use. There have been scattered reports of pseudoephedrine-associated hypertension (Mariani, 1986), coronary artery spasm (Weiner et al., 1990), cardiomyopathy (To et al., 1980), and intracranial hemorrhage in association with ephedrine and pseudoephedrine overdose (Rutstein, 1963; Loizou et al., 1982; Wooten et al., 1983; Nadeau, 1984; Stoessl et al., 1985; Bruno et al., 1993), but the incidence seems to be much lower with ephedrine than with other agents such as phenylpropanolamine, and there is a paucity of autopsy studies. More often than not, toxicology results were not even recorded, and the victims were known to have long-term histories of polydrug use (Bruno et al., 1993). There are no case reports in the peer review literature linking ephedrine, phenylpropanolamine (although case reports linking phenylpropanolamine and stroke were once common), or pseudoephedrine to myocardial infarction. Toxicology tests were not performed in any of the three cases listed in the FDA monograph, and those cases were, in any event, so poorly documented that no conclusions are possible.

Cardiac arrhythmia is known as a complication of catecholamine excess (Lermann et al., 1999), and chronic exposure to high levels of catecholamines can induce a type of myocardial fibrosis that favors arrhythmias, but a linkage with ephedrine and its isomers has never been shown. The literature contains one case report (Weesner et al., 1982). The report described arrhythmias occurring in a 14-yr-old who overdosed on cold medications, taking a total of 3300 mg of caffeine, 825 mg of phenylpropanolamine, and 412 mg of ephedrine. Clearly, large doses of ephedrine, and its enantiomers, are capable of exerting toxicity.

The problem in relating ephedrine to heart disease is that with so many people taking ephedrine-based products, it is inevitable that some ephedrine users will become ill; some may even have preexisting cardiac malformations. Thus, the 1998 death of a child in California was attributed, by a coroner, to use of an ephedra-containing food supplement, even before toxicology testing had been completed. When toxicology testing was done, no ephedrine was detected, but the heart, when finally examined, was found to be diseased (Bland–White–Garland syndrome, with anomalous origin one of the coronary arteries, a congenital disorder). A similar case was reported in 1997 (Theoharides, 1999). A body building college student who died suddenly was found to have areas of myocardial necrosis and cellular infiltration. There was no ephedrine in the blood and only nanogram quantities in the urine. The pattern, at least as described in the journal article, could have been the result of many other disorders, including steroid or stimulant abuse.

### *1.7.4 Other Medical Problems and Effects*

Ma huang has traditionally been used to treat cough and respiratory infection. However, the latest studies suggest that there may be other reasons for treating respiratory infections with ephedra; it contains a compound that, in the test tube at least, has antibiotic properties. It is a quinoline alkaloid (4-quinolone-2-carboxylic acid), isolated from the aerial part of *Ephedra transitoria* by column chromatography, and called transtorine. It inhibits growth of common bacteria, such as *Enterobacter cloacae*, *Escherichia coli*, *Pseudomonas aeruginosa*, and *Staphylococcus aureus* (Al-Khalil et al., 1998). Unfortunately, there have been no clinical trials.

In addition to possessing antibiotic activity, extracts of *Ephedra sinica* cause a partial inhibition of serum complement activity, specifically inhibiting C2 complement (Ling et al., 1995). Traditional Chinese herbalists have always claimed that ma huang could be used to treat arthritis, and although clinical trials are still lacking, it appears that these claims could have a solid scientific foundation. One problem in establishing efficacy is that traditional herbalists usually combine ephedra with other herbs. In vitro studies have shown that an ephedrine containing remedy called *shinpi-to*, which also contains *Prunus armeniaca, Magnolia obovata, Citrus unshiu, Glycyrrhiza uvalensis*, and *Bupleurum falcatan*, inhibits immunoglobulin E (IgE) mediated leukotriene synthesis, another action that could prove to be effective in the treatment of arthritis (Hamasaki et al., 1997).

An area of very major interest is weight loss. Appetite control is impaired in the obese, especially when diets are fat rich and energy dense. Many obese people have a lower than expected resting metabolic rate, a deficiency that may be genetically controlled. Agents that stimulate adrenergic neurons inhibit hunger and stimulate energy expenditure, lipolysis, and fat oxidation, which is why combinations of ephedrine and caffeine have been evaluated in clinical trials. In most of the trials, the combination has been shown to induce weight loss (Astrup and Lundsgaard, 1998). The mechanism by which this reduction occurs is not known, but it is believed to involve the stimulation of a family of β-receptors, thereby causing increased energy expenditure (and therefore calorie consumption). The most exciting new work in this area suggests that stimulation of some β-receptors may lead to the production of a group of proteins (called uncoupling protein, or UCP1,2, and 3) that can uncouple ATP production from mitochondrial respiration, resulting in the dissipation of energy as heat. Studies with Pima Indians have shown that the greater the degree of UCP3 expression, the lower the body mass index (Schrauwen et al., 1999). Obviously, much more needs to be known.

## *1.8 Postmortem Toxicology*

Very few fatalities have ever been reported (or studied), but it appears that the therapeutic index for ephedrine is very great indeed. A 1997 case report described a 28-yr-old woman with two prior suicide attempts, who died after ingesting amitriptyline and ephedrine. The blood ephedrine concentration was 11,000 ng/mL, and the liver concentration was twice that value (kidney, 14 mg/kg; brain, 8.9 mg/kg). The amitriptyline concentration was 0.33 mg/kg in blood and 7.8 mg/kg in liver (Backer et al., 1997). Values in a second case report (where methylephedrine concentrations was nearly 6000 ng/mL) may or may not be relevant to the problem of ephedrine toxicity, as the individual in question took massive quantities of a calcium channel blocker, and it is not know whether methylephedrine exerts all the same effects as ephedrine (Levine et al., 1993). Baselt and Cravey mention the case of a young woman who died several hours after ingesting 2.1 g of ephedrine combined with 7.0 g of caffeine, but tissue findings were not described. Her blood ephedrine level was 5 mg/L, while the concentration in the liver was 15 mg/kg (Baselt and Cravey, 1989).

Pseudoephedrine concentrations, but not measurements for ephedrine or any of the other enantiomers, have been published by the National Association of Medical Examiners in their Annual Registry report. In 15 children diagnosed with sudden infant death syndrome, the mean blood pseudoephedrine concentration was 3.55 mg/L, the median 2.3 mg/L, with a range of 0.07–13.0 mg/L (SD = 3.36 mg/L). The authors of the study take pains to point out that "The data do not allow definitive statements about the toxicity of pseudoephedrine at a given concentration" (Hanzlick, 1995). Nor is it at all clear that any meaningful inferences can be drawn about ephedrine (as opposed to pseudoephedrine) toxicity!

## 1.9 Analytic Considerations

Reliable techniques exist for liquid–liquid extraction of ephedrine from alkaline tissue samples. Gas chromatography–mass spectrometry measurement requires pentafluoropropionic acid derivatization. Blood and tissue measurements have been reported in several ephedrine-related deaths, and in clinical trials with therapeutic doses of the drug (Backer et al., 1997). More recently capillary electrophoresis has been used to separate and identify all 10 stereoisomers of the ephedrine family found in nutritional supplements. Chiral discrimination is effected by using hydroxypropyl-β-cyclodextrin (Flurer et al., 1995).

## 1.10 Methamphetamine Manufacture

In Japan, in the remote past, ephedrine abuse was a real and considerable public health problem. That is no longer the case, except in the rare instances in which ephedrine is promoted as "herbal ecstasy," and large quantities of the drug are taken in hopes of getting "high." Such products are no longer on the market and are really not an issue. Today, the only concern about abuse is the diversion of ephedrine to make methamphetamine. Either (–)-ephedrine or (+)-pseudoephedrine can be used to make methamphetamine by reductive dehalogenation using red phosphorus as a catalyst (Irvine and Chen, 1991). If (–)-ephedrine is used as the starting material, the process will generate (+)-methamphetamine. If pseudoephedrine is used, the result will be dextromethamphetamine. As this synthetic route has become more popular, there has been increasing demand for ephedrine, and many states have moved to restrict sales (Karch, 1996).

## 1.11. Commission E Recommendations

Commission E recommends ephedra for "diseases of the respiratory tract with mild bronchospasms in adults and children over the age of six." According to the Commission, use is contraindicated in patients with high blood pressure, glaucoma, "impaired circulation of the cerebrum, adenoma of the prostate with residual urine accumulation, pheochromocytoma, and thyrotoxicosis." "Anxiety and restlessness" are also considered contraindications (Blumenthal, 1998). Ephedra is regulated as a dietary supplement in the United States. The FDA has proposed a dosage limit of 8 mg every 6 h, and a daily maximum dose of 24 mg (Anonymous 1997).

## REFERENCES


Al-Khalil S, Alkofahi A, et al. Transtorine, a new quinoline alkaloid from *Ephedra transitoria*. J Nat Prod 1998;61:262–3.

Anonymous. Adverse events associated with ephedrine-containing products—Texas, December 1993–September 1995. MMWR Morb Mortal Wkly Rep 1996a;45:689–93.

Anonymous. Dietary supplements containing ephedrine alkaloids; proposed rule. 21 CFR 111. Fed Register 1997;62(107):30677-–724.

Anonymous. From the Centers for Disease Control and Prevention. Adverse events associated with ephedrine-containing products—Texas, December 1993–September 1995. JAMA 1996b;276:1711–2.

Astrup A, Lundsgaard C. What do pharmacological approaches to obesity management offer? Linking pharmacological mechanisms of obesity management agents to clinical practice. Exp Clin Endocrinol Diabetes 1998;106(Suppl 2):29–34.

Backer R, Tautman D, et al. Fatal ephedrine intoxication. J Forensic Sci 1997;42:157–9.

Baselt R, Cravey B. Disposition of toxic drugs and chemicals in man. 3rd edit., Chicago, London: Year Book Medical Publishers, 1989.

Blau JJ. Ephedrine nephrolithiasis associated with chronic ephedrine abuse. J Urol 1998;160(3 Pt 1):825.

Blumenthal M. (ed.) Complete German Commission E monographs, therapeutic guide to herbal medicines. Austin, TX, American Botanical Council, 1998.

Bories H. [Kidney stones]. Infirm Fr 1976;179:13–8.

Brater DC, Kaojarern S, et al. Renal excretion of pseudoephedrine. Clin Pharmacol Ther 1980;28:690–4.

Bruno A, Nolte KB, et al. Stroke associated with ephedrine use. Neurology 1993;43:1313–6.

Chen K, Schmidt C. Ephedrine and related substances. Medicine 1930;9:1–94.

Chicharro M, Zapardiel A, et al. Direct determination of ephedrine and norephedrine in human urine by capillary zone electrophoresis. J Chromatogr 1993;8,622:103–108.

Chung YT, Hung DZ et al. Intracerebral hemorrhage in a young woman with arteriovenous malformation after taking diet control pills containing phenylpropanolamine: a case report. Chung Hua I Hsueh Tsa Chih (Taipei) 1998;61:432–5.

Clarkson P, Thompson H. Drugs and sport. Research findings and limitations. Sports Med 1997;24:366–84.

Dawson J, Earnshaw S, et al. Dangerous monoamine oxidase inhibitor interactions are still occurring in the 1990s. J. Accid Emerg Med 1995;12:49–51.

Deverall R. Red China's dirty drug war. The story of opium, heroin, morphine, and philopon traffic, 3rd edit., New York, American Federation of Labor, 1954.

Doyle H, Kargin M. Herbal stimulant containing ephedrine has also caused psychosis. Br Med J 1996;312:1441.

ElSohly M, Jones A. Drug testing in the workplace: could a positive test for one of the mandated drugs be for reasons other than illicit use of the drug? J Analyt Toxicol 1995;19:450–458.

Flurer CL, Lin LA, et al. Determination of ephedrine compounds in nutritional supplements by cyclodextrin-modified capillary electrophoresis. J Chromatogr B Biomed Appl 1995;669:133–9.

Forman HP, Levin S, et al. Cerebral vasculitis and hemorrhage in an adolescent taking diet pills containing phenylpropanolamine: case report and review of literature. Pediatrics 1989;83:737–41.

Garriott JC, Simmons LM, et al. Five cases of fatal overdose from caffeine-containing "look-alike" drugs. J Analyt Toxicol 1985;9:141–3.

Gaultieri J. Cardiomyopathy in a heavy ephedrine abuser. J Toxicol Clin Toxicol 1996;34:581–582.

Glick R, Hoying J, et al. Phenylpropanolamine: an over-the-counter drug causing central nervous system vasculitis and intracerebral hemorrhage. Case report and review. Neurosurgery 1987;20:969–74.

Glidden RS, DiBona FJ. Urinary retention associated with ephedrine. J Pediatr 1977;90:1013–4.

Grinspoon L, Hedblom P. The speed culture: amphetamine use and abuse in America. Cambridge, MA, and London, England: Harvard University Press, 1995.

Gruber A, Pope JH. Ephedrine abuse among 36 female weight lifters. Am J Addict 1998;7:40.

Hamasaki Y, Kobayashi I, et al. The Chinese herbal medicine, shinpi-to, inhibits IgE-mediated leukotriene synthesis in rat basophilic leukemia-2H3 cells. J Ethnopharmacol 1997;56:123–31.

Hanzlick R. National Association of Medical Examiners Pediatric Toxicology (PedTox) Registry Report 3. Case submission summary and data for acetaminophen, benzene, carboxyhemoglobin, dextromethorphan, ethanol, phenobarbital, and pseudoephedrine. Am J Forensic Med Pathol 1995;16:270–7.

Herridge CF, Brook MF. Ephedrine psychosis. Br Med J 1968;2:160.

Holmstedt, B. Historical perspective and future of ethnopharmacology. J Ethnopharmacol 1991;32:7–24.

Hurlbut J, Carr J, et al. Solid-phase extraction cleanup and liquid chromatography with ultraviolet detection of ephedrine alkaloids in herbal products. JAOAC Int 1998;81:1121–7.

Irvine G, Chen L. The environmental impact and adverse health effects of clandestine manufacture of methamphetamine. In NIDA Research Monograph 115, Miller, M. and Kozel, N. (eds.) pp 33–47, 1991.

Ishigooka J, Yoshida Y, et al. Abuse of "BRON": a Japanese OTC cough suppressant solution containing methylephedrine, codeine, caffeine and chlorpheniramine. Prog Neuropsychopharmacol Biol Psychiatry 1991;15:513–21.

Jackson C, Hart A, et al. Fatal intracranial hemorrhage associated with phenylpropanolamine, pentazocine, and tripelenamine overdose. J Emerg Med 1985;3:127–32.

Jawad SS, Eccles R. Effect of pseudoephedrine on nasal airflow in patients with nasal congestion associated with common cold. Rhinology 1998;36:73–6.

Johnson DA, Etter HS, et al. Stroke and phenylpropanolamine use [letter]. Lancet 1983;ii:970.

Jovanovic Z. [Risk factors for stroke in young people]. Srp Arh Celok Lek 1996;124:232–5.

Kalix P. The pharmacology of psychoactive alkaloids from ephedra and catha. J Ethnopharmacol 1991;32:201–8.

Kanfer I, Dowse R, et al. Pharmacokinetics of oral decongestants. Pharmacotherapy 1993;13(6 Pt 2):116S-128S; discussion 143S–6S.

Karch S. The pathology of drug abuse, 2nd edit., Boca Raton, Florida: CRC Press, 1996.

Karch S. Comments on "ma haung toxicity" letter by Dr. Theoharides. J Clin Psychol Pharmacol 1999;19:196–199.

Karch S, Green G, et al. Myocardial hypertrophy and coronary artery disease in male cocaine users. J Forensic Sci 1995;40:591–595.

Kunsman GW, Jones R, et al. Methylephedrine concentrations in blood and urine specimens. J Analyt Toxicol 1998;22:310–3.

Lake C, Rosenberg D, et al. Phenylpropanolamine increases plasma caffeine levels. Clin Pharmacol Ther 1990a;47:675–85.

Lake CR, Gallant S, et al. Adverse drug effects attributed to phenylpropanolamine: a review of 142 case reports. Am J Med 1990b;89:195–208.

Lefebvre RA, Surmont F, Bouckaert J, Moerman E. Urinary excretion of ephedrine after nasal application in healthy volunteers. J Pharm Pharmacol 1992;44:672–5.

Lermann B, Sten K, et al. Catecholamine facilitated reentrant ventricular tachycardia: uncoupling of adenosine's antiadreneregic effects. J Cardiovasc Electrophysiol 1999;10:17–26.

Levine B, Jones R, et al. An intoxication involving BRON and verapamil. J Analyt Toxicol 1993;17:381–3.

Lietava J. Medicinal plants in a Middle Paleolithic grave Shanidar IV. J Ethnopharmacol 1992;35:263–6.

Lindberg AW. [Urinary retention caused by Elsinore pills]. Ugeskr Laeger 1988;150:2086–7.

Ling M, Piddlesden SJ, et al. A component of the medicinal herb ephedra blocks activation in the classical and alternative pathways of complement. Clin Exp Immunol 1995;102:582–8.

Liu YL, Toubro S, et al. Contribution of beta 3–adrenoceptor activation to ephedrine-induced thermogenesis in humans. Int J Obes Relat Metab Disord 1995;19:678–85.

Loizou L, Hamilton J, et al. Intracranial hemorrhage in association with pseudoephedrine overdose. J Neurol Neurosurg Psychiatry 1982;45:471–2.

Lyon CC, Turney JH. Pseudoephedrine toxicity in renal failure. Br J Clin Pract 1996;50:396–7.

Mariani PJ. Pseudoephedrine-induced hypertensive emergency: treatment with labetalol. Am J Emerg Med 1986;4:141–2.

Martin W, Sloan J, et al. Physiologic, subjective and behavioral effects of amphetamine, methamphetamine, ephedrine, phenemetrazine and methylphenidate in man. Clin Pharmacol Ther 1971;12:245–8.

Max B. This and that: the ethnopharmacology of simple phenethylamines, and the question of cocaine and the human heart. Trends Pharm Sci 1991;12:329–33.

Nadeau SE. Intracerebral hemorrhage and vasculitis related to ephedrine abuse [letter]. Ann Neurol 1984;15:114–5.

Nakahara Y, Kikura R. Hair analysis for drugs of abuse. XIX. Determination of ephedrine and its homologs in rat hair and human hair. J Chromatogr B Biomed Sci Appl 1997;700:83–91.

Namba T, Kubo M, et al. Pharmacognostical studies of ephedra plants part I — the comparative histological studies on ephedra rhizomes from Pakistan and Afghanistan and Chinese crude drugs "Ma-Hung-Gen." Planta Med 1976;29:216–25.

Neve KA, Molinoff PB. Effects of chronic administration of agonists and antagonists on the density of beta-adrenergic receptors. Am J Cardiol 1986;57:17F-22F.

Pomerantz B, O'Rourke R. The Stokes–Adams syndrome. Am J Med 1969;46:941–60.

Powell T, Hsu FF, et al. Ma-huang strikes again: ephedrine nephrolithiasis. Am J Kidney Dis 1998;32:153–9.

Ramsey JJ, Colman RJ, et al. Energy expenditure, body composition, and glucose metabolism in lean and obese rhesus monkeys treated with ephedrine and caffeine. Am J Clin Nutr 1998;68:42–51.

Rosene JM, Rosene JA, et al. Decongestant effects on hemodynamics at rest, exercise, and recovery from exercise during 6 degrees of head down tilt. Aviat Space Environ Med 1999;70:15–21.

Roxanas MG, Spalding J. Ephedrine abuse psychosis. Med J Aust 1977;2:639–40.

Rutstein H. Ingestion of pseudoephedrine. Hypertension and unconsciousness following: report of a case. Arch Otolaryngol 1963;77:145–6.

Ryu SJ, Lin SK. Cerebral arteritis associated with oral use of phenylpropanolamine: report of a case. J Formos Med Assoc 1995;94:53–55.

Sagara K, Oshima T, et al. A simultaneous determination of norephedrine, pseudoephedrine, ephedrine and methylephedrine in *Ephedrae herba* and oriental pharmaceutical preparations by ion-pair high-performance liquid chromatography. Chem Pharmacol Bull (Tokyo)1983;31:2359–65.

Schafers M, Dutka D, et al. Myocardial presynaptic and postsynaptic autonomic dysfunction in hypertrophic cardiomyopathy. Circ Res 1998;82:57–62.

Schrauwen P, Walder K, et al. Human uncoupling proteins and obesity. Obes Res 1999;7:97–1105.

Schweisheimer W. [Kidney stones]. Krankenpflege (Frankf) 1976;30:194–5.

Shufman NE, Witztum E, et al. [Ephedrine psychosis]. Harefuah 1994;127:166–8, 215.

Sidney K, Lefcoe NM. The effects of ephedrine on the physiological and psychological responses to submaximal and maximal exercise in man. Med Sci Sports 1977;9:95–99.

Smith D, Perry P. The efficacy of ergogenic agents in athletic competition. Part II: Other performance-enhancing agents. Ann Pharmacother 1992;26:653–9.

Stoessl AJ, Young GB, et al. Intracerebral haemorrhage and angiographic beading following ingestion of catecholaminergics. Stroke 1985;16:734–6.

Strand OA, Lund-Tonnesen S, et al. [Cerebral hemorrhage associated with phenylpropanolamine]. Tidsskr Nor Laegeforen 1991;111:1490–2.

Suwanwela C, Poshyachinda V. Drug abuse in Asia. Bull Narc 1986;38:41–53.

Sweeney S, Kelly R, et al. Amphetamines in hair by enzyme-linked immunosorbent assay. J Analyt Toxicol. 1998;22:418–24.

Takahashi T, Minakami H, et al. Hyperamylasemia in response to ritodrine or ephedrine administered to pregnant women. J Am Coll Surg 1997;184:31–6.

Takayasu T, Ohshima T, et al. False identification of urinary ephedrine as methamphetamine by gas chromatography/mass spectrometry with a DB-17 column. Nippon Hoigaku Zasshi 1997;51:235–40.

Tapia J. [Cerebral hemorrhage associated with the use of phenylpropanolamine. Clinical cases]. Rev Med Chil 1996;124:1499–503.

Taylor E, Oertli E, et al. Accuracy of five on-site immunoassay drugs-of-abuse testing devices. J Analyt Toxicol 1999;23:119–24.

Tekol Y, Tercan E, et al. Ephedrine enhances analgesic effect of morphine. Acta Anaesthesiol Scand 1994;38:396–7.

Theoharides T. Reply to Comments by Dr. Karch. J Clin Psychol Pharmacol 1999;19:198–9.

Thomas SH, Clark KL, et al. A comparison of the cardiovascular effects of phenylpropanolamine and phenylephrine containing proprietary cold remedies. Br J Clin Pharmacol 1991;32:705–11.

To L, Sangster J, et al. Ephedrine-induced cardiomyopathy. Med J Aust 1980;2:35–6.

Tokunaga I, Takeichi S, et al. Electroencephalographical analysis of acute drug intoxication—SS Bron solution-W. Arukoru Kenkyuto Yakubutsu Ison 1989;24:471–9.

Upton R. Pharmacokinetic interactions between theophylline and other medication (Part I). Clin Pharmacokinet 1991;20:66–80.

Vanakoski J, Seppala T. Heat exposure and drugs. A review of the effects of hyperthermia on pharmacokinetics. Clin Pharmacokinet 1998;34:311–22.

Waluga M, Janusz M, et al. Cardiovascular effects of ephedrine, caffeine, and yohimbine measured by thoracic electrical bioimpedance in obese women. Clin Physiol 1998;18:69–76.

Webb AA, Shipton EA. Re-evaluation of i.m. ephedrine as prophylaxis against hypotension associated with spinal anaesthesia for Caesarean section. Can J Anaesth 1998;45:367–9.

Weesner K, Denison M, et al. Cardiac arrhythmias in an adolescent following ingestion of an over-the-counter stimulant. Clin Pediatr 1982;21:700–1.

Weiner I, Tilkian A, et al. Coronary artery spasm and myocardial infarction in a patient with normal coronary arteries: temporal relationship to pseudoephedrine ingestion. Cath Cardiovas Diag 1990;20:51–3.

White LM, Gardner SF, et al. Pharmacokinetics and cardiovascular effects of ma-huang (*Ephedra sinica*) in normotensive adults. J Clin Pharmacol 1997;37:116–22.

Whitehouse AM, Duncan JM. Ephedrine psychosis rediscovered. Br J Psychiatry 1987;50:258–61.

Wilkinson G, Beckett A. Absorption, metabolism, and excretion of the ephedrines in man. II. Pharmacokinetics. J Pharm Sci 1968;57:1933–8.

Wooten MR, Khangure MS, et al. Intracerebral hemorrhage and vasculitis related to ephedrine abuse. Ann Neurol 1983;13:337–40.

Yap JC, Critchley LA, et al. A comparison of three fluid-vasopressor regimens used to prevent hypotension during subarachnoid anaesthesia in the elderly. Anaesth Intensive Care 1998;26:497–502.

Yin PA. Ephedrine-induced intracerebral hemorrhage and central nervous system vasculitis. Stroke 1990;21:1641.

Zhang J, Tian Z, et al. [Quality evaluation of twelve species of Chinese Ephedra]. Yao Hsueh Hsueh Pao 1989;24:865–871.

# Chapter 2

# Kava


## Shawn Reeder and Melanie Johns Cupp


*Piper methysticum*, kava-kava, awa, kew, tonga (Anonymous, 1996), kawa, yaqona, sakau (Norton and Ruze, 1994), ava, ava pepper, intoxicating pepper (Heiligenstein and Guenther, 1998)

## 2.1 History and Traditional Uses

Kava is a term used to describe both *Piper methysticum* and the preparation made from its dried rhizome and root (Anonymous, 1996). This South Pacific plant is a robust, branching, perennial shrub with heart-shaped, green, pointed leaves (Singh, 1992) that grow up to 28 cm long and flower spikes that grow up to 9 cm long (Anonymous, 1996). The shrub grows best in warm, humid conditions with lots of sunlight, at altitudes of 150–300 m above sea level (Singh, 1992), where it forms dense thickets (Norton and Ruze, 1994). Kava reproduces vegetatively, without fruit or seeds, usually under cultivation (Norton and Ruze, 1994). There are reports of up to 72 varieties of the kava plant which differ in appearance, and chemical analysis has shown differences in their composition as well which may lead to differences in physiologic activity (Singh, 1992). Kava has been described in the European literature since the early 1600s when it was taken there by the Dutch explorers LeMaire and Schouten, who had acquired it while seeking new passages across the Pacific (Norton and Ruze, 1994). Captain James Cook was the first to describe the use of kava during the religious and cultural ceremonies of the people of the South Sea Islands, where it was, and still is, prepared as a beverage and consumed for its intoxicating, calming effects that promote sociability (Norton and Ruze, 1994). Thus, kava is used for the purposes that Western society uses alcohol,


From Forensic Science: *Toxicology and Clinical Pharmacology of Herbal Products*
Edited by: M. J. Cupp © Humana Press Inc., Totowa, New Jersey

the Native American populations use peyote, and the people of the Middle or Far East use opium (Singh, 1992). Events typically accompanied by kava ceremonies included weddings, funerals, births, religious occasions, seasonal feasts, reconciliations, welcoming of royalty or other guests, and the exchange of gifts (Norton and Ruze, 1994). Women and commoners seldom participated in these ceremonies because that was viewed as unacceptable; however, some cultures did permit use by commoners to relax after a hard day's work (Norton and Ruze, 1994). The beverage was traditionally made by mixing grated, crushed, or chewed fresh or dried root with cool water or coconut milk and then straining the mixture through plant fibers to isolate the liquid, which was consumed (Norton and Ruze, 1994). Today the beverage is most often prepared by crushing dried roots with a large mortar and pestle, then straining the mixture in the traditional way or through cotton cloth (Norton and Ruze, 1994). Other folk uses of kava have included treatment of headaches, colds, rheumatism, sexually transmitted diseases, and inflammation of the uterus (Anonymous, 1996). It has also been used as a sedative, aphrodisiac, urinary antiseptic (Heiligenstein and Guenther, 1998), wound healing agent, and a treatment for asthma (Anonymous, 1996). Several substances extracted from the roots were also used briefly in Europe as diuretics (Norton and Ruze, 1994).

## 2.2 Current Promoted Uses

Kava is currently promoted for relief of anxiety and stress.

## 2.3 Products Available

Kava is available from a variety of manufacturers in most health food stores under a variety of names. Kavatrol® is a popular brand found in retail outlets in the United States. Kava is marketed in Europe under a variety of names including Laitan® or Kavasporal® in Germany, Potter's antigian tablets in the United Kingdom, Viocava® in Switzerland, and Mosaro® in Austria (Schelosky et al., 1995).

## 2.4 Pharmacologic/Toxicologic Effects

### 2.4.1 Neurologic Effects

The neurologic effects of kava are attributed to a group of substituted dihydropyrones called kava lactones (Anonymous, 1996). The main bioactive constituents include yangonin, desmethoxyyangonin, 11-methoxyyangonin, kavain (kawain), dihydrokavain, methysticin, dihydromethysticin, and 5,6-dehydromethysticin (Keller and Klohs, 1963). It is believed that the components present in the lipid-soluble kava extract, or kava resin, are responsible for the central nervous system (CNS) activities of kava including sedation, hypnosis, analgesia, and muscle relaxation (Jamieson et al., 1989). Aqueous kava extract was not active orally in mice or rats.

A randomized 25-wk placebo-controlled study by Volz and Kieser showed a significant benefit from the use of kava-kava extract WS 1490 over placebo in treating anxiety disorders of nonpsychotic origin. One hundred one patients suffering from agoraphobia, specific phobia, generalized anxiety disorder, or adjustment disorder with anxiety—as per the Diagnostic and Statistical Manual of Mental Disorders, Third edition, revised (DSM-III-R)—were randomized to placebo or WS 1490 containing 90–100 mg dry extract per capsule three times daily. The main outcome criterion, the patients' score on the Hamilton Anxiety Scale (HAMA), was significantly better ($p<0.001$) for the WS 1490 patients compared to placebo at 24 wk. Few adverse effects were judged to be related or possibly related to kava administration. Two patients in the WS 1490 group experienced stomach upset, two experienced vertigo, and one experienced vertigo and palpitations. These results support use of kava as an alternative to antidepressants and benzodiazepines (Volz and Kieser, 1997). Another study compared the cognitive effects of this same kava extract at a dose of 200 mg three times daily for 5 d to oxazepam 15 mg, followed by 75 mg on the experimental day (Heinze et al., 1994). The results suggest that kava is less likely to affect cognitive function than oxazepam, but the oxazepam dosing regimen used was not typical of that seen in practice. Nevertheless, kava is purported to promote relaxation and sleep without dampening alertness, causing heavy sedation, or causing a "hangover" effect the morning after consumption (Anonymous, 1998). The limbic structures of the brain might represent the site of action of kava, explaining its ability to promote relaxation and sleep without cognitive effects (Jussofie et al., 1994).

The mechanism of the anxiolytic effect of kava is unclear. Studies of kava's effects in vitro, in vivo, and ex vivo show conflicting results in regard to kava's effects on benzodiazepine or $\gamma$-aminobutyric acid (GABA) receptors (Davies et al., 1992; Jussofie et al., 1994; Heiligenstein and Guenther, 1998). This disparity may be explained by differences in GABA receptor subtypes among the different regions of the brain studied (Jussofie et al., 1994). It is thought that kavapyrones elicit a tranquilizing effect by enhancing GABA binding in the amygdala, but do not act directly as agonists at GABA receptors (Jussofie et al., 1994).

One study has suggested that a nonstereoselective inhibition of [$^3$H]noradrenaline uptake may be responsible for, or at least contribute to, kava's anxiolytic effect (Seitz et al., 1997). This study tested the effects of naturally occurring (+)-kavain, (+)-methysticin, and a synthetic racemic mixture of kavain on synaptosomes from the cerebral cortex and hippocampus of rat brain. Both forms of kavain inhibited [$^3$H]noradrenaline uptake more than methysticin, but the concentrations necessary to achieve this effect were about 10 times higher than those in mouse brains after a dose of kavain high enough to cause significant sedation. This indicates that inhibition of noradrenaline uptake is probably only part of the psychotropic effects of kava. No effects were seen on the uptake of [$^3$H]serotonin. A subsequent study (Baum et al., 1998) in rats showed that (+)-kavain and other kavapyrones affect serotonin levels in the mesolimbic area. The authors postulated that this effect could explain kava's hypnotic action. Dopamine levels in the nucleus accumbens were decreased by yangonin and low-dose (+)-kavain, but were increased by higher doses of (+)-kavain and desmethoxyyangonin. The investigators attributed kava's anxiolytic and euphoric effects to its action on mesolimbic dopaminergic pathways.

A study conducted in Germany indicates that kava may have neuroprotective properties primarily due to its constituents methysticum and dihydromethysticum (Backhauβ and Krieglstein, 1992). The investigators studied the effects of kava extract WS 1490 and the individual pyrones kavain, dihydrokavain, methysticin, dihydromethysticin, and yangonin on the size of infarction in mouse brains. The extract as well as the individual pyrones methysticin and dihydromethysticin showed significant reductions in infarct area similar to those produced by memantine, an anticonvulsive agent known to have neuroprotective qualities (Backhauβ and Krieglstein, 1992).

Kava lactones are also centrally acting skeletal muscle relaxants (Tyler et al., 1981). A study by Kretzschmar et al. compared the antagonistic effects of kavain, dihydrokavain, methysticin, and dihydromethysticin to those of mephenesin and phenobarbital in preventing convulsions and death caused by strychnine. All the kava pyrones showed an antagonistic effect, with methysticin being the most potent; however, kavain and dihydrokavain doses required to produce an effect approached the toxic range (Kretzschmar et al., 1970). In contrast to mephenesin and phenobarbital, all the pyrones tested protected against strychnine at doses up to 5 mg/kg without causing impairment of motor function.

Kava also produces analgesic effects that appear to be mediated through a nonopiate pathway. A study conducted by Jamieson and Duffield compared the activity of an aqueous and a lipid extract of kava as well as eight purified pyrones on two tests for antinociception in mice. Both the aqueous and lipid extracts were effective analgesics, as were four of the eight purified pyrones (lactones): methysticin, dihydromethysticin, kavain, and dihydrokavain (Jamieson and Duffield 1990a). In hopes of discovering the mechanism of analgesia, the investigators attempted to antagonize the effects of kava with naloxone, a known inhibitor of opiate-mediated pathways of analgesia. Naloxone failed to inhibit kava's effects at doses high enough to inhibit the action of morphine, indicating that kava works through a nonopiate pathway to produce analgesia.

In humans, kava is reported to produce a mild euphoria characterized by happiness, fluent and lively speech, and increased sensibility to sounds (Anonymous, 1996). It has also been reported to cause visual changes such as reduced near-point accommodation and convergence, increase in pupil diameter, and oculomotor balance disturbances (Garner and Klinger, 1985). It might even have an antipyretic effect (Tyler et al., 1981). Although kava is a centrally acting agent, it is unclear if tolerance and physical dependence occur with usual oral doses of commercially available kava products (Duffield and Jamieson, 1991). Its effects on the peripheral nervous system are limited to a local anesthetic effect, resulting in numbness in the mouth if kava is chewed (Anonymous, 1996). Lipid-soluble kava extract, or resin, is also capable of causing anesthesia of the oral mucosa, while the water-soluble fraction is not (Jamieson et al., 1989).

### *2.4.2 Dermatological Effects*

There have been many reports of skin disturbances associated with the use of kava that date as far back as the 1700s (Norton and Ruze, 1994). Chronic ingestion of kava may cause a temporary yellowing of the skin, hair, and nails (Blumenthal, 1997). Two yellow pigments, flavokawains A and B, have been isolated from the kava plant (Keller and Klohs, 1963) and may be responsible for this discoloration (Anonymous, 1996). Chronic ingestion may also lead to a temporary condition known as kava dermopathy (Norton and Ruze, 1994) or kawaism, characterized by dry, flaking, discolored skin and reddened eyes which is reversible with discontinuation (Jappe et al., 1998). In the early 19th century, Peter Corney, a lieutenant on a fur-trading vessel, described this phenomenon in great detail as it applied to the use of this side effect in treating other skin disturbances. "When a man first commences taking it, he begins to break out in scales about the head, and it makes the eyes very sore and red, then the neck and breasts, working downwards, till it approaches the feet, when the dose is reduced. At this time the body is covered all over with white scruff, or scale, resembling the dry scurvy. These scales drop off in the order of their formation, from the head, neck, and body, and finally leave a beautiful, smooth, clear skin, and the frame clear of all disease" (Norton and Ruze, 1996). The exact mechanism for this dermopathy is unknown but it has been speculated that kava may interfere with cholesterol metabolism, leading to a reversible, acquired ichthyosis similar to that seen with the use of lipid lowering agents such as triparanol (Norton and Ruze, 1996). Skin biopsies of two recent cases associated with use of the commercially available product have revealed lymphocytic attacks on sebaceous glands, with subsequent destruction and necrosis caused by CD8+ cells (*see* Section 2.5) (Jappe et al., 1998). Yet another theory involves interference with B vitamin metabolism or action (Mathews et al., 1988).

### *2.4.3 Musculoskeletal Effects*

As mentioned in Section 2.4.1, kava is a centrally acting skeletal muscle relaxant. The kava lactones kavain, dihydrokavain, methysticin, and dihydromethysticin isolated from kava rootstock were shown to antagonize strychnine-induced convulsions in mice (Kretzschmar et al., 1970).

### *2.4.4 Antimicrobial Activity*

Kava has been used traditionally as an antibacterial in the treatment of urinary tract infections (Locher et al., 1995); however, no clinical trials have established that it is truly effective. Kava extracts were not able to inhibit growth of *Candida*, *Pseudomonas*, *E. coli*, *Streptococcus pyogenes*, or *Staphylococcus aureus* (Locher et al., 1995).

### *2.4.5 Hepatotoxicity*

*See* Section 2.6.

### *2.4.6 Antiplatelet Effects*

Racemic kavain, a component of kava, has been shown to have antiplatelet effects, presumably due to inhibition of cyclooxygenase, and thus inhibition of thromboxane synthesis (Gleitz et al., 1997). Antiplatelet effects have not been observed in vivo.

## 2.5 Case Reports of Toxicity Due to Commercially Available Products

Kava dermatopathy in association with traditional use of kava is well described in the literature (Norton and Ruze, 1994). In addition, two cases of dermopathy have recently been associated with commercially available kava products (Jappe et al., 1998). A 70-yr-old man who had been using kava as an antidepressant for 2–3 wk experienced itching, and later erythematous, infiltrated plaques on his chest, back, and face after several hours of sun exposure. Skin biopsy revealed CD8 lymphocytic infiltration with destruction of the sebaceous glands and lower infundibula. A 52-yr-old woman presented with papules and plaques on her face, chest, back, and arms after taking a kava extract for 3 wk. Skin biopsy revealed an infiltrate in the reticular dermis with disruption and necrosis of the sebaceous gland lobules. A kava extract patch test was strongly positive after 24 h.

There have also been four cases of extrapyramidal effects associated with kava use (Schelosky et al., 1995). A 28-yr-old man with a history of antipsychotic-induced extrapyramidal effects experienced torticollis and oculogyric crisis 90 min after a single 100-mg dose of Laitan® (kava extract). These effects resolved spontaneously after 40 min. A 22-yr-old woman experienced oral and lingual dyskinesia, painful twisting movements of the trunk, and torticollis 4 h after a 100 mg dose of the same product taken by the previously described male. The symptoms did not resolve spontaneously, so after 45 min, a 2.5 mg intravenous dose of beperiden was given, with immediate relief. A third patient, a 63-yr-old female, also presented with oral and lingual dyskinesia after taking Kavasporal Forte® (150 mg of kava extract) three times a day for 4 d. A single 5 mg intravenous dose of beperiden was immediately effective. Finally, a 76-yr-old woman experienced worsening of Parkinson's disease symptoms after taking Kavasporal Forte® for 10 d. Improvement was noted 2 d after discontinuation of the product. These extrapyramidal side effects suggest cautious use of kava in the elderly, in patients with Parkinson's disease, and in patients taking antipsychotics.

## 2.6 Toxicity Associated with Traditional Use by Native Populations

Chronic use of the kava beverage has been associated with a wide range of abnormalities. A study (Mathews et al., 1988) of an Australian Aboriginal community revealed malnutrition and weight loss associated with kava use. Red blood cell volume increased in proportion to kava use, while bilirubin, plasma protein, platelet volume, B-lymphocyte count, and plasma urea were inversely proportional to kava consumption. Although these values were not outside the normal range, it was hypothesized that malnutrition and/or reduced hemoglobin turnover might explain these observations. Other findings included hematuria and difficulty acidifying and concentrating the urine, suggesting an effect on the renal tubules; and increased serum transaminases and increased high-density lipoprotein (HDL) cholesterol, suggesting some effect on the liver. Transaminase elevations were greater in the kava-using Aboriginal community compared to those in a community where alcohol, but not kava, was consumed. This suggests that kava might be more hepatotoxic than alcohol. Shortness of breath and EKG abnormalities (tall P waves) consistent with pulmonary hypertension were seen and are interesting in that like kava, the prescription anorexiants fenfluramine and dexfenfluramine withdrawn from the US market in 1998 were associated with pulmonary hypertension. It was also noted by the authors of this observational study that sudden death in relatively young men is more common in kava-using Aboriginal communities than in non-using communities.

## 2.7 Drug Interactions

Alcohol appears to at least add to the hypnotic effect of kava in mice, and was also observed to increase the lethality of kava (Jamieson and Duffield, 1990b). These findings may be of importance because some Australian Aboriginal populations now frequently consume kava with alcohol. Concomitant use of barbiturates, melatonin, and other psychopharmacological agents might potentiate the effects of kava as well (Thorndyke and Rhyne, 1998). The hepatotoxic potential of kava (Mathews et al., 1988) also raises concerns about concomitant alcohol use.

Although a Web site (Anonymous, 1998) promoting a kava product states that it is safe to use kava in combination with benzodiazepines, a case report (Almeida and Grimsley, 1996) suggests otherwise. The combination of kava and alprazolam was believed to be responsible for hospitalizing a 54-yr-old man. The patient's semicomatose (lethargic and disoriented) state improved after several hours. He had been taking an undisclosed brand of kava purchased in a health food store in combination with alprazolam for 3 d. Other medications taken included cimetidine and terazocin.

## 2.8 Pharmacokinetics/Toxicokinetics

### 2.8.1 Absorption

In mice and rats, the aqueous kava extract is inactive when administered orally (Jamieson et al., 1989).

### 2.8.2 Metabolism/Elimination

Several kava lactones have been identified in human urine samples after ingestion of a kava beverage prepared from a commercial 450-g sample of *Piper methysticin* extracted with 3 L of room temperature water (Duffield et al., 1989). Observed metabolic transformations include reduction of the 3,4 double bond and/or demethylation of the 4-methoxyl group on the α-pyrone ring system. Demethylation of the 12-methoxy substituent in yangonin and hydroxylation at carbon 12 of desmethoxyyangonin have also been observed. Chemical structures for these kava components and metabolites can be seen in the cited reference.

## 2.9 Analysis of Biofluids

Methane chemical ionization (CI) gas chromatography–mass spectrometry (GC–MS) and high-performance liquid chromatography (HPLC) (diode array detector) have been utilized to identify kava metabolites in human urine (Duffield et al., 1989). A detailed description of these analyses can be found in the cited reference.

## 2.10 Chemical Analysis

Duffield and colleagues performed methane CI GC–MS on three kava extracts obtained from a Samoan root piece, a dry powdered sample from Sydney, and ground plant from the United States. Similar results were obtained from all samples with the major components kavain, dihydrokavain, dihydromethysticin, yangonin, and desmethoxyyangonin being easily identifiable (Duffield et al., 1986). Several trace components were also identified. A detailed description of these analyses can be found in the cited reference. Additional information pertaining to GC–MS analysis of kava is available (Duve, 1981; Duffield and Lidgard 1986; Duffield et al., 1986; Cheng et al., 1988).

## 2.11 Regulatory Status

Kava is currently sold as a dietary supplement in the United States (Blumenthal, 1997). It has been approved as a nonprescription drug in Germany and is classified as a drug in Sweden.

## References

Almedia JC, Grimsley EW. Coma from the health food store: interaction between kava and alprazolam. Ann Intern Med 1996;125:940–1.

Anonymous. Kava-kava. In: The review of natural products. St. Louis, MO: Facts and Comparisons, 1996.

Anonymous. Topic of the month. Available from: URL: www.ownhealth.com/Topic.html. Accessed 1998 Oct. 29.

Backhauβ C, Krieglstein J. Extract of kava (*Piper methysticum*) and its methysticin constituents protect brain tissue against ischemic damage in rodents. Eur J Pharmacol 1992;215:265–9.

Baum SS, Hill R, Rommelspacher H. Effect of kava extract and individual kavapyrones on neurotransmitter levels in the nucleus accumbens of rats. Prog Neuropsychopharmacol Biol Psychiatry 1998;22:1105–20.

Blumenthal M. Popular Herbs in the U.S. Market. Kava-kava rhizome. American Botanical Council. Austin, TX, 1997.

Cheng D, Lidgard RO, Duffield PH, Duffield AM, Brophy JJ. Identification by methane chemical ionization gas chromatography/ mass spectrometry of the products obtained by steam distillation and aqueous acid extraction of commercial *Piper methysticum*. Biomed Environ Mass Spectrom 1988;17:371–6.

Davies LP, Drew CA, Duffield P, Johnston GAR, Jamieson DD. Kava pyrones and resin: studies on $GABA_A$, $GABA_B$, and benzodiazepine binding sites in rodent brain. Pharmacol Toxicol 1992;71:120–6.

Duffield AM, Jamieson DD, Lidgard RO, Duffield PH, Bourne DJ. Identification of some human urinary metabolites of the intoxicating beverage kava. J Chromatogr 1989;475:273–81.

Duffield PH, Jamieson D. Development of tolerance to kava in mice. Clin Exp Pharmacol Physiol 1991;18:571–78.

Duffield AM, Lidgard RO. Analysis of kava resin by gas chromatography and electron impact and methane negative ion chemical ionization mass spectrometry. Biomed Environ Mass Spectrometry 1986;13:621–6.

Duffield AM, Lidgard RO, Low GKC. Analysis of the constituents of Piper methysticum by gas chromatography methane chemical ionization mass spectrometry. Biomed Environ Mass Spectrometry 1986;13:305–13.

Duve RN. Gas–liquid chromatographic determination of major contituents of *Piper methysticum*. Analyst 1981;106:160–5.

Garner LF, Klinger JD. Some visual effects caused by the beverage kava. J Ethnopharamacol 1985;13:307–11.

Gleitz J, Beile A, Wilkens P, Ameri A, Peters T. Antithrombotic action of kava pyrone (+)-kavain prepared from *Piper methysticum* on human platelets. Planta Med 1997;63:27–30.

Heiligenstein E, Guenther G. Over-the counter psychotropics: a review of melatonin, St. John's wort, valerian, and kava-kava. J Am Coll Health 1998;46:271–6.

Heinze HJ, Munthe TF, Steitz J, Matzke M. Pharmacopsychological effects of oxazepam and kava-extract in a visual search paradigm assessed with event-related potentials. Pharmacopsychiatry 1994;27:224–30.

Jamieson DD, Duffield PH. The antinociceptive actions of kava components in mice. Clin Exp Pharmacol Physiol 1990a;17:495–508.

Jamieson DD, Duffield PH. Positive interaction of ethanol and kava resin in mice. Clin Exp Pharmacol Physiol 1990b;17:509–14.

Jamieson DD, Duffield PH, Cheng D, Duffield AM. Comparison of the central nervous system activity of the aqueous and lipid extract of kava (*Piper methysticum*). Arch Int Pharmacodyn 1989;301:66–80.

Jappe U, Franke I, Reinhold D, Gollnick HPM. Sebotropic drug interaction resulting from kava-kava extract therapy: a new entity? J Am Acad Dermatol 1998;38:104–6.

Jussofie A, Schmiz A, Hiemke C. Kavapyrone enriched extract from *Piper methysticum* as modulator of the GABA binding site in different regions of rat brain. Psychopharmacology 1994;116:469–74.

Keller F, Klohs MW. A review of the chemistry and pharmacology of the constituents of *Piper methysticum*. Lloydia 1963;26:1–15.

Kretzschmar R, Meyer HJ, Teschendorf HJ. Strychnine antagonistic potency of pyrone compounds of the kavaroot (*Piper methysticum* Forst). Experientia 1970;26:283–4.

Locher CP, Burch MT, Mower HF, Berestecky J, Davis H, Van Pool B, et al. Antimicrobial activity and anti-complement activity of extracts obtained from selected Hawaiian medicinal plants. J Ethnopharmacol 1995;49:23–32.

Mathews JD, Riley MD, Fejo L, Munoz E, Milns NR, Gardner ID, et al. Effects of the heavy usage of kava on physical health: summary of a pilot survey in an Aboriginal community. Med J Aust 1988;148:548–55.

Norton S, Ruze P. Kava dermopathy. J Am Acad Dermatol 1994;31:89–97.

Schelosky L, Raffauf C, Jendroska K, Poewe W. Kava and dopamine antagonism. J Neurol Nerosurg Psychiatry 1995;58:639–40.

Seitz U, Schule A, Gleitz J. [$^{3}$H]-Monoamine uptake inhibition properties of kava pyrones. Planta Med 1997;63:548–9.

Singh YN. Kava: an overview. J Ethnopharmacol 1992;37:13–45.

Singh YN. Effects of kava on neuromuscular transmission and muscle contractility. J Ethnopharmacol 1983;7:267–76.

Thorndyke A, Rhyne H. Kava. Available from: URL: www.unc.edu/~cebradsh/kava.html. Accessed 1998 Oct. 29.

Tyler VE, Brady LR, Robbers JE. Pharamcognosy, 8th edit., Philadelphia: Lea and Febiger, 1981.

Volz HP, Kieser M. Kava-kava extract WS 1490 versus placebo in anxiety disorders-a randomized placebo-controlled 25–week outpatient trial. Pharmacopsychiatry 1997;30:1–5.

# Chapter 3

# Ginkgo biloba

*Forouzandeh Mahdavi and Melanie Johns Cupp*

## 3.1 History and Traditional Use

The ginkgo tree, *Ginkgo biloba* (L.), is the last remaining member of the Ginkgoaceae family, which once included many species (Tyler, 1993). It has survived unchanged in China for more than 200 million yr, and was brought to Europe in 1730 and to America in 1784. Since then it has become a popular ornamental tree worldwide. Individual trees may live as long as 1000 yr, and grow to a height of about 125 ft (Anonymous, 1998). Ginkgo fruits and seeds have been used in China for their medicinal properties since 2800 BC (Tyler, 1993). Traditional Chinese physicians used ginkgo leaves to treat asthma and chilblains (swelling of the hands and feet from exposure to damp cold) (Anonymous, 1998). The ancient Chinese and Japanese ate roasted ginkgo seeds as a digestive aid and to prevent drunkenness (Anonymous, 1998). Ginkgo use had spread to Europe by the 1960s.

## 3.2 Current Promoted Use

*Ginkgo biloba* (GB) is sold as a dietary supplement in the United States. It is purported to improve blood flow to the brain and to improve peripheral circulation. It is promoted mainly to sharpen mental focus in otherwise healthy adults as well as in those with dementia. Other conditions for which it is currently used are diabetes-related circulatory disorders, impotence, and vertigo.

## 3.3 Products Available

An acetone–water mixture is used to extract the dried and milled leaves (Tyler, 1993). After the solvent is removed, the extract is dried and standard-

From Forensic Science: *Toxicology and Clinical Pharmacology of Herbal Products*
Edited by: M. J. Cupp © Humana Press Inc., Totowa, New Jersey

ized. Most commercially prepared dosage forms contain 40 mg of this extract (GBE) (Tyler, 1993), and are standardized to contain approx 24% flavonoids (mostly flavone glycosides, or ginkgoflavone glycosides) and 6% terpenes (ginkgolides and bilobalide) (Amri et al, 1996; Hasenohrl et al., 1996; Nemecz and Combest, 1997). Twelve ginkgo products analyzed in the March 1999 issue of *Consumer Reports* contained approx 24% flavone glycosides and 6% terpene lactones, percentages that were chosen based on a study (Le Bars, 1997) that showed benefit in Alzheimer's disease. On average, the brands were within 2% of meeting this standard, but within individual bottles, the content often varied. Of the brands tested, Natural Brand® by General Nutrition and Ginkoba® by Pharmaton contained 24.3% and 23.7% flavone glycosides, respectively, and were closest to the designated amounts. Nature Made® by Pharmavite and Ginkgold® by Nature's Way were closest to the designated amounts of terpene lactones, with 6.4% and 6.9%, respectively (Anonymous, 1999).

GB formulations include:

Ginkoba®, 40-mg tablet
ginkgo, 40-mg tablet, capsule, or softgels
ginkgo biloba, 120-mg extract caplets
ginkgo leaf, 400-mg tablet
Ginkai®, 50-mg tablet
Ginkogin® (ginkgo, ginseng, and garlic) caplets
Bioginkgo®, 60-mg tablet

Other formulations include sublingual sprays, which deliver 40 mg per spray, and concentrated liquid extracts (Nemecz and Combest, 1997). The usual dosage recommended is 120 mg of standardized extract per day for treatment periods of up to 6 wk (Nemecz and Combest, 1997).

## 3.4 Pharmacologic/Toxicologic Effects

The effects of GB are attributed to several chemical constituents of the whole plant rather than to any one individual component. These chemicals include many flavonoids (also called flavonol, flavone, or flavonoid glycosides; ginkgo flavone glycosides; dimeric bioflavones), and the terpene lactones (also called terpenoids; diterpenes; terpenes), including the ginkgolides and bilobalide (Ramassamy et al., 1990; Houghton, 1994; Nemecz and Combest, 1997; Anonymous, 1998).

### 3.4.1 Nervous System Effects

The pharmacologic basis of the effects of GBE on brain function has been addressed in a number of studies. One study (Ramassamy et al., 1990) showed that dietary GBE 761 (prepared by the Henri Baeufour Institute) protected striatal dopaminergic neurons of male Sprague–Dawley rats from damage caused by *N*-methyl-4–phenyl-1,2,3,6-tetrahydropyridine (MPTP). MPTP, which has caused Parkinsonism in young drug abusers, is thought to damage these neurons through formation of free radicals. The mechanism of GBE's protective effect was attributed to an antioxidant action, rather than to prevention of neuronal uptake of MPTP. Whether chronic GBE ingestion could prevent development of idiopathic Parkinson's disease in humans remains to be seen.

This same extract has been investigated for the treatment of dementia. In one study (Le Bars et al., 1997), 40-mg EGb 761 (Murdock, Springville, UT) tablets taken three times daily before meals was compared to placebo in a double-blind, randomized trial in patients with mild to severe Alzheimer type or multiinfarct dementia, diagnosed according to the *Diagnostic and Statistical Manual of Mental Disorders*, 3rd edit., *Revised* (DSM-III-R) and *International Statistical Classification of Diseases, 10th Revision* (ICD-10) criteria. The study lasted 52 wk, and patients were assessed at weeks 3, 26, and 52 using the cognitive subscale of the Alzheimer's Disease Assessment Scale (ADAS-Cog), the Geriatric Evaluation by Relative's Rating Instrument (GERRI), and the Clinical Global Impression of Change (CGIC), three validated rating instruments. Thus, participants' cognitive impairment, daily living and social behavior, and general psychopathology were objectively evaluated. Modest improvement was appreciated using ADAS-Cog and GERRI, but the CGIC score did not reveal improvement compared to placebo. Adverse effects did not differ from those of placebo. The relatively large number of dropouts (only 202 of 309 patients were assessed at week 52) raises questions about the validity of the results. In addition, a meta-analysis of four double-blind, placebo-controlled studies including a total of 424 Alzheimer's patients found a small (3%) but clinically significant improvement on the ADAS-Cog with 120–240 mg of *Ginkgo biloba* administered for 3–6 mo (Oken et al., 1998). Given such small benefits in light of ginkgo's association with spontaneous bleeding (*see* Section 3.5), more data are needed before ginkgo can be recommended for the treatment of Alzheimer's disease.

The cognitive effects of ginkgo have also been assessed in non-Alzheimer's patients. In 18 nondemented elderly men with slight age-related memory loss based on immediate recall of three lists of words, EGb 761 improved the speed of information processing based on ability to recall presented word and pictures (Allain et al., 1993).

Anxiolytic effects have been demonstrated in animal models. The effect of Zingicomb® (Mattern et Partner, Starnberg, Germany), a combination product containing 24% ginkgo flavonoids and 23.5% gingerols, administered orally to rats at a dose of 0.5–100 mg/kg was compared to the effects of placebo and diazepam administered intraperitoneally at a dose of 1 mg/kg on anxiety-associated behaviors (Hasenöhrl et al., 1996). The rats were subjected to an elevated plus-maze consisting of enclosed and open arms. The 0.5 mg/kg dose of Zingicomb® was associated with rats spending more time in the open arms and with more excursions toward the ends of the open arms as compared to placebo. At a dose of 100 mg/kg, excursions to the ends of the open arms and scanning (protruding the head over the edge of an open arm and looking around) were fewer. These results were interpreted to mean that the preparation exhibited anxiolytic effects at a dose of 0.5 mg/kg, but anxiogenic effects at 100 mg/kg. Both the herbal product at a 0.5 mg/kg dose and diazepam increased the number of entries into the open arms, but unlike diazepam, Zingicomb® did not increase open arm scanning, nor did it attenuate risk assessment (protruding the forepaws and head from an enclosed arm). These effects of the herbal preparation were attributed to blockade of 5-hydroxytryptamine$_3$ (5-HT$_3$; serotonin) receptors, which has been shown in previous studies to produce similar results in the elevated plus-maze. In addition, components of both ginger and ginkgo have been shown in several animal studies to exert 5-HT$_3$ receptor-blocking effects.

Vertigo and tinnitus have been successfully relieved with ginkgo at doses of 16–160 mg/d for 3 mo (Kleijnen and Knipschild, 1992).

### 3.4.2 Cardiovascular Effects

EGb 761 at a dose 200 mg administered to 60 patients intravenously for 4 d improved skin perfusion and decreased blood viscosity without affecting plasma viscosity (Kleijnen and Knipschild, 1992). Another GB extract, LI 1730, increased blood flow in nailfold capillaries and decreased erythrocyte aggregation compared to placebo in 10 volunteers at a dose of 112.5 mg (Jung et al., 1990). Blood pressure, heart rate, packed cell volume, and plasma viscosity were unchanged.

Many studies have demonstrated that ginkgolides are capable of inhibiting platelet activating factor (PAF), which is involved in platelet aggregation and inflammatory processes such as are seen in asthma, ulcerative colitis, and allergies. These studies have been reviewed elsewhere (Kleijnen and Knipschild, 1992; Nemecz and Combest, 1997; Chavez and Chavez, 1998).

### 3.4.3 Carcinogenicity/Mutagenicity/Teratogenicity

No mutagenic, carcinogenic, or teratogenic effects have been noted in studies performed using commercially available ginkgo products containing 22–27% flavone glycosides and 5–7% terpene lactones (Blumenthal, 1998).

### *3.4.4 Endocrine Effects*

A study (Amri et al., 1996) of GB extract 761 in rats demonstrated that high doses (10–100 mg/kg) of the extract, as well as isolated ginkgolides A and B at doses of 2 mg/kg, decreased corticosteroid synthesis by up to 50% and 60%, respectively. An associated increase in adrenocorticotropic hormone (ACTH) levels was also seen.

## *3.5 Case Reports of Toxicity Due to Commercially Available Products*

Spontaneous intracerebral hemorrhage occurred in a 72-yr-old woman who had been taking ginkgo 50 mg three times daily for 6 mo (Gilbert, 1997).

Bilateral subdural hematomas were discovered in a 33-yr-old woman who had been taking 60 mg of GB twice daily for 2 yr, acetaminophen, and occasionally an ergotamine/caffeine preparation (Rowin and Lewis, 1996). Bleeding time was elevated, but had normalized when checked approx 1 mo after discontinuation of the product.

In a similar case, a 61-yr-old man presented with a subarachnoid hemorrhage after taking 40 mg GB tablets three or four times daily for >6 mo (Vale, 1998). Bleeding time was elevated (6 min, normal 1–3), but normalized with discontinuation of the product.

A 78-yr-old woman suffered a left parietal hemorrhage after taking a ginkgo preparation for 2 mo (Matthews, 1998). Other medications included warfarin, which she had been taking for 5 yr after undergoing coronary bypass. Prothrombin time was unchanged.

A 70-yr-old man experienced bleeding from the iris into the anterior chamber after self-medicating with 40 mg of Ginkoba® twice daily for 1 wk (Rosenblatt and Mindel, 1997). Other medications included 325 mg of aspirin daily for 3 yr post-coronary bypass. Ginkgo, but not aspirin, was discontinued, and no further bleeding problems occurred.

"Gin-nan" food poisoning, a toxic syndrome associated with ingestion of 50 or more ginkgo seeds, can result in loss of consciousness, tonic/clonic seizures, and/or death (Anonymous, 1998). Seventy cases were reported between 1930 and 1960, with a 27% mortality rate. Infants were at greatest risk. Although ginkgotoxin (4-*O*-methylpyridoxine), which is found mostly in the seeds, has been implicated as the responsible neurotoxin, its concentrations in several commercially available ginkgo products tested were deemed too low to have a toxic effect (Arenz et al., 1996). If used as directed, the maximum daily intake of 4-*O*-methylpyridoxine would be approx 60 μg; however, the presence of this neurotoxin raises questions about the herb's ability to lower the seizure threshold in patients with seizure disorders (Arenz et al., 1996). The authors of this study cite evidence that bilobalide present in the formulations may decrease the severity of convulsions, thus counteracting any neurotoxic effects of 4-*O*-methylpyridoxine.

Adverse effects listed in the German Commission E Ginkgo biloba leaf extract monograph include gastrointestinal upset, headache, and rash (Blumenthal, 1998).

## 3.6 Drug Interactions

In two of the five spontaneous bleeding episodes described in Section 3.4, medications that can affect platelet function or prothrombin time (i.e., aspirin and warfarin) were involved. Because ginkgo is known to be an inhibitor of PAF (Chung et al., 1987), an interaction between antiplatelet drugs (e.g., aspirin, nonsteroidal antiinflammatory drugs [NSAIDS], clopidogrel, ticlopidine, dipyridamole) or anticoagulants (e.g., warfarin, heparin) and ginkgo would appear possible. In fact, EGb 761 was shown to potentiate the antiplatelet effect of ticlopidine in rats (Kim et al., 1998). The dosages of both drugs used were higher on a milligram per kilogram basis compared to the usual human dose.

A study in which 400 mg of EGb was administered to 24 healthy volunteers for 13 d demonstrated that ginkgo is not an inducer of hepatic microsomal enzymes (Duche et al., 1989).

## 3.7 Pharmacokinetics/Toxicokinetics

### 3.7.1 Absorption

In humans, absolute bioavailability is 98–100% for ginkgolide A, 79–93% for ginkgolide B, and at least 70% for bilobalide (Blumenthal, 1998). In two healthy volunteers, flavonol glycosides administered as the product LI 1370 at doses of 50 mg, 100 mg, and 300 mg were absorbed in the small intestine with peak plasma concentration attained within 2–3 h (Kleijnen and Knipschild, 1992). Additional data from human experiments from the manufacturer of 80-mg EGb 761 solution show that the absolute bioavailabilities of ginkgolides A and B were >80%, while that of ginkgolide C was very low. Bioavailability of bilobalide was 70% after administration of 120 mg of the extract. Corroborating these results was a later pharmacokinetic study (Fourtillan et al., 1995) that found mean bioavailabilities of 80%, 88%, and 79% for ginkgolide A, ginkgolide B, and bilobalide, respectively. Food intake did increase the time to peak concentration, but did not affect bioavailability.

A study in rats using radiolabeled EGb 761 revealed a bioavailability of at least 60% (Kleijnen and Knipschild, 1992). Peak blood concentrations occurred at 1.5 h. At 3 h, the highest radioactivity was measured in the stomach and small intestine, indicating that these are the sites of absorption.

### *3.7.2 Distribution*

Rat studies using radiolabeled EGb 761 have revealed that the extract follows a two-compartment model of distribution (Kleijnen and Knipschild, 1992). The radiolabeled extract was distributed into glandular and neuronal tissues, as well as the eyes.

The volumes of distribution of ginkgolide A, ginkgolide B, and bilobalide are 40–60 L, 60–100 L, and 170 L, respectively (Kleijnen and Knipschild, 1992).

### *3.7.3 Metabolism/Elimination*

The half-life of the flavonol glycosides administered as the product LI 1370 is 2–4 h (Kleijnen and Knipschild, 1992). Similar results were obtained using 80 mg of the product EGb 761; half-lives of ginkgolides A and B were 4 h and 6 h, respectively. The half-life of bilobalide was 3 h after administration of 120 mg of this extract. Similar results were reported in another study (Fourtillan et al., 1995) using this same product; mean half-lives of ginkgolide A, ginkgolide B, and bilobalide were 4.5 h, 10.57 h, and 3.21 h, respectively.

A study in rats using radiolabeled EGb 761 reveled a half-life of 4.5 h, with elimination following first-order (linear) kinetics (Kleijnen and Knipschild, 1992).

Approximately 70% of ginkgolide A, 50% of ginkgolide B, and 30% of bilobalide is excreted unchanged in the urine (Kleijnen and Knipschild, 1992). Metabolites isolated from human urine after administration of EGb include a 4-hydroxybenzoic acid conjugate, 4-hydroxyhippuric acid, 3-methoxy-4-hydroxyhippuric acid, 3,4-dihydroxybenzoic acid, 4-hydroxybenzoic acid, hippuric acid, and 3-methoxy-4-hydroxybenzoic acid (vanillic acid) (Pietta et al., 1997). In accord with previous data, these metabolites accounted for <30% of the administered EGb dose. Metabolites were not detectable in blood samples.

## 3.8 Chemical Analysis

Identification and chemical analysis can be found in the *National Formulary* (USP, 1998).

## 3.9 Analysis of Biofluids

Urine and blood samples were analyzed for EGb metabolites after administration to healthy volunteers (Pietta et al., 1997). Urine was collected for 3 d, and blood samples were collected every 30 min for 5 h. Samples were analyzed using SPE C18 cartridges and reverse-phase liquid chromatography with a diode array detector.

Twelve healthy volunteers were administered 0.9–3.36 mg EGb 761 intravenously or orally on three separate occasions (Fourtillan et al., 1995). Blood and urine samples were collected for up to 36 h and 48 h, respectively. Plasma and urine concentrations of ginkgolide A, ginkgolide B, and bilobalide were quantitatively measured using gas chromatography–mass spectrometry (GC–MS) with negative chemical ionization. Measurement of plasma concentrations as low as 0.2 ng/mL was possible using this sensitive method.

## 3.10 Regulatory Status

GB leaf extract is approved by the German Commission E for memory deficits, disturbances in concentration, depression, dizziness, vertigo, headache, dementia, and intermittent claudication (Blumenthal, 1998). It is regulated as a dietary supplement in the U.S.

## References

Allain H, Raoul P, Lieury A, LeCoz F, Gandon J. Effect of two doses of Ginkgo biloba extract (EGb 761) on the dual-coding test in elderly subjects. Clin Ther 1993;15:549–57.

Amri H, Ogwuegbu SO, Boujrad N, Drieu K, Papadopoulos V. In vivo regulation of peripheral-type benzodiazepine receptor and glucocorticoid synthesis by Ginkgo biloba extract EGb 761 and isolated ginkgolides. Endocrinology 1996;137:5707–18.

Anonymous. Ginkgo. In: The review of natural products. St. Louis, Missouri: Facts and Comparisons, 1998.

Anonymous. Ginkgo biloba active ingredients meet proper levels—*Consumer Reports*. F-D-C Reports. "The Tan Sheet." March 8, 1999, p. 8.

Arenz A, Klein M, Fiehe K, Groβ J, Drewke C, Hemscheidt T, Leistner E. Occurrence of neurotoxic 4'-*O*-mehtylpyridoxine in Ginkgo biloba leaves, Ginkgo medications, and Japanese ginkgo food. Planta Med 1996;62:548–51.

Blumenthal M. Ginkgo biloba. The complete German commission E monographs. Austin, TX, American Botanical Council, 1998.

Chavez ML, Chavez PI. Ginkgo (Part I): History, use, and pharmacologic properties. Hosp Pharm 1998;33:658–72.

Chung KF, McCusker M, Page CP, Dent G, Guinot P, Barnes PJ. Effect of ginkgolide mixture (BN 52063) in antagonizing skin and platelet responses to platelet activating factor in man. Lancet 1987;1:248–51.

Duche JC, Barre J Guinot P, Duchier J, Cournot A, Tillement JP. Effect of Ginkgo biloba extract on microsomal enzyme induction. Int J Clin Pharmacol Res 1989;9:165–8.

Fourtillan JB, Brisson AM, Girault J, Ingrand I, Decourt JP, Drieu K, et al. Pharmacokinetic properties of bilobalide and ginkgolides A and B in healthy subjects after intravenous and oral administration of Ginkgo biloba extract (EGb 761). Therapie 1995;50:137–44.

Gilbert GJ. Ginkgo biloba [letter]. Neurology 1997;48:1137.

Hasenohrl RU, Nichau CH, Frisch CH, De Souza Silva MA. Huston JP, Mattern CM, Hacker R. Anxiolytic-like effect of combined extracts of Zingiber officinale and Ginkgo biloba in the elevated plus-maze. Pharmacol Biochem Behav 1996;53:271–5.

Houghton P. Ginkgo. Pharm J 1994;253:122–3.

Kim YS, Pyo MK, Park PH, Hahn BS, Wu SJ, Yun-Choi HS. Antiplatelet and antithrombotic effects of a combination of ticlopidine and Ginkgo biloba extract (EGb 761). Thrombos Res 1998;91:33–8.

Kleijnen J, Knipschild P. Ginkgo biloba. Lancet 1992;340:1136–9.

Jung F, Mroweitz C, Kiesewetter H, Wenzel E. Effect of Ginkgo biloba on fluidity of blood and peripheral microcirculation in volunteers. Arzneim Forsch 1990;40:589–93.

Le Bars PL, Katz MM, Berman N, Itil TM, Freedman AM, Schatzberg AF, et al. A placebo controlled, double-blind, randomized trial of an extract of Ginkgo biloba for dementia. JAMA 1997;278:1327 -32.

Matthews MK. Association of Ginkgo biloba with intracranial hemorrhage [letter]. Neurology 1998;50:1933–4.

Nemecz G, Combest WL. Ginkgo biloba. US Pharmacist 1997(Sept):144,147–8,151.

Oken BS, Storzbach DM, Kaye JA. The efficacy of Ginkgo biloba on cognitive function in Alzheimer's disease. Arch Neurol 1998;55:1409–15.

Pietta PG, Gardana C, Mauri PL. Identification of Ginkgo flavonol metabolites after oral administration to humans. J Chromatogr Biomed Sci Appl 1997;693:249–55.

Ramassamy C, Clostre F, Christen Y, Costentin J. Prevention by a ginkgo extract (GBE 761) of the dopaminergic neurotoxicity of MPTP. J Pharm Pharmacol 1990;42:785–9.

Rosenblatt M, Mindel J. Spontaneous hyphema associated with ingestion of Ginkgo biloba extract [letter]. N Engl J Med 1997;336:1108.

Rowin J, Lewis SL. Spontaneous bilateral subdural hematomas associated with chronic Ginkgo biloba ingestion [letter]. Neurology 1996;46:1775–76.

Tyler VE. The honest herbal. 3rd edit., Binghamton, NY: Pharmaceutical Products Press, 1993.

United States Pharmacopoeia (USP). National Formulary. 18th edit., Suppl 9. Rockville, MD: United States Pharmacopeial Convention, 1998.

Vale S. Subarachnoid hemorrhage associated with Ginkgo biloba [letter]. Lancet 1998;352:36.

# Chapter 4

# Valerian

*Marlea Givens and Melanie Johns Cupp*

*Valeriana officinalis* (L.), *V. wallichii* DC. (Indian valerian), *V. alliariifolia* Vahl, *V. sambucifolia* Mik, radix valerianae, red valerian (*Centranthus ruber* [L.] DC) (Anonymous, 1991), valerian root, valerianae radix (USP, 1998), garden heliotrope, all heal, amantilla, and setwall (Heiligenstein and Guenther, 1998)

## 4.1 History and Traditional Uses

Valerian is a perennial herb comprised of grooved hollow stems and saw-toothed green leaves. White, pale pink, or reddish flowers appear from June to August. Valerian grows to heights of 3–5 ft in the temperate climates of North America, western Asia, and Europe, often in moist soil along riverbanks. The vertical rhizome and attached roots of valerian are parts used medicinally, and are best harvested in the autumn of the second year (Combest, 1997). Although the fresh drug has no distinctive odor, over time hydrolysis of compounds present in the volatile oil produces isovaleric acid, which has an offensive, somewhat putrid odor (Anonymous, 1991). Fortunately, the smell can be removed from the skin and utensils by washing with sodium bicarbonate (Houghton, 1994). Even though valerian has a disagreeable odor, people in the 16th century considered it a fragrant perfume (Anonymous, 1991). Traditional uses include treatment of migraine headache, anxiety, fatigue, and seizures (USP, 1998). It has also been applied externally on cuts, sores, and acne. Traditional Chinese uses include treatment of headache, numbness due to rheumatic conditions, colds, menstrual difficulties, and bruises.

## 4.2 Current Promoted Uses

Valerian is promoted in the United States for treatment of insomnia (USP, 1998).

From Forensic Science: *Toxicology and Clinical Pharmacology of Herbal Products*
Edited by: M. J. Cupp, ed. © Humana Press Inc., Totowa, New Jersey

## 4.3 Products Available

Crude valerian root, rhizome, or stolon is dried and used either "as is" or used to prepare an extract. Valerian is available as a capsule, tablet, oral solution, or tea (USP, 1998). Valerian is also administered externally as a bath additive (Blumenthal, 1998). The following are a few examples of valerian products found in retail outlets:

- Yourlife® valerian is standardized to 0.8% valerenic acid. The recommended dose is two 100-mg softgels at bedtime with a full glass of water.
- NaturaLife® valerian is standardized to 0.15% valerenic acid. The recommended dose is 2–4 mL of the 0.15 mg/mL liquid extract 30–60 min before going to sleep. It can be added to food or beverages.
- Twinlab TruHerbs® timed release valerian is standardized to 0.8% valerenic acid. Each capsule contains 450 mg of valerian (300 mg of valerenic acid and 150 mg of valerian root). The capsules are designed to release the herb over 12 h. The recommended dose is one capsule daily.
- Nature's Resource® standardized valerian root capsules contain 530 mg of valerian. The recommended dose is one or two capsules 1 h prior to bedtime.
- Sundown® Herbals valerian root complex contains 400 mg of valerian root and 180 mg of a kava/passion flower blend. The recommended dose is two capsules up to four times daily as needed.
- Quanterra™ Sleep conains valerian 150 mg and lemon balm 75 mg. Consumers are instructed to take 2–3 tablets one-half hour to one hour before bedtime. The manufacturer claims this product is unique because it is odor-controlled.

## 4.4 Pharmacologic/Toxicologic Effects

### 4.4.1 Central Nervous System Effects

Several studies have examined the effects of valerian on sleep (Leathwood et al., 1982; Leathwood and Chauffard, 1985; Balderer and Borbely, 1985; Lindahl and Lindwall, 1989; Schulz et al., 1994). Leathwood and colleagues demonstrated valerian's effect on sleep quality. A freeze dried aqueous extract of valerian root (*Rhizoma valeriana officinalis* [L.]) 400 mg was compared to two Hova® (valerian 60 mg and hop flower extract 30 mg per tablet) tablets and placebo (finely ground brown sugar) in this crossover study involving 128 volunteers. Study participants took the study medication 1 h before retiring, and filled out a questionnaire the following morning. This was repeated on nonconsecutive nights, such that each of the three treatments, identified only by a code number, was administered in random order three times to each patient. Valerian caused a significant improvement in subjectively evaluated sleep quality and a significant decrease in perceived sleep latency. The self-reported improvement in sleep quality was especially notable in smokers, those patients who considered themselves poor or irregular sleepers, and those who reported having difficulty falling asleep on a prestudy questionnaire. Hova® did not demonstrate any beneficial effect, but it was reported to cause a "hangover effect" the next morning. Because subjective sleep questionnaires may not correlate with sleep EEG results, a parallel EEG sleep study was performed comparing valerian to placebo in 10 young men. There was not a statistically significant difference between valerian and placebo in this small study. The authors hypothesized that the results of this experiment might have differed from the questionnaire-assessed study because of small sample size and differences in study populations. The larger study involved young and old individuals, men and women, and good and poor sleepers, while the EEG study involved young men with no reported sleep abnormalities. Rather than place more credence on the objective study, the investigators concluded that the questionnaire provides a more sensitive means of detecting mild sedative effects.

A double-blind, placebo-controlled study (Leathwood and Chauffard, 1985) was performed in eight volunteers recruited from among the research staff at Nestle Products and their families who reported that they "usually have problems getting to sleep." Sleep latency was measured using an activity monitor and questionnaire. The investigators documented a small (7 min) but statistically significant decrease in sleep latency with 450 mg of an extract of valerian (*Valeriana officinalis* [L.]). No further improvement was demonstrated with a 900-mg valerian dose; however, patients receiving the higher dose were more likely to feel sleepy the next morning. Sleep quality, sleep latency, and sleep depth also improved according to a nine-point subjective rating scale. However, the appropriateness of the statistical analysis used to interpret the results of the subjective portion of the study is questionable.

A more objective double-blind, placebo-controlled trial (Balderer and Borbely, 1985) evaluated the effect of 450-mg and 900-mg doses of an aqueous valerian extract (*Valeriana officinalis* [L.]) on two groups of healthy, young (21–44 yr of age) volunteers at home and in a laboratory setting. The effect of valerian on sleep was measured using a questionnaire and night-time motor activity recordings in both settings. The effects of valerian on the volunteers in the sleep laboratory were also measured using polysomnography and spectral analysis of the sleep EEG. Both groups demonstrated the mild hypnotic effects of valerian; however, the benefits of valerian were statistically significant only under home conditions. No difference in efficacy between the lower and higher valerian dose was appreciated, as in the study by Leathwood and Chaffaurd. Also, as with Leathwood and colleagues, these investigators were not able to confirm the results of subjective questionnaires using more objective methods. The authors attributed these results to the unfamiliar, artificial conditions of the laboratory, or to the young age of the study subjects.

Another double-blind, placebo-controlled crossover study (Lindahl and Lindwall, 1989) evaluated Valerina Natt®, a preparation equivalent to 400 mg of valerian root composed mainly of sesquiterpenes from *Valeriana officinalis* [L.], on subjective sleep quality assessed using a three-point rating scale. Study subjects were 27 consecutive patients seen in a medical clinic for evaluation of sleep difficulty and fatigue who were willing to participate in the investigation. Statistically significant improvement in sleep in quality was noted with the valerian preparation. Twenty-one subjects rated valerian as better than placebo, two rated the preparations equally, and four preferred placebo. No adverse effects were reported. Although some study subjects had experienced nightmares when using conventional hypnotics, nightmares were not reported in the study.

The effects of repeated doses (three tablets thrice daily) for eight days of Valdispert Forte® (135 mg of dried extract of *Valeriana officinalis* [L.]) in 14 elderly women with sleeping difficulties was assessed using polysomnography in a particularly well-designed study (Schulz et al., 1994). Inclusion criteria were well defined: sleep latency longer than 30 min, more than three nocturnal awakenings per night with inability to go back to sleep within 5 min, and total sleep time less than 5 h. Subjects could not have medical, psychological, or weight-related causes of sleep difficulty, and had to have normal health status for their age. Sedatives, hypnotics, and other central nervous system (CNS)-active drugs were discontinued 2 wk prior to the study, and drug screening for morphine, benzodiazepines, barbiturates, and amphetamine was done prior to study commencement. Results showed an increase in slow-wave-sleep (SWS), and a decrease in sleep stage 1. There was no effect on REM sleep, sleep latency, time awake after sleep onset, or self-rated sleep quality.

In aggregate, the results of these clinical studies suggest that at doses of approx 450 mg of the aqueous extract, valerian has mild hypnotic effects, possibly by affecting non-REM sleep in patients with reduced SWS. Unlike benzodiazepines, valerian appears not to adversely affect slow-wave or REM sleep, and does not appear to cause nightmares or hangover. Further well-designed studies are needed to objectively evaluate valerian.

Results of animal studies reflect the clinical data. Sedative properties of Valdispert® (dried aqueous extract of *Valeriana officinalis* [L.]) in mice were documented based on reduced spontaneous movement and an increase in thiopental-induced sleep time; however, these effects were slightly less than those of diazepam and chlorpromazine. No significant anticonvulsant effect was observed (Leuschner et al., 1993).

Hendriks and colleagues tested several components of the volatile oil, obtained by steam distillation of *Valeriana officinalis* [L.], on mice. The essential oil, its hydrocarbon fraction, its oxygen fraction, valeranone, valerenal, valerenic acid, and isoeugenyl-isovalerate were injected intraperitoneally at various doses ranging from 50 to 1600 mg/kg, with three mice receiving each dose. The mice were observed between 15 and 30 min post-injection for various symptoms suggestive of CNS stimulation or depression, analgesia, sympathomimetic or sympatholytic activity, vasodilation, or vasoconstriction. It was concluded that components of the essential oil, particularly valerenic acid and valerenal, which are present in the oxygen fraction, have a sedative and/or muscle relaxant effect.

A later study by these same authors (Hendriks et al., 1985) tested the effect of intraperitoneal valerenic acid compared to diazepam, chlorpromazine, and pentobarbital on ability to walk on a rotating rod and grip strength in mice. The effects of valerinic acid on spontaneous motor activity and on pentobarbital-induced sleeping time were also assessed. Diazepam, a muscle relaxant, affected the grip test but not the rotarod test, while chlorpromazine, a neuroleptic, affected the rotarod test but not the grip test. Valerenic acid, like pentobarbital, decreased performance in both the rotarod and grip tests. The authors concluded that valerenic acid, like pentobarbital, has general CNS depressant activity. Valerenic acid also decreased spontaneous motor activity and prolonged pentobarbital-induced sleeping time. Dose–response effects of valerenic acid were also observed by the investigators. At a dose of 50 mg/kg, a decrease in spontaneous motor activity occurred. At 100 mg/kg, mice exhibited ataxia, then remained motionless. Muscle spasms occurred at 150–200 mg/kg and convulsions at 400 mg/kg, followed by death in six of seven mice within 24 h.

Sedation is mediated predominantly through the inhibitory neurotransmitter γ-aminobutyric acid (GABA). Dihydrovaltrate, hydroxyvalerenic acid, a hydroalcoholic extract containing 0.8% valerenic acid; a lipid extract; an aqueous extract of the hydroalcoholic extract, and another aqueous extract of *Valeriana officinalis* (L.) were assessed for in vitro binding to rat GABA, benzodiazepine, and barbiturate receptors (Mennini et al., 1993). The results indicated that an interaction of some component of the hydroalcoholic extract, the aqueous extract derived from the hydroalcoholic extract, and the other aqueous extract had affinity for the $GABA_A$ receptor. Because hydroxyvalerenic acid (a volatile oil sesquiterpene) and dihydrovaltrate (a valepotriate) did not show any notable activity, the investigators could not identify the specific constituents responsible for this activity. The lipophilic extract derived from the hydroalcoholic extract as well as dihydrovaltrate showed affinity for barbiturate receptors, and some affinity for peripheral benzodiazepine receptors.

Other in vitro studies have also yielded results that suggest GABA-mediated activity; however, the active constituent was unidentified. Cavadas and colleagues verified that valerenic acid (0.1 mmol/L) was not able to displace

[$^3$H] muscimol from the $GABA_A$ receptor, although both an aqueous and a hydroalcoholic extract were able to do so. The investigators then attempted to identify other compounds in the extracts capable of displacing [$^3$H] muscinol. Both glutamate and glutamine, amino acids present in the aqueous extract, had little inhibitory effect on [$^3$H] muscinol binding. However, glutamine can cross the blood–brain barrier and can be taken up by nerve terminals and converted to GABA inside GABAergic neurons. Thus, glutamine could be responsible for the sedative effect of the aqueous extract, but not the hydroalcoholic extract, in which it is not present. GABA is found in both extracts, but GABA itself cannot explain the sedative effects of valerian because it is unlikely to cross the blood–brain barrier in amounts significant to cause sedation (Cavadas et al., 1995). However, the amount of GABA present in the aqueous extract is sufficient to have effects on peripheral GABA receptors, perhaps resulting in muscle relaxation (Santos et al., 1994b). Another study (Santos et al., 1994a) suggests a different mechanism of action involving inhibition of neuronal GABA uptake and stimulation of GABA release from synaptosomes. These investigators did not attempt to elucidate which constituent of the aqueous extract was responsible for these effects.

The CNS depressant component of valerian is still unknown. Thus far, three major constituents of valerian have been identified: the volatile or essential oil, containing sesquiterpenes and monoterpenes, nonglycosidic iridoid esters (valepotriates), and a small number of alkaloids (Anonymous, 1991). Valepotriates are unstable compounds and are easily hydrolyzed by heat and moisture (Wagner et al., 1998). In addition, valepotriates are not water soluble, and aqueous extracts contain small amounts (Wagner et al., 1998). For example, the aqueous extract used in the study by Balderer and Borbely, described previously, was analyzed using thin-layer chromatography (TLC), and no valepotriates were detectable. Furthermore, valepotriates are not well absorbed orally (Tyler, 1993). Therefore, the likelihood that valepotriates are a major contributor to valerian's effects is questionable. Because of the low amount of alkaloid present in preparations, their contribution is also questionable (Houghton, 1988). It is postulated that a combination of volatile oils, valepotriates, and possibly certain water-soluble constituents that have not yet been identified are responsible for valerian's sedative effects (Tyler, 1993).

Antidepressant effects of valerian were identified by Oshima and associates using a methanol extract of *Valeriana fauriei* roots (Oshima et al., 1995). They found a strong antidepressant activity in mice as measured by the forced swimming test. One active component isolated was α-kessyl alcohol, a volatile oil component. At 30 mg/kg intraperitoneally, α-kessyl alcohol exhibited an effect similar to imipramine, a commonly used antidepressant. Kessanol and cyclokessyl acetate, guaiane-type sesquiterpenoids, also exhibited antidepressant activity. Kanokonol, kessyl glycol, and kessyl glycol diacetate, valerane-type sesquiterpenoids, did not exhibit an effect.

A 30% ethanol extract of the Japanese valerian root ("Hokkai-Kisso") extract (4.1 g/kg and 5.7 g/kg) and imipramine (20 mg/kg) also demonstrated statistically significant antidepressant effects compared to placebo as measured by the forced swimming test in rats (Sakamoto et al., 1992). As in the Oshima study, kessyl glycol diacetate exhibited no antidepressant activity in the forced swimming test. Because the forced swimming test can be affected by stimulants, anticholinergics, and antihistamines as well as antidepressants, the effect of the valerian extract on reserpine-induced hypothermia, a test for antidepressant activity and inhibition of neuronal reuptake of monoamines, was measured. Both valerian (11.2 g/kg) and imipramine (20 mg/kg) reversed reserpine-induced hypothermia, suggesting that the antidepressant effect of valerian is due to reuptake of monoamine neurotransmitters, as with conventional antidepressants.

### *4.4.2 Musculoskeletal Effects*

(*See also* Section 4.4.1 for a discussion of the possible mechanisms of musculoskeletal effects.)

Isovaltrate and valtrate (valepotriates) and valeronone, an essential oil component, isolated from *Valeriana edulis* ssp. *procera* Meyer (Valeriana "mexicana") caused suppression of rhythmic contractions in guinea pig ileum in vivo at a dose of 20 mg/kg administered intravenously via the jugular vein. The investigators also demonstrated that the same compounds as well as dihydrovaltrate isolated from the same valerian species produced relaxation of carbachol-stimulated guinea pig ileum preparations in vitro. They concluded that these compounds have a musculotropic action in concentrations from $10^{-5}$ to $10^{-4}$ *M* (Hazelhoff et al., 1982).

### *4.4.3 Reproduction*

There has been a theoretical concern with regard to pregnant women taking valerian because of possible effects on uterine contractions (Combest, 1997), but no problems were noted in three cases of intentional overdose with 2–5 g of valerian during wk 3–10 of pregnancy (Czeizel et al., 1997). A mentally retarded child was born to a woman who overdosed on valerian 3 g, phenobarbital, glutethamide, amobarbital, and promethazine at 20 wk gestation, but this same woman delivered a mentally retarded child 2 yr later after an overdose attempt with glutethamide, amobarbital, and promethazine (Czeizel et al., 1988).

*Valeriana officinalis* (L.) was tested on rats and their offspring. A mixture, containing three valepotriates (80% dihydrovaltrate, 15% valtrate, and 5% acevaltrate), was orally administered to female rats for 30 d at 6 mg/kg, 12 mg/kg, and 24 mg/kg doses. Ten rats received each dose, and 10 received placebo. No changes were noted in the average length of the estrus cycle, nor the number of estrus phases during the 30-d observation period. Forty pregnant rats were also administered the valepotriate mixture or placebo in the manner described previously from the first through the 19th day of pregnancy. Valerian did not increase the risk of fetotoxicity or external malformation. However, internal examination revealed a significant increase in the number of fetuses with retarded ossification with the 12 mg/kg and 24 mg/kg doses. No developmental changes were detected in the offspring after treatment during pregnancy (Tufik et al., 1994).

### 4.4.4 Cardiovascular Effects

Pharmacological investigations using a particular valepotriate fraction called $V_{pt2}$ extracted from the roots of *Valeriana officinalis* (L.) have shown antiarrhythmic activity and ability to dilate coronary arteries in experimental animals. Moderate positive inotropic and a negative chronotropic effect were also observed. $V_{pt2}$ contains valtratum (50%), valeridine (25%), and valechlorin (3%), with trace amounts of acevaltrate, dihydrovaltratum, and epi-7-desacetylisovaltrate (Petkov, 1979).

Alcoholic extracts of *Valeriana officinalis* (L.) root (labeled V103 and V115) demonstrated hypotensive effects in rats, cats, and dogs. The V115 fraction showed greater potency and was extracted by a countercurrent distribution to yield three fractions. The first two fractions demonstrated hypotensive effects in rats, with the first fraction showing a hypotensive effect at 30 mg/kg. The third fraction produced hypertensive effects at a dose of 200 mg/kg. The authors noted that apparently, with each succeeding extraction, less of the hypotensive principle was extracted. The hypotensive effect of the V103 fraction in rats was demonstrated at a dose of 500 mg/kg, and was hypothesized to act via a parasympathomimetic effect, blockade of the carotid sinus reflex, and CNS depression (Rosecrans et al., 1961).

### 4.4.5 Cytotoxicity

The valepotriates valtrate/isovaltrate and dihydrovaltrate were isolated from *Valeriana mexicana* and *Valeriana wallichii*, respectively. The valepotriates tested were cytotoxic to granulocyte/macrophage colony forming units (GM-CFCUs), lymphocytes, and erythrocyte colony forming units (E-CFCUs).

Valtrate was found to be a more potent inhibitor of GM-CFCUs ($ID_{50}$ ~ $3.7 \times 10^{-6}$ *M* vs ~ $1.7 \times 10^{-5}$ *M*) and T-lymphocytes ($ID_{50}$ ~$2.8 \times 10^{-6}$ *M* vs ~ $3 \times 10^{-5}$ *M*) than dihydrovaltrate. Valtrate and dihydrovaltrate were similar in their activity against E-CFCUs ($ID_{50}$ ~ $2.3 \times 10^{-8}$ vs ~ $4.2 \times 10^{-8}$ *M*). Because pharmaceutical products containing valepotriates are orally administered, their cytotoxicity to gastrointestinal mucosal cells is of concern (Tortarolo et al., 1982).

The effects of valtrate, dihydrovaltrate, and deoxido-dihydrovaltrate, valepotriates extracted from *Valeriana wallichii* (DC.), on cultured rat hepatoma cells have been studied. Valtrate killed 50% of the cell population at a concentration of 5 μ*M*, Deoxido-dihydrovaltrate and dihydrovaltae demonstrated this same toxicity at double the dose. Valtrate was also the most potent inhibitor of DNA and protein synthesis (Bounthanh et al., 1983). These results suggest a mechanism by which valerian may cause hepatotoxicity.

## 4.5 Case reports of Toxicity Due to Commercially Available Products

Four cases of women who sustained liver damage after taking valerian-containing herbal medicines to relieve stress have been described (MacGregor et al., 1989). These cases are discussed in detail in the Scullcap chapter. In addition, valerian was used by a patient who exhibited hepatotoxicity attributed to Chaparral (*see* Chaparral chapter).

Twenty-three patients were admitted to hospitals for treatment of intentional overdose with Sleep-Qik® (75 mg of valerian dry extract, 0.25 mg of hyoscine hydrobromide 2 mg of cyproheptadine hydrochloride) between 1988 and 1991. Nine men and 14 women, mean age of 23.8 yr (range 15–37 yr) were treated. They were previously healthy, except for two patients with histories of psychiatric illness. The mean number of Sleep-Qik® tablets taken per patient history was 33 (range 6–166), for an average of 2.5 g (range 0.5–12 g) of valerian. Four patients were asymptomatic. The other 19 patients reported drowsiness ($n$ = 11), dilated pupils ($n$ = 11), tachycardia ($n$ = 6), nausea ($n$ = 4), confusion ($n$ = 3), urinary retention ($n$ = 3), visual hallucination ($n$ = 2), flushing ($n$ = 2), dry mouth ($n$ = 1), and dizziness ($n$ = 1). Coingestants were alcohol ($n$ = 2), a pesticide ($n$ = 1), and Pansedan® ($n$ = 1) (*Passiflora* extract, *Viscum album* extract, *Uncaria rhyncophylla* extract, and *Humulus lupulus*). One patient who was drowsy had also taken Panseden®, and one who was confused had ingested alcohol. Most patients received gastric lavage ($n$ = 14), and one received syrup of ipecac. The patient who took 60 tablets of Sleep-Qik® required ventillary support. Liver function tests were performed on 12 patients approx 6–12 h after ingestion with normal results. Drowsiness and confusion resolved within 24 h. All patients recovered completely and were discharged after an average of 1.7 d (range 1–6 d). At an average of 43 mo (range 27–65 mo) after presentation, 10 patients were contacted by telephone. They had all remained well after discharge and none continued taking Sleep-Qik®. Delayed onset of severe liver damage was ruled out via telephone interview, but subclinical disease could not be ruled out (Chan et al., 1995).

Subsequently, Chan reported on twenty-four cases of overdose of a product containing valerian dry extract 75 mg, hyoscine hydrobromide 0.25 mg, and cyproheptadine hydrochloride 2 mg. Six patients developed vomiting, and fifteen underwent gastric lavage. Co-ingestants included alcohol ($n = 10$), cold products ($n = 3$), hypnotics ($n = 2$), unknown drugs ($n = 2$), and gasoline ($n = 1$). Symptoms were mainly central nervous system depression and anticholinergic symptoms. One patient required ventilatory support. Liver function tests performed in seventeen, and all were normal. Over the next 22–48 mo post-ingestion, none of the patients returned to the hospital or clinic for any reason, suggesting that serious hepatotoxicity did not occur. The author points out that gastric lavage and spontaneous vomiting may have limited the amount of valerian absorbed in these patients, thus decreasing the risk of any delayed adverse effects (Chan, 1998). Other adverse effects attributed to overdose or chronic use of valerian include headaches, excitability, restlessness, uneasiness, blurred vision, and cardiac disturbances (USP, 1998).

In another reported suicide attempt, an 18-yr female ingested between 40 and 50 470-mg capsules (18.8–23.5 g valerian) of 100% powered valerian root (Nature's Way®, Springville, UT). Thirty minutes after ingestion, the patient complained of fatigue, crampy abdominal pain, chest tightness, tremor of the hands and feet, and lightheadedness. She presented to the emergency room 3 h post-ingestion. Her vital signs were blood pressure 111/64 mm Hg, pulse 72 beats/min, respiratory rate 14 breaths/min, and temperature 37.6°C. Physical exam was unremarkable except for mydriasis (6 mm bilaterally). EKG, complete blood count (CBC), and chemistry profile including liver function tests were normal. Toxicology screen was positive for marijuana, which she admitted using 2 wk previously. She denied ingesting anything else. After two doses of activated charcoal, her symptoms resolved within 24 h (Willey et al., 1995).

Subsequently, Chan reported on twenty-four cases of overdose of a product containing valerian dry extract 75 mg, hyoscine hydrobromide 0.25 mg, and cyproheptadine hydrochloride 2 mg. Six patients developed vomiting, and fifteen underwent gastric lavage. Co-ingestants included alcohol ($n = 10$), cold products ($n = 3$), hypnotics ($n = 2$), unknown drugs ($n = 2$), and gasoline ($n = 1$). Symptoms were mainly central nervous system depression and anticholinergic symptoms. One patient required ventilatory support. Liver function tests performed in seventeen, and all were normal. Over the next 22–48 mo post-ingestion, none of the patients returned to the hospital or clinic for any reason, suggesting that serious hepatotoxicity did not occur. The author points out that gastric lavage and spontaneous vomiting may have limited the amount of valerian absorbed in these patients, thus decreasing the risk of any delayed adverse effects (Chan, 1998).

A withdrawal syndrome was described after abrupt discontinuation of valerian root extract in a 58-yr-old man who had taken 530–2000 mg/dose five times daily as an anxiolytic and hypnotic for many years. Withdrawal symptoms included sinus tachycardia of up to 150 beats/min, tremulousness, and delirium after recovery from general anesthesia (propofol, nitrous oxide, isoflurane, and thiopental) for open biopsy of a lung nodule. Medical history included coronary artery disease, hypertension, and congestive heart failure with an ejection fraction of 30–35%. Medications included isosorbide dinitrate, digoxin, furosemide, benazepril, aspirin, lovastatin, ibuprofen, potassium, zinc supplement, and vitamins. The biopsy was complicated by multiple episodes of oxygen desaturation, and after extubation, the patient experienced tacycardia, oliguria, and increasing oxyen requirement. Naloxone was administered, with worsening of symptoms. Swan–Ganz catheterization revealed high-output heart failure. At this time, interview with family members revealed the patient's long-standing valerian use. Because valerian withdrawal was suspected, midazolam 1 mg each hour (total dose 11 mg in 17 h) was administered. Signs and symptoms improved, and stabilized by the third postoperative day. He was switched to lorazepam 1 mg each hour as needed (total dose 5 mg in 24 h), and then to a tapering dose of clonazepam. He was discharged on postoperative day 7, and was stable at 5-mo follow-up. Other causes of high output heart failure were ruled out, but because of the patient's multiple medical problems, postsurgical status, and medications administered, the cause of the patient's symptoms is unclear (Garges et al., 1998). The authors of this case report note that valerian has been shown to attenuate benzodiazepine withdrawal in rats (Andreatini and Loire, 1994).

## 4.6 Drug Interactions

Two alcoholic valerian extracts were found to potentiate pentobarbital sleeping time in mice (Rosecrans et al., 1961), and Valdispert®, an aqueous extract prepared from *Valeriana officinalis* (L.), increased the thiopental sleeping time in a dose-dependent manner in rats (Leuschner et al., 1993). Based on these animal studies, in vitro studies of valerian's effect on GABAergic transmission, as well as the case series reported by Chan and colleagues, valerian would be expected to have at least an additive effect with barbiturates, alcohol, benzodiazepines, and other CNS depressants.

Also *see* Chapter 5, St. John's wort, section 5.6 Drug Interactions.

## 4.7 Chemical Analysis

Isolation and identification of the essential oil components valeranone, valerenal, valerenic acid and isoeugenyl-isovalerate (Hazelhoff et al., 1979a; Hendriks et al., 1981) and the valepotriates valtrate, isovaltrate, and didrovaltrate (Hazelhoff et al., 1979b; Tittel and Wagner, 1978; Tittel et al., 1978).

## 4.8 Regulatory Status

Valerian was included as an official drug in the *US Pharmacopeia* until 1936 and in the *National Formulary* until 1946. Currently, the USP advisory panel does not recommend valerian's use owing to lack of adequate scientific evidence and conflicting study results. They encourage further research (USP, 1998). Valerian is generally recognized as safe (GRAS) as a food and beverage flavoring by the FDA (Anonymous, 1991). The German Commission E has approved valerian as a sleep-promoting and calmative agent to be used in the treatment of unrest and sleep disturbances caused by anxiety (Blumenthal, 1998). In Australia, valerian is acceptable as an active ingredient in the "listed products" category of the *Therapeutic Goods Administration*. In Belgium, subterranean parts, powder extract, and tincture are allowed for use as traditional tranquilizers. The Health Protection Branch of Health Canada allows products containing valerian as a single agent in the form of crude dried root in tablets, capsules, powders, extracts, tinctures, drops, or tea bags intended for use as sleeping aids and sedatives. In the United Kingdom, valerian is included on the General Sale List of the Medicines Control Agency and is allowed in "traditional herbal remedies" as a sedative to promote natural sleep (USP, 1998).

## References

Andreatini R, Loire JR. Effect of valepotriates on the behavior of rats in the elevated plus-maze during diazepam withdrawal. Eur J Pharmacol 1994;260:233–5.

Anonymous. Valerian. Lawrence Review of Natural Products. St. Louis, MO: Facts and Comparisons, 1991.

Balderer G, Borbely AA. Effect of valerian on human sleep. Psychopharmacology 1985;87:406–9.

Blumenthal M. Valerian root. The complete German Commission E monographs. Austin, TX: American Botanical Council, 1998.

Bounthanh C, Richert L, Beck JP, Haag-Berrurier M, Anton R. The action of valepotriates on the synthesis of DNA and proteins of cultured hepatoma cells. Planta Med 1983;49:138–142.

Cavadas C, Araujo I, Cotrim MD, Amaral T, Cunha AP, Macedo T, et al. *In vitro* study on the interaction of *Valeriana officinalis* L. extracts and their amino acids on $GABA_A$ receptor in rat brain. Arzneim Forsch 1995;45:753–5.

Chan TYK. An assessment of the delayed effects associated with valerian overdose [letter]. Int J Clin Pharmacol Ther 1999;36:569.

Chan TYK, Tang CH, Critchley J. Poisoning due to an over-the-counter hypnotic, Sleep-Qik (hyoscine, cyproheptadine, valerian). Postgrad Med J 1995;71:227–8.

Combest WL. Valerian. US Pharmacist 1997;22:62,64,66,68.

Czeizel A, Szentesi I, Szekeres H, Molnar G, Glauber A, Bucski P. A study of adverse effects on the progeny after intoxication during pregnancy. Ach Toxicol 1988;62:1–7.

Czeizel AE, Tomcsik M, Timar L. Teratologic evaluation of 178 infants born to mothers who attempted suicide by drugs during pregnancy. Obstet Gynecol 1997; 90:195–201.

Garges HP, Varia I, Doraiswamy PM. Cardiac complications and delirium associated with valerian root withdrawal [letter]. JAMA 1998;280:1566–7.

Hazelhoff B, Malingre TM, Meijer DKF. Antispasmodic effects of valeriana compounds: an in-vivo and in-vitro study on the guinea-pig ileum. Arch Int Pharmacodyn 1982;257:274–87.

Hazelhoff B, Smith D. Malingre TM, Hendriks H. The essential oil of Valeriana officinalis L. s.l. Pharm WeeKbl Sci Ed 1979a;114:71–7.

Hazelhoff B, Weert B, Denee R, Malingre TM. Isolation and analytical aspects of valeriana compounds. Pharm Wkbl 1979;114:140–8.

Heiligenstein E, Guenther G. Over-the counter psychotropics: a review of melatonin, St. John's wort, valerian, and kava-kava. J Am Col Health 1998;46:271–6.

Hendriks H, Bos R, Allersma DP, Malingre TM, Koster AS. Pharmacological screening of valerenal and some other components of essential oil of *Valeriana officinalis*. Planta Med1981;42:62–8.

Hendriks H, Bos R, Woerdenbag HJ, Koster AS. Central nervous depressant activity of valerenic acid in the mouse. Planta Medica 1985;1:28–31.

Houghton P. The biological activity of valerian and related plants. J Ethnopharmacol 1988;22:121–42.

Houghton P. Valerian. Pharm J 1994;253:95–96.

Leathwood PD, Chauffard F. Aqueous extract of valerian reduces latency to fall asleep in man. Planta Med 1985;2:144–8.

Leathwood PD, Chauffard F, Heck E, Munoz-Box R. Aqueous extract of valerian root (*Valeriana officinalis* L.) improves sleep quality in man. Pharmacol Biochem Behav 1982;17:65–71.

Leuschner J, Muller J, Rudmann M. Characterization of the central nervous depressant activity of a commercially available valerian root extract. Arzneim Forsch 1993;43:638–41.

Lindahl O, Lindwall L. Double blind study of a valerian preparation. Pharmacol Biochem Behav 1989;32:1065–6.

MacGregor FB, Abernethy VE, Dahabra S, Cobden I, Hayes PC. Hepatotoxicity of herbal remedies. Br Med J 1989;299:1156–7.

Mennini P, Bernasconi P, Bombardelli E, Morazzoni P. *In vitro* study on the interaction of extracts and pure compounds from *Valeriana officinalis* roots with GABA, benzodiazepine and barbiturate receptors in rat brain. Fitoterapia 1993;64:291–300.

Oshima Y, Matsuoka S, Ohizumi Y. Antidepressant principles of *Valeriana fauriei* roots. Chem Pharmacol Bull 1995;43:169–70.

Petkov V. Plants with hypotensive, antiatheromatous and coronarodilatating action. Am J Chin Med 1979;7:197–236.

Rosecrans JA, Defeo JJ, Youngken HW. Pharmacological investigation of certain *Valeriana officinalis* L. extracts. J Pharmaceut Sci 1961;50:240–4.

Sakamoto T, Mitani Y, Nakajima K. Psychotropic effects of Japanese valerian root extract. Chem Pharmacol Bull 1992;40:758–61.

Santos MS, Ferreira F, Cunha AP, Carvalho AP, Macedo T. An aqueous extract of valerian influences the transport of GABA in synaptosomes. Planta Med 1994a;60:278–79.

Santos MS, Ferreira F, Faro C, Pires E, Carvalho AP, Cunha AP, Macedo T. The amount of GABA present in aqueous extracts of valerian is sufficient to account for [$^3$H] GABA release in synaptosomes. Planta Med 1994b;60:475–6.

Schulz H, Stolz C, Muller J. The effect of valerian extract on sleep polygraphy in poor sleepers: a pilot study. Pharmacopsychiatry 1994;27:147–51.

Tittel G, Chari VN, Wagner H. HPLC-analyse von valeriana mexicana extrakten. Planta Med 1978;34:305–10.

Tittel G, Wagner H. [High-performance liquid chromatographic separation and quantitative determination of valepotriates in valeriana drugs and preparations]. J Chromatogr 1978;148:459–68.

Tortarolo M, Braun R, Hubner GE, Maurer HR. In vitro effects of epoxide-bearing valepotriates on mouse early hematopoietic progenitor cells and human T-lymphocytes. Arch Toxicol 1982;51:37–42.

Tufik S, Fujita K, Seabra MDV, Leticia LL. Effects of a prolonged administration of valepotriates in rats on the mothers and their offspring. J Ethnopharmacol 1994;41:39–44.

Tyler VE. The honest herbal, 3rd edit., Binghamton, NY: Pharmaceutical Products Press, 1993.

Wagner J, Wagner ML, Hening WA. Beyond benzodiazepines: alternative pharmacologic agents for the treatment of insomnia. Ann Pharmacother 1998;32:680–91.

Willey LB, Mady SP, Cobaugh DG, Wax PM. Valerian overdose: a case report. Vet Hum Toxicol 1995;37:364–5.

United States Pharmacopeial Convention (USP). Valerian. Botanical monograph series. Rockville, MD: United States Pharmacopeial Convention, 1998.

# Chapter 5

# St. John's Wort

*John T. Schwarz and Melanie Johns Cupp*

*Hypericum perforatum*, goat weed, klamath weed, rosin rose, amber touch and heal, tipton weed (Bradshaw et al. 1998); blutdkraut, Johnswort, qian ceng lou, Sankt Hans urt, St. Jan's kraut, St. Johnswort, toutsaine, tupfelhartheu, walpurgiskraut, zweiroboij, amber, chassediable, corazoncillo, hardhay, hartheu, herbe de millepertuis, herrgottsblut, hexenkraut, hierba de San Juan, hipericon, hypericum, iperico, Johannesort, pelatro, perforata, Johannisblut, Johanniskraut (USP, 1998a)

## 5.1 History and Traditional Uses

*Hypericum* is a perennial aromatic shrub with bright yellow flowers that bloom from June to September (Wincor and Gutierrez, 1997). The flowers are said to be at their brightest and most abundant around June 24th, the day traditionally believed to be the birthday of John the Baptist. The plant is native to Europe and can also be found in the United States and Canada. It grows in the dry ground of fields, roadsides, and woods.

Historically, St. John's wort has been used to treat neurologic and psychiatric disturbances (anxiety, insomnia, bed-wetting, irritability, migraine, excitability, exhaustion, fibrositis, hysteria, neuralgia, and sciatica), gastritis, gout, hemorrhage, pulmonary disorders, and rheumatism, and has been used as a diuretic (USP, 1998a). Some forms of the herb have been used topically as an astringent and to treat blisters, burns, cuts, hemorrhoids, inflammation, insect bites, itching, redness, sunburn, and wounds.

## 5.2 Current Promoted Uses

St. John's wort is promoted for treatment of mood disorders, particularly depression, and promotion of emotional well being. It has also been promoted

From Forensic Science: *Toxicology and Clinical Pharmacology of Herbal Products*
Edited by: M. J. Cupp © Humana Press Inc., Totowa, New Jersey

in combination with ma huang (ephedra) for weight loss, but use of such products has been discouraged by the FDA (USP, 1998a).

## 5.3 PRODUCTS AVAILABLE

Most commercially available preparations of hypericum in the United States are dried alcoholic extracts in a solid oral dosage form. Other preparations include the dried herb or liquid extracts. The following is a list of a few of the available formulations:

Movana® — tablet containing 0.3% hypericin extract (300 mg)
Kira® — tablet containing 0.3% hypericin extract (300 mg)
Dr. Art Ulene's Herbal Formulas® — capsule containing 150 mg of hypericin
Nature's Fingerprint® — 500-mg capsule and 300-mg tablet containing extract
NaturaLife® — grain alcohol extract (250 mg of hypericin/mL)
Celestial Seasoning® — capsule containing 0.3% hypericin extract (300 mg) with Siberian ginseng, vitamins $B_6$, $B_3$, $B_{12}$, zinc, and folic acid
One A Day® — tablet with 225 mg of hypericin and 100 mg of kava kava
Harmonex® — 450 mg of hypericin from a flower extract and 90 mg ginseng
Sundown® Herbals — 300 mg of hypericin with ginkgo biloba, ginseng, and ginger

## 5.4 PHARMACOLOGIC/TOXICOLOGIC EFFECTS

### 5.4.1 Neurological Effects

Many studies have been done comparing St. John's wort to placebo or to tricyclic antidepressants (Linde et al., 1996). However, problems with inclusion criteria, diagnostic criteria, antidepressant dosing, and study duration do not permit definitive conclusions about the safety and efficacy of St. John's wort for treatment of depression.

Studies indicate that St. John's wort may be effective in treating depression (Linde et al., 1996). However, the exact chemical entity that causes this effect and the mechanism of action is unknown. St. John's wort contains compounds from several chemical classes. These include naphthodianthrones (hypericin, pseudohypericin, protopseudohypericin, cyclopseudohypericin), flavonoids (quercetin, hyperosid, quercitrin, isoquercitrin, campherol, rutin, luteolin, and I3-II8-biapigenin), ethereal oil, phenol carbonic acids (e.g., chlorogenic acid), procyanidins, 1,3,6,7-tetrahydroxyxanthone, and hyperforin. Of these, hyperforin, the hypericins, and tetrahydroxyxanthone are characteristic of St. John's wort, while the other constituents are found in many plants (Wagner and Bladt, 1994). Interestingly, melatonin, a human pineal gland hormone, has been identified in St. John's wort flower and leaf at concentrations of 4.39 μg/g and 1.75 μg/g, respectively (Murch et al., 1997), but its role in the pharmacological effects of St. John's wort have yet to be investigated.

Most of the research regarding the antidepressant action of St. John's wort has focused on the hypericins (Wagner and Bladt, 1994). Research has been done to examine the possibility of monoamine oxidase (MAO) or catechol-*O*-methyltransferase (COMT) inhibition, and inhibition of serotonin and norepinephrine reuptake (Perovic and Muller, 1995; Raffa, 1998). In one study, the effects of hypericum total extract, hypericum fractions, and hypericin on MAO and COMT activity were examined in vitro (Thiede and Walper, 1994). It was concluded that the in vitro concentrations of these preparations required to inhibit MAO were in excess of that attained through ingestion, and thus MAO inhibition could not be an explanation of the herb's antidepressant activity. In addition, COMT inhibition appeared to be associated with flavonols and xanthones rather than hypericins. Another study (Cott, 1997) showed that pure hypericin did not bind to MAO, and confirmed that concentrations of the crude extract required for MAO inhibition exceeded those attained after oral administration.

Raffa found that hypericin had no significant affinity for dopamine $D_1$, $\gamma$-aminobutyric acid (GABA), opioid, benzodiazepine, 5-hydroxytryptamine$_{1B}$ (5-HT$_{1B}$; serotonin), or norepinephrine receptors. It also did not inhibit serotonin or norepinephrine reuptake at the concentrations studied. However, binding affinity at muscarinic cholinergic receptors (mAChRs) and $\sigma$-receptors was relatively good, and hypericin displayed some affinity for 5-HT$_{1A}$ receptors and minor inhibition of dopamine reuptake. These findings may indicate that St. John's wort has different mechanisms of action than traditional antidepressants. Another component of St. John's wort that has been hypothesized to be involved in its central nervous system effects is amentoflavone. The concentration of amentoflavone in *Hypericum* sp. flower extracts correlates with the extracts' abilities to inhibit binding of radiolabeled flumazenil to benzodiazepine receptors, while hypericin concentration does not correlate (Baureithel et al., 1997).

St. John's wort extract may help to enhance sleep quality. In a study of 12 volunteers, hypericum extract LI 160 (Jarsin®) 300 mg, three times daily, did not improve sleep onset, intermittent wakenings, or total sleep duration. However, EEG analysis showed an increase in the mean percentage of time spent in deep (stages 3 and 4; slow wave) sleep (Schulz and Jobert, 1994). Human and animal studies suggest these EEG effects may be due to hyperforin (Schellenberg et al., 1998).These effects on sleep are not consistent with the effects observed with the use of traditional antidepressants, and are striking because a deficit in slow-wave sleep has been associated with affective disorders (Schulz and Jobert, 1994).

### 5.4.2 Antimicrobial Effects

In a pilot study of HIV-infected adults, hypericin was administered at doses of 0.25 mg/kg or 0.5 mg/kg intravenously twice weekly, 0.25 mg/kg intravenously thrice weekly, or 0.5 mg/kg/d orally for up to 24 wk. No regimen displayed antiretroviral activity based on CD4 lymphocyte counts, p24 antigen, or HIV RNA titers (Gulick et al., 1999). In vitro studies suggest that St. John's wort may have activity against cytomegalovirus (CMV), herpes simplex, influenza A (USP, 1998a), and methicillin resistant *Staphylococcus aureus* (Schempp et al., 1999).

### 5.4.3 Mutagenicity

Quercetin, a flavonoid component of St. John's wort and several other medicinal plants, has been implicated as a mutagen. However, St. John's Wort aqueous ethanolic extract showed no mutagenic effects in mammalian cells. Tests used included the HGPRT (hypoxanthine guanidine phosphoribosyl transferase) test, the UDS (unscheduled DNA synthesis) test, the cell transformation test uring Syrian hamster embryo cells, the mouse fur spot test, and the chromosome aberration test using Chinese hamster bone marrow cells (Okpanyi et al., 1990).

### 5.4.4 Reproduction

A report describes two pregnant women self-medicated with St. John's wort at a dose of 900 mg/d. Both had a history of recurrent major depressive disorder. One patient discontinued her prescribed fluoxetine and methylphenidate and began taking St. John's wort due to concerns about the effects of the medications on her fetus. The gestational week during which this change was made and pregnancy outcome were not reported. The other patient began taking St. John's wort at gestational wk 24. The pregnancy was unremarkable, except for a maternal platelet count of 88,000 cells/mm$^3$, and neonatal jaundice at d 5, requiring phototherapy. The woman discontinued the St. John's wort 24 h prior to delivery, but resumed the product at a dose of 300 mg/d when her infant was 20-d-old. Behavioral assessment of the neonate, who was being breastfed, was normal at 4 and 33 d of age (Grush et al., 1999). The authors note that although animal studies suggest that St. John's wort may have uterine stimulating effects, no adverse reproductive effects have been documented in rats or dogs at doses up to 2700 mg/kg.

## 5.5 Adverse Effects and Toxicity

Although the adverse effect profile of St. John's wort appears to be better than that of standard prescription antidepressants, side effects have been reported. For example, USP lists the following: allergic reaction (itching, hives, skin rash), fatigue (unusual tiredness), gastrointestinal symptoms (abdominal pain, bloated feeling or gas, constipation, nausea or vomiting), restlessness, dizziness, dry mouth, phototoxicity, and sleep disturbances.

A study found that hypericin inhibits bovine choroidal endothelial cell proliferation in vitro (Kimura et al., 1997). The effect was found to be dose dependent. Further studies in other animal models are needed to investigate this potential effect.

Phototoxicity manifested as elevated, itching, erythematous lesions has been described (Golsch et al., 1997). Phototoxicty may also present as neuropathy, presumably caused by demyelination of cutaneous axons by photoactivated hypericins (Bove, 1998). After taking ground St. John's wort extract for 4 wk, a 35-yr-old woman complained of stinging pain on sun-exposed areas, worsened by cold, minimal mechanical stimuli, and sun exposure. The neuropathy improved over 2 mo after she discontinued the product (Bove, 1998).

In a study (Gulick et al., 1999) using both intravenous and oral hypericin (*see* Section 5.4.2 for doses used), 26 of 30 enrolled patients experienced phototoxicity manifested as erythema, numbness, pain, and temperature sensitivity requiring analgesic use. Other adverse effects reported in this study included fever, diarrhea, decreased hemoglobin < 8 mg/dL, and glucose > 250 mg/dL (one patient each). Two patients had alkaline phosphatase levels greater than five times normal, and aminotransferase greater than five times normal was experienced by three patients. Although the patients in this study were HIV infected, those taking antiretrovial, phototoxic, or hepatotoxic drugs were excluded.

A 47-yr-old woman diagnosed with panic disorder and major depressive disorder experienced a hypomanic episode characterized by distorted and racing thoughts, irritability, hostility, aggressive driving, and decreased need for sleep after taking a 0.1% St. John's wort tincture for 10 d. These symptoms resolved 2 d after she discontinued using St. John's wort. She had discontinued 50 mg of sertraline 1 wk prior to taking the St. John's wort product because of sexual side effects. Prior to taking 50 mg of sertraline, she had taken 75 mg of sertraline for several months, but required dosage reduction after experiencing irritability and insomnia, demonstrating a vulnerability to activation. This hypomanic episode appears to be an adverse effect of St. John's wort, rather than an interaction between sertraline and St. John's wort (Schneck, 1998).

An additional report describes two cases of hypomania occurring after 6 wk and after 3 mo of St. John's wort use. Hypomania was characterized by irritability, disinhibition, agitation, anger, insomnia, and difficulty concentrating and required treatment with antimanic drugs (O'Breasail and Argouarch, 1998).

## 5.6 Drug Interactions

A 50-yr-old woman with a history of chronic depression experienced central nervous system symptoms after taking a single dose of 20 mg of paroxetine in addition to her usual daily dose of 600 mg of St. John's wort. Ten days earlier she discontinued paroxetine (40 mg/d), which she had been taking for 8 mo for treatment of depression, and initiated self-therapy with 600 mg of St. John's wort powder. No side effects were noticed at that time. On d 10 of St. John's wort therapy, she took a single 20 mg dose of paroxetine because she was experiencing difficulty sleeping. The next day, she was found to be groggy, lethargic, and incoherent, but her Mini Mental Status examination, chemistry panel, and blood count were normal. She complained of fatigue, nausea, and weakness. Physical exam revealed limp muscle tone and slow response time, but was otherwise normal. Mental, neurologic, and physical exams were normal the following day (Gordon, 1998). This patient experienced problems when paroxetine was added to established St. John's wort therapy, but had not experienced adverse effects when discontinuing paroxetine and starting St. John's wort. Because it takes up to 2 wk for MAO to regenerate after inhibition, the time course of this patient's symptoms suggests that some component of St. John's wort might have clinically significant MAO inhibition.

Other authors have also reported evidence that St. John's wort may have the potential for clinically significant monoamine oxidase inhibition. In this case report, disorientation, agitation, and confusion in association with use of St. John's wort, valerian, and loperamide in a 39-yr-old white female is documented. On physical exam, pupils were unreactive and dilated at 6 mm. She was afebrile, with a respiratory rate of 24 breaths per minute, blood pressure 140/100 mm Hg, and pulse of 140 beats per minute. Abnormal blood chemistry results included mildly elevated glucose (139 mg/dL), and low serum potassium (2.9 mmol/L). Toxicology screen was positive for opiods. EKG and CT of the brain were normal. Empiric treatment included thiamine 100 mg to prevent neurotoxicity due to thiamine deficiency, naltrexone 2 mg for possible opioid intoxication, ceftriaxone 1 gram for possible infection, and lorazepam 8 mg as a sedative. Intubation was required briefly. The patient recovered from her delerium 2 d later. The patient revealed a history of depression and migraine headaches, and reported having taken a combination product containing St. John's wort and valerian for the past 6 mo, with the recent addition of loperamide to treat diarrhea, possibly caused by St. John's wort. The authors did not report doses. Loperamide use explained the positive urine opiate screen, but whether the patient's delirium was caused by loperamide, the herbal product, an interaction between one or both herbs and loperamide, or another etiology is unclear. Operating under the assumption that St. John's wort can inhibit monoamine oxidase after oral administration in humans, the authors hypothesized that loperamide, like meperidine, might be capable of interacting with monoamine oxidase inhibitors, causing delirium and hypertension (Khawaja et al., 1999).

A single-blind, placebo-controlled pharmacokinetic study examined the effects of St. John's wort extract LI 160 on digoxin concentrations. Healthy volunteers received digoxin 0.25 mg twice daily for 2 d, then daily for 5 d, followed by 10 d of concomitant placebo ($n = 12$) or LI 160 900 mg ($n = 13$) daily. By d 15, trough digoxin plasma concentrations (IMx Digoxin Assay, Abbott Laboratories) had decreased by a mean of 33% ($p = 0.0023$), and peak concentrations had decreased by a mean of 26% ($p = 0.0095$) in the LI 160 group compared to the placebo group. The LI 160 group experienced a mean decrease in trough concentration of 37% ($p = 0.0001$) between d 5 and 16, and a decrease in peak concentration of 26% ($p = 0.0013$) between d 5 and 15. The mechanism of decreased digoxin concentration was thought to be induction of p-glycoprotein, a protein pump responsible for transport of digoxin into the renal tubules for elimination (Johne et al., 1999).

A case report (Nebel et al., 1999) describes an interaction between St. John's wort and theophylline. A patient taking 300 mg of theophylline (Theo-Dur) twice daily required a dosage increase to 800 mg twice daily to maintain a theophylline level of 9.2 mg/L after she began taking a St. John's wort preparation standardized to 0.3% hypericin. Other medications included furosemide, potassium, morphine, zolpidem, valproic acid, ibuprofen, amitriptyline, albuterol, prednisone, zafirlukast, and inhaled triamcinolone acetonide. She also smoked one-half pack of cigarettes each day. Other than the addition of St. John's wort, there had been no other changes in her medication regimen or smoking habits when she required an increase in theophylline dose. St. John's wort was discontinued, and 7 d later, her theophylline level was 19.6 mg/L. The authors note that hypericin and pseudohypericin are polycyclic aromatic hydrocarbons, like the hydrocarbons in cigarette smoke that are known to induce the drug metabolizing enzymes CYP1A2 and glutathione-*S*-transferase. Using an in vitro model of hepatic enzyme induction, hypericin at a concentration of 12.5–125 m*M* was found to be an enzyme inducer. Other drugs that are metabolized by CYP1A2 and thus might interact with St. John's wort include R-warfarin, clozapine, olanzapine, clomipramine, and imipramine.

Concerns that St. John's wort may potentiate the cardiovascular effects of local and general anesthetics have been voiced by some authors, but adverse outcomes are poorly documented.

Some authors caution that tannins in St. John's wort (as well as those in fever few, borage, saw palmetto, and chamomile) might inhibit iron absorption. Study is needed to determine if this is a concern.

## 5.7 Pharmacokinetics/Toxicokinetics

Two pharmacokinetic studies have examined the pharmacokinetics of hypericin and pseudohypericin (Staffeldt et al., 1994; Kerb et al., 1996). Standardized hypericum extract LI 160 (Jarsin 300®, Lichtwer Pharma GmbH, Berlin) was used in both trials. In Part I of the studies, subjects in both trials were administered a single dose of either 300 mg, 900 mg, or 1800 mg of the extract (one, three, or six coated tablets) at 10–14-d intervals. Each dose contained 250 µg, 750 µg, or 1500 µg of hypericin and 526 µg, 1578 µg, or 3156 µg of pseudohypericin, respectively. The doses were administered on an empty stomach in the morning after a 12-h fast. Subjects fasted for an additional 2 h after administration. Multiple plasma levels of hypericin and pseudohypericin were measured for up to 120 h after administration. In addition, urine samples were collected in the study performed by Kerb and colleagues. After a 4-wk washout from Part I, subjects were given one coated tablet containing 300 mg of hypericum extract three times a day (8 am, 1 pm, and 6 pm) before meals for 14 d. Blood samples were obtained over the 2-wk dosing period.

### 5.7.1 Absorption

For single doses of 300 mg, 900 mg, or 1800 mg of dried hypericum extract in humans, the median time that elapsed from taking the dose and detectable plasma concentration ($t_{lag}$) in hours is as follows:

Hypericin: 2.6, 2.0, and 2.6 (Staffeldt et al., 1994)
2.1, 1.9, and 1.9 (Kerb et al., 1996)
Pseudohypericin: 0.6, 0.4, and 0.4 (Staffeldt et al., 1994)
0.5, 0.4, and 0.4 (Kerb et al., 1996)

A difference is observed between the $t_{lag}$ of hypericin compared to pseudohypericin. These differences may be a function of the dosage form given. Pseudohypericin may be released from the dosage form more quickly than hypericin. Also, hypericin and pseudohypericin may be absorbed in different locations in the gastrointestinal tract. Another explanation may be that hypericin may undergo first-pass hepatic metabolism (Staffeldt et al., 1994).

The median maximum plasma concentrations ($C_{max}$) in (g/L for the respective doses are as follows:

Hypericin: 1.5, 7.5, and 14.2 (Staffeldt et al., 1994)
1.3, 7.2, and 16.6 (Kerb et al., 1996)

Pseudohypericin: 2.7, 11.7, and 30.6 (Staffeldt et al., 1994)
3.4, 12.1, and 29.7 (Kerb et al., 1996)

The maximum plasma concentrations increased in a nonlinear fashion (Staffeldt et al., 1994; Kerb et al., 1996).

The median time to peak plasma concentration ($T_{max}$) in hours for the corresponding doses are as follows:

Hypericin: 5.2, 4.1, and 5.9 (Staffeldt et al., 1994)
5.5, 6.0, and 5.7 (Kerb et al., 1996)
Pseudohypericin: 2.7, 3.0, and 3.2 (Staffeldt et al., 1994)
3.0, 3.0, and 3.0 (Kerb et al., 1996)

Overall no correlation is observed between dose and $T_{max}$. However, hypericin takes longer to reach maximum plasma concentration. This corresponds with the lag time data (Staffeldt et al., 1994).

After multiple dosing of 300 mg of hypericum extract three times daily, the data for median $C_{max}$ and trough plasma concentration ($C_{min}$) were as follows:

Hypericin: $C_{max}$ 8.5 μg/L (Staffeldt et al., 1994)
$C_{max}$ 8.8 μg/L (Kerb et al., 1996)
$C_{min}$ 5.3 μg/L* (Staffeldt et al., 1994)
$C_{min}$ 7.9 μg/L (Kerb et al., 1996)
Pseudohypericin: $C_{max}$ 5.8 mg/L (Staffeldt et al., 1994)
$C_{max}$ 8.5 mg/L (Kerb et al., 1996)
$C_{min}$ 3.7 mg/L* (Staffeldt et al., 1994)
$C_{min}$ 4.8 mg/L (Kerb et al., 1996)
*mean.

### *5.7.2 Distribution*

For oral doses, the volume of distribution appears to be approx 162 L for hypericin and 63 L for pseudohypericum (Kerb et al., 1996).

### *5.7.3 Metabolism/Elimination*

The median half-lives in hours for single 300-mg, 900-mg, and 1800-mg oral doses are as follows:

Hypericin: 24.8, 26.0, and 26.5 (Staffeldt et al., 1994)
24.5, 43.1, and 48.2 (Kerb et al., 1996)
Pseudohypericin: 16.3, 36.0, and 22.8 (Staffeldt et al., 1994)
18.2, 24.8, 19.5 (Kerb et al., 1996)

After multiple doses of hypericum extract 300 mg three times daily, median half-lives in hours were:

Hypericin: 28.0* (Staffeldt et al., 1994)
41.3 (Kerb et al., 1996)
Pseudohypericin: 23.5* (Staffeldt et al., 1994)
18.8 (Kerb et al., 1996)
*mean.

The data in these two studies differ in regard to the elimination half-life of hypericin. It is difficult to ascertain whether half-life for either hypericin or pseudohypericin is dose related.

Neither hypericin, pseudohypericin, their glucuronic acid conjugates, nor their sulfate conjugates were detected in the urine (Kerb et al., 1996). The chemical structure and molecular size (>500 Da) of hypericin and pseudohypericin suggest metabolism via hepatic glucuronidization followed by biliary excretion (Kerb et al., 1996).

## 5.8 Chemical Analysis

Identification and chemical analysis of St. John's wort are detailed in the *National Formulary* (USP, 1998b).

## 5.9 Analysis of Biofluids

Hypericin and pseudohypericin content of plasma and urine has been measured using HPLC with a spectrofluorometric detector (Kerb et al., 1996; Liebes et al., 1991). HPLC with a UV photometric detector has also been used to analyze plasma (Staffeldt et al., 1994).

## 5.10 Regulatory Status

The German E Commission has approved St. John's wort for internal consumption for psychogenic disturbances, depressive states, sleep disorders, anxiety and/or nervous excitement, particularly that associated with menopause. Oily *Hypericum* preparations are approved for stomach and gastrointestinal complaints, including diarrhea. Oily *Hypericum* preparations are also approved by the Commission E for external use for the treatment of incised and contused wounds, muscle aches, and first degree burns (Blumenthal, 1998).

The USP advisory panel recognizes that St. John's wort has a long history of use. However, because of a lack of well-controlled clinical trials its use is not recommended (USP, 1998a).

The National Institutes of Health (NIH) is conducting the first clinical trial of St. John's wort in the United States. NIH's Office of Alternative Medicine (OAM) is performing the study. The 3-yr trial will include 336 patients with major depression randomized to receive St. John's wort, placebo, or a selective serotonin re-uptake inhibitor (SSRI). The treatment period will last 8 wk (NIH, 1998).

## REFERENCES


Baureithel KH, Buter KB, Engesser A, Burkard W, Schaffner W. Inhibition of benzodiazepine binding in vitro by amentoflavone, a constituent of various species of Hypericum. Pharm Acta Helv 1997;72:153–7.

Blumenthal M. St. John's wort. The complete German Commission E monographs. Austin, TX: American Botanical Council, 1998.

Bove GM. Acute neuropathy after exposure to sun in a patient treated with St. John's wort [letter]. Lancet 1998;352:1121–2.

Bradshaw C, Nguyen A, Surles J. Available from URL: www.unc.edu/~cebradsh/stjohn.html. Accessed 1998 Oct 28.

Johne A, Brockmöller J, Bauer S, Maurer A, Langheinrich M, Roots I. Pharmacokinetic interaction of digoxin with an herbal extract from St. John's wort (*Hypericum perforatum*). Clin Pharmacol Ther 1999;66:338–45.

Cott JM. In vitro receptor binding and enzyme inhibition by *Hypericum perforatum* extract. Pharmacopsychiatry 1997;30(Suppl 2):108–12.

Golsch S, Vocks E, Rakoski J, Brockow K, Ring J. Reversible increase in photosensitivity to UV-B caused by St. John's wort extract [German]. Hautarzt 1997; 48:249–52.

Gordon J. SSRI's and St. John's wort: possible toxicity? [letter] Am Fam Phys 1998;57:950, 953.

Grush LR, Nierenberg A, Keefe B, Cohen LS. St. John's wort during pregnancy [letter]. JAMA 1998;280:1566.

Gulick RM, McAuliffe V, Holden-Wiltse J, Crumpacker C, Liebes L, Stein DS for the AIDS Clinical Trials Group 150 and 258 Protocol Teams. Phase I studies of hypericin, the active compound in St. John's wort, as an antiretroviral agent in HIV-infected adults. Ann Intern Med 1999;130:510–4.

Kerb R, Brockmoller J, Staffeldt B, Ploch M, Roots I. Single-dose and steady state pharmacokinetics of hypericin and pseudohypericin. Antimicrob Agents Chemother 1996;40:2087–193.

Khawaja IS, Marotta RE, Lippmann S. Herbal medicines as a factor in delirium [letter]. Psychiatr Serv 1999;50:969–70.

Kimura H, Harris MS, Sakamoto T, Gopalakrishna R, Gundimeda U, Cui JZ, et al. Hypericin inhibits choroidal endothelial cell proliferation and cord formation in vitro. Curr Eye Res 1997;16:967–72.

Liebes L, Mazur Y, Freeman D, Lavie D, Lavie G, Kudler N, Mendoza S, Levin B, Hochster H, Meruelo D. A method for the quantification of hypericin, an antiviral agent, in biological fluids by high-performance liquid chromatography. Analyt Biochem 1991;195:77–85.

Linde K, Ramirez G, Mulrow CD, Pauls A, Weidenhammer W, Melchart D. St. John's wort for depression - an overview and meta-analysis of randomized clinical trials. Br Med J 1996;313:253–8.

Murch SJ, Simmons CB, Saxena PK. Melatonin in feverfew and other medicinal plants. Lancet 1997;350:158–9.

National Institute of Mental Health. Available from URL: http://www.nih.gov/events/prsjw.htm. Accessed Oct 26 1998.

Nebel A, Schneider BJ, Kroll DJ. Potential metabolic interaction between St. John's wort and theophylline [letter]. Ann Pharmacother 1999;33:502.

O'Breasail AM, Argouarch S. Hypomania and St. John's wort [letter]. Can J Psychiatry 1998;43:746–7.

Okpanyi SN, Lidzba H, Scholl BC, Miltenburger HG. Genotoxicity of a standardized hypericum extract. Arzneimittelforschung 1990;40:851–5

Perovic S, Muller WE. Pharmacological profile of hypericum extract. Effect on serotonin uptake by postsynaptic receptors. Arzneim Forsch 1995;451145–8.

Raffa R. Screen of receptor and uptake-site activity of hypericin component of St. John's wort reveals σ receptor binding. Life Sci 1998;62:PL265–70.

Schellenberg R, Sauer S, Dimptel W. Pharmacodynamic effects of two different hypericum extracts in healthy volunteers measured by quantitative EEG. Pharmacopsychiatry 1998;31(Suppl 1):44–53.

Schempp CM, Pelz K, Wittmer A, Schopf E, Simon JC. Antibacterial activity of hyperforin from St. John's wort, against multiresistant *Staphylococcus aureus* and gram-positive bacteria. Lancet 1999;353:2129.

Schneck C. St. John's wort and hypomania. J Clin Psychiatry 1998;59:689.

Schulz H, Jobert M. Effects of hypericum extract on the sleep EEG in older volunteers. J Geriatr Psychiatry and Neurol 1994;7(Suppl 1):S39–43.

Staffeldt B, Kerb R, Brockmoller J, Ploch M, Roots I. Pharmacokinetics of hypericin and pseudohypericin after oral intake of *Hypericum perforatum* extract LI 160 in healthy volunteers. J Geriatr Psychiatry Neurol 1994;7(Suppl 1):S47–53.

Thiede HM, Walper A. Inhibition of MAO and COMT by hypericum extracts and hypericin. J Geriatr Psychiatry Neurol 1994;7(Suppl 1):S54–6.

United States Pharmacopeial Convention (USP). Hypericum (St. John's wort). Botanical monograph series. Rockville, MD: United States Pharmacopeial Convention, 1998a.

United States Pharmacopoeia (USP). National Formulary. 18th edit., Suppl. 9. Rockville, MD: United States Pharmacopeial Convention, 1998b.

Wagner H and Bladt S. Pharmaceutical quality of *Hypericum* extracts. J Geriatr Psychiatry Neurol 1994:7(Suppl 1):S65–8.

Wincor MZ, Gutierrez, MA. St. John's wort and the treatment of depression. US Pharmacist 1997;22:88–97.

# Chapter 6

# Chamomile

*Melanie Johns Cupp*

*Matricaria chamomilla* (L.) (German chamomile, Hungarian chamomile, genuine chamomile), *Anthemis nobilis* (English chamomile, Roman chamomile, common chamomile); sometimes called *Chamaemelum nobile* (L.) (Anonymous, 1991)

## 6.1 History and Traditional Uses

Chamomile has been used medicinally since ancient Rome for its purported sedative, antispasmodic, and antirheumatic effects (Anonymous, 1991).

## 6.2 Current Promoted Uses

Chamomile is used topically to treat a variety of inflammatory conditions involving the mouth, skin, respiratory tract (via inhalation), and gastrointestinal tract. It is also used internally as a gastrointestinal antispasmodic and anti-inflammatory (Blumenthal, 1998). Chamomile is purported to have sedative, hypnotic, analgesic, and immunostimulant effects (Yamada et al., 1996).

## 6.3 Products Available

The flowers of *M. chamomilla* and *A. nobilis* are used in teas and extracts (Anonymous, 1991). Chamomile oil is used in aromatherapy (Yamada et al., 1996).

## 6.4 Pharmacologic/Toxicologic Effects

### 6.4.1 Neurologic Effects

The effects of chamomile oil vapor were studied in ovariectomized rats, which served as an experimental menopausal model (Yamada et al., 1996).

From Forensic Science: *Toxicology and Clinical Pharmacology of Herbal Products*
Edited by: M. J. Cupp © Humana Press Inc., Totowa, New Jersey

Inhalation of chamomile vapor attenuated restriction stress-induced adrenocorticotropic hormone (ACTH) secretion, and was superior to diazepam in this regard. The effects of chamomile vapor were blocked by pretreatment with flumazenil, a benzodiazepine antagonist. The investigators concluded that chamomile might act via the γ-aminobutyric acid-ergic (GABAergic) system in a manner similar to the benzodiazepines; however, properly designed studies of chamomile's sedative effects in humans are lacking.

### 6.4.2 *Antineoplastic Effects*

Apigenin, a flavonoid found in chamomile, has been found to suppress 12-*O*-tetradecanoyl-phorbol-13-acetate (TPA)-induced tumor promotion in mouse skin. Inhibition of protein kinase C, and thus proto-oncogene expression, by competing with ATP is the proposed mechanism of action (Huang et al., 1996). Apigenin has also been noted to cause reversible $G_2$/M arrest (Lepley et al., 1996).

Apigenin at a 5 μ*M* concentration applied topically reduces the number of UVB-induced squamous cell carcinomas in mice and may prove to be a useful sunscreen ingredient (Lepley et al., 1996).

### 6.4.3 *Anti-Inflammatory Activity*

Chamomile is purported to have antiinflammatory effects, but studies of chamomile cream have not proven its efficacy. Chamomile mouthwash was noted to be well-tolerated and appeared to be beneficial in the treatment and prevention of radiation or chamotherapy-induced mucositis in a case series of ninety-eight patients (Carl and Emrich, 1991). These results prompted a double-blind, placebo-controlled trial for the prevention of 5-fluorouracil-induced stomatitis (Fidler et al., 1996). One hundred and sixty-five patients were randomized to receive chamomile or placebo mouthwash. The patients were stratified based on smoking history, chemotherapy regimen, and institution. Stomatitis severity was rated on a scale of 0 to 4 by the attending physician and by the patient. There was no difference in stomatitis scores between the two groups, with a wide 95% confidence interval (–23% to +15%), suggesting no benefit. Subset analysis revealed that men tended to benefit, while the chamomile tended to have a detrimental effect in women. No biologically plausible explanation for this finding was found. Chamomile mouthwash was without toxicity.

## 6.5 Case Reports of Toxicity Due to Commercially Available Products

A 35-yr-old pregnant woman was administered an enema containing glycerol and Kamillosan®, an oily chamomile flower extract, during labor. Ten minutes later, she experienced nausea. Twenty-five minutes after administration, she developed urticaria, laryngeal edema, tachycardia, and hypotension. Intravenous fluids, corticosteroids, and antihistamines were administered. Forty-four minutes after enema administration, a cesarean delivery was performed. The uterus was atonic and bloodless. The newborn had an Apgar score of 0, and a pH of 6.85. Although initially responding to sodium bicarbonate, the newborn died the next day after suffering a tonic–clonic seizure. The woman suffered a hematoma of the abdominal wall, a bleeding gastric ulcer, paralytic ileus, and sepsis, but recovered with laparogastrotomy and a 3-wk course of antibiotics. Skin prick tests were negative for latex, glycerol, and common airborne allergens. A skin prick test with Kamillosan® was postitive, and immunoglobulin E (IgE) specific for chamomile was detected by radioallergosorbent test (RAST). Although the extraction of dried chamomile plants for the production of Kamillosan® yields a low amount of protein in the product, it is apparently enough to trigger anaphylaxis when the product is applied to a large area of the colonic mucosa. The investigators attempted to identify the protein responsible for antibody production using electrophoresis (Jensen-Jarolim et al., 1998).

Anaphylaxis to chamomile tea has also been reported (Benner and Lee, 1973; Casterline, 1980). A 35-yr-old woman experienced abdominal cramps, tongue "thickness," a tight sensation in her throat, angioedema of the lips and eyes, diffuse itching, and a full sensation in her ears after a few sips of chamomile tea. Her symptoms resolved over 1–2 h after treatment with diphenhydramine and a corticosteroid. A scratch test with chamomile produced a large wheal-and-flare with pseudopod formation. She had a history of ragweed hay fever and a strong positive reaction to ragweed on skin testing. Five of 15 additional patients with a history of positive reactions to ragweed developed positive skin test reactions to chamomile tea. These patients were not challenged with chamomile tea orally because of the risk of anaphylaxis (Benner and Lee, 1973).

In another case report (Casterline, 1980), a 54-yr-old woman experienced generalized hives, upper airway obstruction, and pharyngeal edema 20 min after drinking a cup of chamomile tea and taking two aspirin tablets. She was treated with epinephrine and diphenhydramine in the emergency room with complete symptom resolution. The patient had no history of aspirin allergy, but reported mild seasonal allergic rhinitis. Total IgE was elevated, and RAST was 2+ for ragweed. Graded oral aspirin challenges produced no immediate or delayed reaction.

In addition to being used as a beverage, chamomile tea is used as an eye wash to treat conjuctivitis and other ocular conditions. Seven patients ages 21–51 suffered conjunctivitis after eye washing with chamomile tea. The reactions were immediate, and two patients suffered angioedema of the eyelid. One required emergency treatment with epinephrine. All had histories of seasonal allergic rhinitis or asthma. One patient reported allergy to honey (lip swelling and itching of mouth), and one to sunflower seeds (scratchy feeling in the throat). Rechallenge with ocular administration of chamomile tea extract produced an immediate conjuctival reaction in all seven patients, with the patient who had required epinephrine reacting to a very dilute solution. All patients had positive prick tests to chamomile tea extract, but all tolerated oral chamomile tea (Subiza et al., 1990).

One hundred additional patients with hay fever were challenged with chamomile tea extract as a skin test and as a conjuctival provocation test to determine the prevalence of this type of reaction. IgE to chamomile tea was also measured. Only two of the 100 patients had a positive reaction to ocular chamomile tea extract. This ruled out an irritant effect of the tea as a mechanism of the patients' responses, but clinicians must be aware that irritants such as alcohol may be present in chamomile products used in the eye. Twenty-eight patients had specific IgE to antigens contained in the chamomile tea extract (Subiza et al., 1990).

## 6.6 Pharmacokinetics/Toxicokinetics

*See* Section 6.7.

## 6.7 Analysis of Biofluids

Blood and urinary concentrations of the flavonoids apigenin, apigenin-7-glucoside, and herniarin were measured in one patient after a single oral dose of 40 mL of a aqueous/ethanolic chamomile extract (Tschiersch and Holzl J, 1993).

Reversed-phase high-performance liquid chromatography (HPLC) with variable wavelength UV detector (Li et al., 1997) and HPLC-scintillation analysis (Li and Birt, 1996) have been used to determine apigenin content of mouse skin after topical application of apigenin.

## 6.8 Regulatory Status

Chamomile is regulated as a dietary supplement in the United States. Chamomile flower (German) is approved by the German Commission E for external use to treat skin, gum, and mucous membrane inflammation; bacterial skin diseases; inflammation and irritation of the respiratory tract (via inhalation); and ano–genital inflammation. Internally, it is approved for use in treating gastrointestinal spasms and inflammation (Blumenthal, 1998).

## References

Anonymous. Chamomile. The Lawrence review of natural products. St. Louis, MO: Facts and Comparisons,1991.

Benner MH, Lee HJ. Anaphylactic reaction to chamomile tea. J Allergy Clin Immunol 1973;52:307–8.

Blumenthal M. The complete German Commission E monographs. Therapeutic guide to herbal medicnes. Austin, TX: American Botanical Council;1998.

Carl W, Emrich LS. Management of oral musositis during local radiation and systemic chemotherapy: a study of 98 patients. J Prosthet Dent 1991;66:361–9.

Casterline CL. Allergy to chamomile tea. JAMA 1980;244:330–1.

Fidler P, Loprinzi CL, O'Fallon JR, Leitch JM, Lee JK, Hayes DL, et al. Prospective evaluation of a chamomile mouthwash for prevention of 5–FU-induced oral mucositis. Cancer 1996;77:522–5.

Huang Y, Kuo M, Liu J, Huang S, Lin J. Inhibitions of protein kinase C and proto-oncogene expressions in NIH 3T3 cells by apigenin. Eur J Cancer 1996;32A:146–51.

Jensen-Jarolim E, Reider N, Fritsch R, Breiteneder H. Fatal outcome of anaphylaxis to chamomile-containing enema during labor. J Allergy Clin Immunol 1998;102:1041–2.

Lepley D, Li B, Birt DF. The chemopreventive flavonoid apigenin induced $G_2$/M arrest in keratinocytes. Carcinogenesis 1996;17:2367–75.

Li B, Birt DF. *In vivo* and *in vitro* percutaneous absorption of cancer preventive flavonoid apigenin in different vehicles in mouse skin. Pharmacol Res 1996;13:1710–5.

Li B, Robinson DH, Birt DF. Evaluation of properties of apigenin and [G-$^3$H]apigenin and analytic method of development. J Pharmacol Sci 1997;86:721–5.

Subiza J, Subiza JL, Alonso M, Hinojosa M, Garcia R, Jerez M, Subiza E. Allergic conjuctivitis to chamomile tea. Ann Allergy 1990;65:127–32.

Tschiersch K, Holzl J. [Resorption und ausscheidung von apigenin, apegenin-7–glucosid und herniarin ncah peroraler gabe eines extrakts von *Matricaria recutita* (L.) (syn. *Chamomilla recutita* (L.) Rauschert). Pharmazie 1993;48:554–5.

Yamada K, Miura T, Mimaki Y, Sashida Y. Effect of inhalation of chamomile oil vapour on plasma ACTH level in ovariectomized-rat under restriction stress. Biol Pharmacol Bull 1996;19:1244–6.

# Chapter 7

# Echinacea

*Julie Davis and Melanie Johns Cupp*

*Echinacea angustifolia* DC, *E. purpurea* (L.) Moench, *E. pallida* (Nutt.) Britton, American cone flower, black susans, comb flower, hedgehog, Indian head, Kansas snakeroot, narrow-leaved purple cone flower, purple cone flower, scurvy root, snake root (Anonymous, 1996)

## 7.1 History and Traditional Uses

*Echinacea*, a genus including nine species that grow in the United States, is a member of the daisy (Asteraceae; Compositae) family. Three of these species are commonly found in herbal preparations: the dried rhizome and roots of *E. angustifolia*, the narrow-leaved echinacea; *E. pallida*, the pale-flowered echinacea; and *E. purpurea*, the cultivated variety. The latter is the species most commonly found in herbal preparations (Tyler, 1993).

Echinacea was originally utilized by Native Americans for a variety of conditions. The plant was considered to be a "blood purifier" and was used for the treatment of snake bites (Anonymous, 1996), infections, and malignancy (Tyler et al., 1981). In 1871, a Nebraska physician named HCF Meyer learned of the Native Americans' use of echinacea. Meyer informed the pharmaceutical manufacturer Lloyd Brothers of Cincinnati about the purported benefits of echinacea in 1885. Meyer claimed the plant was effective for many conditions, including rheumatism, streptococcal erysipelas, stomach upset, migraines, pain, sores, wounds, eczema, sore eyes, snake bites, gangrene, typhoid, diphtheria, rabies, hemorrhoids, dizziness, herbal poisoning, tumors, syphilis, malaria, and bee stings. The company marketed echinacea as an antiinfective, and by 1920, echinacea was their best-selling plant product. The introduction of

From Forensic Science: *Toxicology and Clinical Pharmacology of Herbal Products*
Edited by: M. J. Cupp © Humana Press Inc., Totowa, New Jersey

modern antiinfectives such as the sulfa drugs led the product to fall out of favor (Tyler, 1993).

## 7.2 Current Promoted Uses

In the United States echinacea is promoted primarily in oral dosage forms as an immune stimulant that helps increase resistance to colds, influenza, and other infections, although topical products for wounds and inflammatory skin conditions are also available.

## 7.3 Products Available

Fresh herb, freeze-dried or dried herb, and alcoholic extracts are available in the United States in the form of tablets, capsules, lozenges, liquid, tea, and salves. Many products combine echinacea with ginseng, goldenseal, or garlic.

Some echinacea-containing products have been found to be contaminated with *Parthenium integrifolium*, a plant of the same family that has no known pharmacologic activity (Anonymous, 1996).

*Consumer Reports* analyzed 12 echinacea products in the March 1999 issue, using a standard set by industry. Although the standard some manufacturers use is 4% phenolic compounds (caffeoyl-tartaric acid, chlorogenic acid, cichoric acid, and echinacoside), only three products, Vita-Smart® by American Fare®, One-A-Day® Cold Season by Bayer, and Echinex® by Sunsource approached this standard at 4.5%, 4%, and 3.9%, respectively. There was also variation among different bottles of the same brand (Anonymous, 1999).

## 7.4 Pharmacologic/Toxicologic Effects

### 7.4.1 Immunologic Effects

The majority of the published literature about echinacea focuses on the plant's activity as an immunostimulant. In many in vitro studies, echinacea extracts have been shown to stimulate phagocytosis, increase leukocyte mobility, and increase cellular respiration. Lipophilic extracts appear to be more active than hydrophilic extracts (Anonymous, 1996).

One constituent of echinacea, the polysaccharide arabinogalactan, has been identified as a macrophage activator in vitro, causing macrophages to attack tumor cells and microorganisms. When injected into mice intraperitoneally, arabinogalactan was able to activate macrophages. Macrophage production of tumor necrosis factor-α (TNF-α), interleukin-1 (IL-1), and interferon-$B_2$ was increased in vitro, and production of oxygen free radicals was increased both in vitro and in vivo (Luettig et al., 1989). An earlier study also showed that a crude polysaccharide extract of E. purpurea also increased macrophage cytotoxicity toward tumor cells and increased macrophage IL-1 production (Stimpel et al., 1984). Echinacea polysaccharide effects on T-cells and B-cells were limited (Luettig et al., 1989; Stimpel et al., 1984).

### *7.4.2 Antimicrobial/Antiviral Effects*

A study assessed ability of an echinacea extract to enhance natural killer cell activity against K562 cells and antibody-dependent cellular cytotoxicity (ADCC) against human herpesvirus infected H9 cells (See et al., 1997). Dried, ground preparations of fresh echinacea were homogenized and filtered to produce an extract that was added in increasing concentrations to peripheral blood mononuclear cells from patients with AIDS, chronic fatigue syndrome (CFS), and healthy volunteers. CFS and AIDS patients were excluded from the study if they were taking corticosteroids, colony-stimulating factors, interleukins, interferons, or cancer chemotherapy. Echinacea extract enhanced the cytotoxicity of natural killer cells, and increased activity against cells infected with human herpesvirus 6 (HH6) in all three groups at concentrations of at least 0.1 μg/mL and 1 μg/mL, respectively.

The ability of an oral echinacea preparation to prolong the time to onset of an upper respiratory infection was compared to that of placebo in 302 volunteers from an industrial plant and several military institutions (Melchart et al., 1998). Volunteers were administered either placebo or 50 drops (2 mL) twice daily of 30% ethanol in water extract of *E. angustifolia* or *E. purpurea* providing approx 200 mg of echinacea daily for 12 wk. Although patients felt they had benefited from echinacea ($p = 0.04$), there was no difference among the three groups in regard to time to the first upper respiratory infection, the main outcome measure. A second outcome measure, the number of patients in each group who developed at least one infection, was not different to a statistically significant degree.

Another study (Grimm and Muller, 1999) also examined the efficacy of echinacea in preventing colds and upper respiratory infections, but used a different preparation. The preparation used in this study was fluid extract of Echinacea purpurea, the juice expressed from whole flowering *E. purpurea* (without the roots) in a 22% alcohol solution. This preparation was identical to Echinacin-Liquidum, a German product. This study was unique because patients were enrolled only if they had a history of more than three colds or respiratory infections in the preceding year. One hundred and eight patients were randomized to receive 4 mL twice daily of study drug or identical placebo for 8 wk. The primary outcome measures were the incidence and severity of colds during the study period. Medical history, physical exam, and hematologic exam were performed by blinded investigators at baseline and at wk 4 and 8. Patients were also instructed to see the investigator if he or she experienced burning or tearing eyes, ear pain, loss of hearing with pressure in the ear, stuffy or runny nose, sore throat, difficulty swallowing, hoarseness, coughing, sputum production, headache, joint pain, myalgia, fever, rigors, sweating, or general weakness/tiredness. If a patient was found to have a respiratory infection, follow-up occurred every 2–3 d to assess its duration and severity. Severity was graded on a scale of 1–3. Results showed that the two groups did not differ in number of colds or respiratory infections per patient ($p = 0.33$), duration of infection ($p = 0.45$), or number of infections in each category of severity ($p = 0.15$). Four echinacea patients and three placebo patients dropped out of the study. Reasons for withdrawal in the echinacea group included nausea, constipation, and "awful taste." Four echinacea patients experienced central nervous system (CNS) effects (tiredness, somnolence, dizziness, headache, aggressiveness), four patients in each group experienced gastrointestinal effects (nausea, heartburn, mild epigastric pain, constipation), one patient in each group experienced increased urge for micturition, one echinacea patient reported eczema, and one echinacea patient experienced hair loss. The incidence of adverse effects was not significantly different ($p = 0.44$) between the two groups.

The investigators in this study (Grimm and Muller, 1999) mention that echinacea has also been used to *treat* colds and upper respiratory infections in adults, but the majority of these studies were uncontrolled, retrospective studies that in some cases used other herbs as well as echinacea; however, in two placebo-controlled trials, 900 mg/d of expressed juice of *E. purpurea* roots (Brauning et al., 1992) and ethanolic extract of *E. pallida* roots (Brauning and Knick, 1993) showed benefit in reducing symptoms (Brauning et al., 1992; Brauning and Knick, 1993), clinical findings (Brauning et al., 1992), and infection duration (Brauning and Knick, 1993) in patients with colds and upper respiratory infections. A more recent randomized, double blind, placebo-controlled study of treatment of the common cold with Echinacea recruited 559 volunteers, 246 of whom caught a cold. Affected volunteers took placebo, Echinaforce (Echinacea purpurea 5% root and 95% herb), a preparation seven times as concentrated as Echinaforce, or an *Echinacea purpurea* root preparation. Two tablets were taken three times daily for 7 d or until symptoms resolved, whichever came first. Echinaforce and the concentrated preparation were superior to placebo in reducing the "complaint index" as defined by twelve symptoms. Adverse effects were comparable to placebo (Brinkeborn et al., 1999). A review of all blinded placebo-controlled randomized trials of Echinacea for prevention or treatment of upper respiratory infection concluded that Echinacea may be effective for early treatment of upper respiratory infections, but evidence supporting efficacy for prevention is sparse (Barrett et al., 1999). Clearly, more study is needed to identify the echinacea dose and preparation that is effective for the treatment or prevention of colds and other upper respiratory infections.

### *7.4.3 Antineoplastic Activity*

*See also* 7.4.1 Immunologic Effects. An investigation details the isolation of (Z)-1,8-pentadecadiene from *E. angustifolia* DC. and E. pallida (Nutt.) Britton. This root oil constituent has inhibitory effects against Walker carcinosarcoma 256 and P-388 lymphocytic leukemia in the mouse and rat, respectively (Voaden and Jacobson, 1972).

A clinical study was conducted to determine the toxicity and immunostimulating effect of echinacin, an extract of *E. purpurea,* in combination with cyclophosphamide and thymostimulin (stimulates IL-2 and interferon production) in patients with progressive colorectal cancer refractory to chemotherapy or radiation (Lersch et al., 1992). Fifteen outpatients with advanced colorectal cancer received 300 mg/m$^2$ of cyclophosphamide IV every 28 d, followed by 30 mg/m$^2$ of thymostimulin and 60 mg/m$^2$ of echinacin IM on d 3–10 of the cycle. Subsequently, the thymostimulin and echinacin were repeated twice weekly. The regimen was continued until the tumor size increased by more than 50%, or CNS metastasis occurred. Because these patients had advanced cancer, tumor response rate was not an outcome measure; however, after 2 mo of therapy, one patient experienced a 50% regression in tumor size and in six patients tumor size stabilized. Mean survival time was 4 mo, with two patients surviving more than 8 mo. Immunological monitoring was performed on days 0, 1, 7, 14, and 21. Total T-cell (CD3+) count, T-helper/inducer (CD4+) count, T-suppressor/cytotoxic (CD8+) count, B-cell (CD19+) count, natural killer cell count and activity (lysis rate), lymphokine activated killer (LAK) cell lysis activity, and phagocytic activity of polymorphonuclear leukocytes were measured. All were increased except CD8+ count and B-cell count. Although the authors attribute these effects to echinacin, the statistical methods used and lack of placebo control make the results difficult to interpret. No adverse effects were noted, but details about echinacin were not provided, limiting the applicability of these results. Injectable echinacea products are no longer available in Germany (Blumenthal, 1998).

### *7.4.4 Wound-Healing*

The wound-healing actions of Echinacea stem from two effects: inhibition of hyaluronidase, an enzyme produced by bacteria that enables them to spread throughout a wound, and stimulation of fibroblasts to produce granulation tissue (Bauer 1996). The specific constituents responsible for antihyaluronidase activity appear to be the caffeic acid derivatives cichloric acid, cafteric acid, cynarin, and chlorogenic acid (Facino et al., 1993).

### *7.4.5 Anti-Inflammatory Effects*

Polyunsaturated alkamides isolated from *Echinacea angustifolia* inhibit cyclooxygenase and 5-lipoxygenase in vitro (Mullr-Jakic et al., 1994). Certain high-molecular weight polysaccharaide components also appear to have anti-inflammatory activity (Tragni et al., 1988).

### *7.4.6 Mutagenicity/Carcinogenicity*

*Echinacea purpurea* gave negative results in bacterial and mammalian cell mutagenicity tests. Hamster embryo cell carcinogenicity studies revealed no malignant transformation (Mengs et al., 1991).

### *7.4.7 Reproduction*

Preliminary results of a prospective cohort study suggest that echinacea does not appear to pose a teratogenic risk. This study cohort was identified through Canada's Motherisk Program. Forty-five pregnancies in which echinacea was used have been followed thus far, with two spontaneous abortions, no stiilbirths, and no malformations. Data on additional pregnancies will be collected (Gallo et al., 1998).

## 7.5 Case Reports of Toxicity Due to Commercially Available Products

A 37-yr-old woman had been taking various dietary supplements, including echinacea, for 2–3 yr. One morning, she took vitamins $B_{12}$, E, vitamin B complex, folate, an herbal iron preparation (FeFol), a multivitamin, zinc, antioxidants, a garlic and onion product, and evening primrose oil, all over a 5–10-min period. Fifteen minutes later, she ingested one teaspoon (twice the amount recommended by the manufacturer) of a 40% ethanol in water solution of echinacea, which she diluted in apple and black currant juice, as directed by the label. The amount ingested was equal to 3825 mg of whole plant extract of *E. angustifolia* and 150 mg of dried root of *E. purpurea.* Immediately, she experienced burning of the mouth and throat, which she had not previously experienced. After eating a few bites of cereal with milk, chest tightness, generalized urticaria, and diarrhea developed within 15 min of taking the echinacea. She self-administered 75 mg of promethazine orally, and was taken to the hospital by ambulance. She was observed in the emergency room for 2 h and recovered with no further treatment. Past medical history was significant for mild wheezing precipitated by respiratory infection, allergic rhinitis, and oral pruritis ("oral allergy syndrome") caused by various raw (not cooked) fruits and vegetables, although apple and black currant juice were tolerated by the patient. Eating bananas resulted in urticaria and angioedema. She had taken echinacea from the same bottle a few weeks prior to this episode with no problems, but declined rechallenge with any of the dietary supplements she had been taking. Skin prick testing with the echinacea extract resulted in a 3-mm wheal and 5-mm flare, with similar results obtained at dilutions of 1:100 and 1:1000 in saline. Radioallergosorbent (RAST) testing of the patient's serum revealed immunoglobulin E (IgE) against echinacea. The patient did not react to skin testing with apple and black currant juice, commercial extracts of rice and soy protein, or crude extracts of the other dietary supplements prepared at 10% (w/v) in saline. Skin prick testing with aqueous or glycerinated echinacea extracts was positive in 19% (16) of 84 subsequent patients with asthma or allergic rhinitis, although only two had ever taken echinacea. In addition, echinacea-binding IgE was identified by RAST in 11 of 15 randomly selected stored serum samples from atopic patients (Mullins, 1998).

The Australian Adverse Drug Reactions Advisory Committee received 11 reports of adverse reactions associated with echinacea use between July 1996 and September 1997. There were three reports of hepatitis; three reports of asthma; one rash; one of rash, myalgia, and nausea; one urticaria; one anaphylaxis (the previously described case); and one of dizziness and tongue swelling. Echinacea was the only reported ingestant in five of the eight reports, resembling hypersensitivity. Onset of symptoms occurred within 24 h in two cases. There are two additional published case reports of echinacea-associated contact dermatitis and anaphylaxis (Mullins, 1998).

Although not documented, cross-sensitivity between echinacea and other members of the daisy family such as feverfew, chamomile, and ragweed might occur.

## 7.6 Chemical Analysis

The thin-layer chromatography (TLC) analysis of echinacea, including identification of the adulterant *Parthenium integrifolium*, has been described (Bisset, 1994).

## 7.7 Regulatory Status

Echinacea is regulated as a dietary supplement in the United States. German Commission E has approved *E. pallida* root and *E. purpurea* herb (above-ground parts). *E. purpurea* root and *E. angustifolia* root are on the Commission's unapproved list. This decision was based on the realization that some pharmacologic studies done before 1988 using *E. angustifolia* actually involved *E. pallida*. Therefore, there is a lack of information on *E. angustifolia* root and the above-ground (aerial) parts of *E. angustifolia* and *E. pallida* (Blumenthal, 1998).

## REFERENCES

Anonymous. Echinacea. The review of natural products. St. Louis, MO: Facts and Comparisons, 1996.

Anonymous. Ginkgo biloba active ingredients meet proper levels—*Consumer Reports*. F-D-C Reports. "The Tan Sheet." March 8, 1999.

Barrett B, Vohmann M, Calabrese C. Echinacea for upper respiratory infection. J Fam Pract 1999;48:628–35.

Bauer R. Echinacea drugs-effects and active ingredients. Z Arztl Fortbild (Jena). 1996;90:111–5.

Bisset NG. Herbal drugs and phytomedicinals. London: CRC Press, 1994;182–4.

Blumenthal M. The complete German Commission E monographs: therapeutic guide to herbal medicines. Austin, TX: American Botanical Council, 1998.

Brauning B, Knick E. [Therapeutische erfahrungen mit *Echinacea pallida* bei grippalen infekten]. Naturheilpraxis 1993;1:72–5.

Brauning B, Dorn M, Knick E. [*Echinacea purpurea* radix: Zur starkung der korpereigenen abwehr bei grippaken infekten]. Z Phytother 1992;13:7–13.

Brinkeborn RM, Shah DV, Degenring FH. Echinaforce and other Echinacea fresh plant preparations in the treatment of the common cold. A randomized, placebo-controlled, double-blind clinical trial. Phytomedicine 1999;6:1–6.

Facino RM, Carini M, Aldini G, Marinello C, Arlandini E. Franzoi L, et al. Direct characterization of caffeoyl esters with a trihyaluronidase activity in crude extracts from *Echinacea angustiflia* roots by fast atom bombardment tandem mass spectrometry. Farmco 1993;48:1447–61.

Gallo M, Au W, Koren G. The safety of echinacea use during pregnancy: a prospective controlled cohort study. Teratology 1998;57:283.

Grimm W, Muller H. A randomized controlled trial of the effect of fluid extract of *Echinacea purpurea* on the incidence and severity of colds and respiratory infections Am J Med 1999;106:138–43.

Lersch C, Zeuner M, Bauer A, Siemens M, Hart R, Drescher M, et al. Nonspecific immunostimulation with low doses of cyclophosphamide (LDCY), thymostimulin, and echinacea purpurea extracts (echinacin) in patients with far advanced colorectal cancers: preliminary results. Cancer Invest 1992;10:343–8.

Leuttig B, Steinmuller C, Gifford GE, Wagner H, Lohmann-Matthes ML. Macrophage activation by the polysaccharide arabinogalactan isolated from plant cell cultures of *Echinacea purpurea*. J Natl Cancer Inst 1989;81:669–75.

Melchart, Walther E, Linde K, Brandmaier R, Lersch C. Echinacea root extracts for the prevention of upper respiratory tract infections. A double-blind, placebo-controlled randomized trial. Arch Fam Med 1998;7:541–5.

Mengs U, Clare CB, Poiley JA. Toxicity of *Echinacea purpurea*. Acute, subacute, and genotoxicity studies. Arzneimittelforschung 1991;41:1076–81.

Muller-Jakic B, Breu W, Probstle A, Redl K, Greger H, Bauer R. In vitro inhibition of cyclooxygenase and 5-lipoxygenase by alkamides from Echinacea and Achillea species. Planta Med 1994;60:37–40.

Mullins RJ. Echinacea-associated anaphylaxis. Med J Aust 1998;168:170–1.

See DM, Broumand N, Sahl L, Tilles JG. In vitro effects of echinacea and ginseng on natural killer and antibody-dependent cell cytotoxicty in healthy subjects and chronic fatigue sysndrome or acquired immunodeficiency syndrome patients. Immunopharmacology 1997;35:229–35.

Stimpel M, Proksch A, Wagner H, lohmann-Matthes ML. Macrophage activation and induction of macrophage cytotoxicity by purified polysaccharide fractions from the plant *Echinacea purpurea*. Infect Immun 1984;46:845–9.

Tragni E, Galli CL, Tubaro A, Del Negro P, Della Loggia R. Anti-inflammatory activity of *Echinacea angustifolia* fractions separated on the basis of molecular weight. Pharmacol Res Comm 1988;20(Suppl 5):87–90.

Tyler VE, Brady LR, Robbers JE. Pharmacognosy, 8th edit., Philadelphia: Lea and Febiger, 1981.

Tyler VE. The honest herbal. A sensible guide to the use of herbs and related remedies. 3rd edit., Binghamton, NY: Pharmaceutical Products Press, 1993.

Voaden DJ, Jacobson M. Tumor inhibitors. 3. Identification and synthesis of an oncolytic hydrocarbon from Americna coneflower roots. J Med Chem 1972;15:619–23.

# Chapter 8

# Feverfew



## Brian Schuller and Melanie Johns Cupp



*Tanacetum parthenium* Schulz-Bip, formerly *Chrysanthemum parthenium* (L.) Bernh, *Leucanthemum parthenium* (L.) Gren and Gordon, *Pyrethum parthenium* (L.) Sm; also described as a member of the genus *Matricaria* (Anonymous, 1994; USP, 1998a); featherfew, altamisa, bachelor's button, featherfoil, febrifuge plant, midsummer daisy, nosebleed, Santa Maria, wild chamomile, wild quinine (Anonymous, 1994), amargosa, flirtwort, manzanilla, mutterkraut, varadika (USP, 1998a)

## 8.1 History and Traditional Uses

Feverfew is a short perennial bush that grows along fields and roadsides. It reaches heights of 15–60 cm. With its yellow-green leaves and yellow flowers, it can be mistaken for chamomile (*Matricaria chamomilla*). The flowers bloom from July to October (Anonymous, 1994). Since the time of Dioscorides in the first century AD, feverfew has been used for the treatment of headache, menstrual irregularities, and fever. The common name is in fact a corruption of the Latin word *febrifugia* (Tyler, 1993). Other traditional uses include treatment of menstrual pain, asthma, arthritis (Anonymous, 1994), psoriasis, threatened miscarriage, toothache, opium abuse, vertigo, (Knight, 1995), tinnitus, anemia, the common cold, and gastrointestinal disturbances (USP, 1998a). It was also used to aid in expulsion of the placenta and stillbirths (Knight, 1995), and in difficult labor (USP, 1998a). Feverfew has been planted around houses to act as an insect repellant, as well as for use as a topical remedy for insect bites (Anonymous, 1994).

## 8.2 Current Promoted Uses

In the 1970s, use of feverfew as an alternative to traditional medicines for relief from arthritis and migraine headache began gaining popularity (Tyler,

From Forensic Science: *Toxicology and Clinical Pharmacology of Herbal Products*
Edited by: M. J. Cupp © Humana Press Inc., Totowa, New Jersey

1993). Prevention of migraine headache is the most commonly promoted indication for feverfew.

## 8.3 Products Available

Feverfew is available as the fresh leaf; dried, powdered leaf; capsules; tablets; fluid extract; dry standardized extract; crystals; and oral drops (USP, 1998a). Brand names include Migracare (600 µg of parthenolide per capsule), Migracin (feverfew extract 1:4 and white willow bark), MigraSpray, MygraFew, Lomigran, 125-mg Migrelief (light green round tablet containing 600 µg of parthenolide), Partenelle, Phytofeverfew, and 125-mg Tanacet (not <0.2% parthenolide). Feverfew contains flavonoid glycosides and sesquiterpene lactones. Parthenolide can constitute up to 85% of the sesquiterpene lactones in feverfew grown in Europe (Anonymous, 1994; USP, 1998a), but is present in lesser amounts or is even totally absent from North American feverfew (USP, 1998a). Parthenolide is concentrated in the flowers and leaves, as opposed to stems and roots, and parthenolide content of the leaves may decrease during storage (Heptinstall et al., 1992; USP, 1998a). The vegetative cycle also influences parthenolide content (USP, 1998a). Although parthenolide is thought to be the active ingredient in feverfew, and preparations are often standardized based on parthenolide content (Tyler, 1994), there may be other active compounds, including the lipophilic flavonol tanetin, other methyl monoterpene ethers, and chrysanthenyl acetate, monoterpene (USP, 1998a).

Most tablet and capsule formulations contain 300 mg of feverfew, and the recommended dose is usually two to six tablets or capsules per day. A dose of 250 µg of parthenolide is considered an adequate daily dose, and 0.2% parthnolide is considered the acceptable minimum parthenolide concentration; therefore, the manufacturer's recommended dose is probably in excess of what is considered therapeutic (Tyler, 1994). In the prevention of migraine headache, doses used in studies have been 50–100 mg of dried feverfew leaves daily (Johnson et al., 1985; Palevitch et al., 1997; Murphy et al., 1988) (60 mg of dried feverfew leaves = 2½ leaves) (USP, 1998a). However, the parthenolide content of the North American plant is low (Tyler, 1994), and parthenolide content in feverfew products varies widely (Heptinstall et al., 1992), and may be lower than stated on the label (Groenewegen and Heptinstall, 1986) or even absent from some preparations (Groenewegen and Hepinstall, 1986; Heptinstall et al., 1992). For example, no parthenolide could be detected in two-thirds of feverfew products purchased in Louisiana health food stores (Tyler, 1994). The parthenolide content of powdered feverfew leaves falls during storage (Heptinstall et al., 1992). Given that the active ingredients of feverfew have yet to be definitively determined, it is difficult to designate a therapeutic or toxic dosage range. (*See* discussion of melatonin content of feverfew products in Section 8.4.1.)

## 8.4 Pharmacology/Toxicology

### 8.4.1 Neurologic Effects

Feverfew's mechanism of action in the prevention of migraine headaches is not known. It is speculated that feverfew affects platelet activity or inhibits vascular smooth muscle contraction, perhaps by inhibiting prostaglandin synthesis (USP, 1998a). Results of in vitro studies suggest that rather than acting as a cyclooxygenase inhibitor, feverfew inhibits phospholipase $A_2$, thus inhibiting release of arachidonic acid from the cell membrane phospholipid bilayer (Collier et al., 1980; Makheja and Bailey, 1981).

Drugs that are serotonin antagonists are used in migraine prevention (e.g., methysergide) (Murphy et al., 1988). During a migraine, serotonin is released from platelets (Murphy et al., 1988), and in vitro studies using a bovine platelet bioassay have shown that parthenolide, as well as other sesquiterpene lactones, inhibits platelet serotonin release (Marles et al., 1992). Both parthenolide and a chloroform extract of dried, powdered leaves were also able to inhibit serotonin release and platelet aggregation in an in vitro study using human platelets and a variety of platelet-activating agents (Groenewegen and Heptinstall, 1990). The effect of these substances on platelet aggregation due to a variety of chemicals was tested, and was similar except that inhibition of platelet aggregation induced by the calcium ionophore A23187 by chloroform extract leveled off at a relatively low concentration and was not complete, while parthenolide inhibited aggregation in a dose-dependent manner, suggesting a different mechanism of action.

Similarly discrepant results were reported in a study comparing chloroform extracts of fresh and dried feverfew, and parthenolide (Barsby et al., 1993b). In this in vitro study, both the fresh extract and parthenolide were able to irreversibly inhibit contraction of rabbit aortic ring and rat anococcygeus muscle in a dose-dependent manner. In contrast, the extract from dried powdered feverfew leaves was spasmogenic, causing a slow, maintained, reversible contraction. The differences in pharmacologic effect were explained by the differences in composition of the extracts; unlike the extract of fresh leaves, the extract of dried powdered leaves did not contain parthenolide or other sesquiterpene lactones. The specific functional group responsible for inhibition of smooth muscle contraction has been identified as the $\alpha$-methylene moiety present on parthenolide and other sesquiterpene lactones (Hay et al., 1994). It has been hypothesized that the irreversible inhibition of platelet aggregation and inhibition of smooth muscle contraction are caused by covalent binding of parthenolide and other lactones to sulfhydryl (SH-) groups on proteins (Barsby et al., 1993b).

Another study using chloroform extract of fresh feverfew leaves demonstrated reversible blockade of open voltage-dependent potassium channels, but not of calcium-dependent potassium channels, in smooth muscle cells in vitro (Barsby et al., 1993a). Inhibition of potassium channels would be expected to increase the excitability of smooth muscle cells, potentiate the effects of depolarizing stimuli, and open voltage-dependent calcium channels, thus leading to muscle contraction. In the study described previously (Barsby et al., 1993a), the extract of dried, powdered feverfew had this very effect, which could be explained by potassium channel blockade; however, the *fresh* extract had the opposite effect (i.e., it irreversibly inhibited contractility). In addition, parthenolide, which was present in fresh but not dried extracts, did not appear to inhibit potassium channels. The substances in feverfew that cause potassium channel blockade and muscle contraction have not been identified, but because voltage-dependent potassium channels present in smooth muscle cells are similar to those present in neurons, it is possible that feverfew interferes with the neurogenic response in migraine (Barsby, 1993a).

One of the first studies to attempt to objectively evaluate the efficacy of feverfew for migraine prophylaxis enrolled 17 patients with common or classical migraine who had been self-medicating with raw feverfew leaves (average 2.44 leaves [60 mg]) daily for at least 3 mo (Johnson et al., 1985). Patients were randomized to receive either 50 mg of freeze-dried feverfew powder or placebo for 6 mo. One patient in each group was taking conjugated equine estrogens (Premarin) and one patient in the feverfew group was taking Orlest® 21, an oral contraceptive. Efficacy was assessed using patient diaries in which patients recorded the duration and severity of headache pain, severity and duration of nausea and vomiting, and analgesic use on an ordinal scale. The frequency of migraine, nausea, and vomiting, was significantly ($p < 0.02$) lower in the feverfew group, but analgesic use was similar. Two patients taking placebo withdrew from the study because of recurrent severe migraine. Patients taking feverfew reported a similar number of migraine attacks during the study compared to before the study when they were self-medicating with feverfew. Conversely, placebo patients reported a frequency of headache that was greater than when they were self-medicating, and similar to the frequency of headache before beginning feverfew self-treatment. At the end of the study, the patients assessed the overall efficacy of the treatment; feverfew had a more favorable rating than placebo ($p < 0.01$). Because there was underreporting of headache in the placebo group, the difference between feverfew and placebo may have been even greater. Adverse events were not reported in the feverfew group, but patients did complain of the product's taste. A potential problem with this study was blinding; most patients guessed correctly which treatment they were receiving. Another criticism of this study is that because the participants were recruited from a population already taking feverfew and who presumably felt they were benefiting from feverfew, the investigators were in effect selecting known "feverfew responders" for their study. Such a selection process limits the extent to which these study results can be extrapolated to the general population.

In a subsequent study, efficacy of feverfew in migraine prophylaxis was further assessed in a double-blind, randomized, crossover design (Murphy et al., 1988). One capsule of dried feverfew leaves (70–114 mg, average 82 mg) was compared to placebo in 72 adult volunteers with classical or common migraine. All subjects had migraine of at least 2 yr duration, and suffered at least one attack per month. Patients were excluded if they were being treated for any other disease, but women taking oral contraceptives were eligible for the study if they had been on the same contraceptive for at least 3 mo. Females of childbearing potential were excluded unless they were using adequate contraception. All migraine-related drugs were stopped at the beginning of the trial, which commenced with a 1-mo single-blind placebo run-in period. Patients were then randomized to placebo or feverfew for 4 mo each. Efficacy was assessed based on a patient diary in which patients recorded the number, severity, and duration of any migraine attacks, as well as the presence of nausea and vomiting, on a scale from 0 to 3. In addition, every 2 mo, the patient's overall impression of migraine control was assessed using a 10-cm visual analog scale. There was a significant difference ($p < 0.05$) between placebo and feverfew in number of attacks only after month 4, but there was a significant difference between the two groups in overall impression after month 4 ($p < 0.05$) and after month 6 ($p < 0.01$) when assessed via the visual analog scale. Feverfew decreased the number of classical migraine attacks by 32% (95% CI 11–53%, $p < 0.05$), but the effect on the number of common migraine attacks was not statistically significant ($p = 0.06$). When assessing the responses of patients who had never used feverfew before study enrollment ($n$ = 42/59) the number of attacks was reduced by 23% (95% CI 10–33%, $p = 0.06$). This nonsignificant result gives credence to the concerns about selection bias in the study by Johnson and colleagues. The overall impression of both common and classical migraineurs was favorable based on the visual analog scale ($p < 0.01$). Vomiting associated with attacks was also decreased with feverfew, and there was a trend toward reduction in migraine severity. Duration of attacks was unchanged. Incidence of adverse effects, including mouth ulceration, indigestion, heartburn, dizziness, lightheadedness, rash, and diarrhea was low and comparable to placebo.

Another randomized, double-blind, crossover study assessed the efficacy of 100 mg of feverfew (0.2% parthenolide) daily compared to placebo in 57 patients (Palevitch et al., 1997). Efficacy was assessed using a questionnaire. Feverfew was superior to placebo in reducing intensity of migraine pain and other symptoms. However, an alcoholic extract of feverfew providing 0.5 mg of parthenolide daily for 4 mo was not superior to placebo in the number of migraine attacks in a randomized, double-blind, crossover study in 44 evaluable patients (DeWeerdt et al., 1996).

Surprisingly, melatonin, a human pineal hormone, has been identified in fresh green feverfew leaves at a concentration of 2.45 μg/g, and in a commercially available feverfew tablet (Tanacet®, Ashbury Biologicals, Inc., Toronto, Canada) at a concentration of 0.143 μg/g. Each Tanacet® tablet contains 70–80 ng of melatonin, and the recommended dose is one or two tablets daily. Freeze-dried green leaf contains 2.19 μg/g of melatonin, fresh golden feverfew leaf contains 1.92 μg/g, oven-dried green leaf contains 1.69 μg/g, freeze-dried golden leaf conatins 1.61 μg/g, and oven-dried golden leaf contains 1.37 μg/g. Because chronic migraine headaches are associated with lower circulating melatonin levels, it is possible that melatonin plays a role in feverfew's purported efficacy in preventing migraine headache. This finding underscores the need to fully characterize the ingredients in herbs and medicinal preparations made from them (Murch et al., 1997).

Larger studies are needed to definitively determine the efficacy of feverfew in the prevention of migraine, and to identify the component or components responsible for its pharmacologic effects.

### *8.4.2 Anti-Inflammatory Effects*

Organic and aqueous feverfew powdered leaf extracts were found to inhibit interleukin-1 (IL-1)-induced prostaglandin $E_2$ ($PGE_2$) release from synovial cells, interleukin-2 (IL-2)-induced thymidine uptake by lymphoblasts, and mitogen-induced uptake of thymidine by peripheral blood mononuclear cells (PBMCs) (O'Neill et al., 1987). Parthenolide also inhibited thymidine uptake by PBMCs. Both parthenolide and the extracts were cytotoxic to the PBMCs and synovial cells; thus, the antiinflammatory effects of feverfew may be secondary to cytotoxicity. These results reflect those of previous researchers who found parthenolide and other sesquiterpene lactones to be cytotoxic to cultures of human fibroblasts, human laryngeal carcinoma cells, and human cells transformed with simian virus 40 (Lee et al., 1971).

The antiinflammatory effect of dried powdered feverfew leaf was compared to placebo in the treatment of rheumatoid arthritis (RA) (Pattrick et al., 1989). This double-blind randomized study utilized dried powdered feverfew leaf 70–86 mg of (mean 76 mg) equivalent to 2–3 μmol of parthenolide. Forty-one female RA patients from a rheumatology clinic participated. Patients were allowed to continue their usual doses of nonsteroidal antiinflammatory drugs (NSAIDs) and other analgesics. If a patient deteriorated acutely during the study, a single intraarticular dose of 20 mg of triamcinolone hexacetonide was allowed at week 3. Efficacy was determined by clinical assessments at weeks 3 and 6, and included duration of early morning stiffness in minutes, inactivity stiffness (present/absent), pain (10 cm visual analog scale), grip strength, and Richie articular index. Patients were also questioned about adverse effects. At weeks 0 and 6, hemoglobin, white blood cell count (WBC), platelet count, urea, creatinine, erythrocyte sedimentation rate (ESR), C reactive protein, immunoglobulin G (IgG), IgM, IgA, latex fixation test, Rose–Waaler titer, C3 degradation products, and Steinbrocker functional capacity were determined. At week 6, a global impression from both the patient and the clinician were recorded as better, same, or worse. One patient in the placebo group dropped out after the third day because of lightheadedness, but complete data were obtained for the remaining 40 patients. One patient receiving feverfew reported minor ulceration and soreness of the tongue. At baseline, hemoglobin and serum creatinine levels were lower in the placebo group than in the feverfew group. By week 3, urea levels had significantly increased ($p = 0.04$) in the feverfew group, but this was not apparent at 6 wk. At 6 wk, grip strength and IgG were increased in the feverfew group compared with baseline ($p = 0.47$ and 0.025, respectively). Overall, the results of this study do not support the efficacy of 76 mg of dried feverfew leaf in the treatment of RA.

### 8.4.3 Mutagenicity/Carcinogenicity/Teratogenicity

In 30 migraine patients who had been taking feverfew leaves, tablets, or capsules for at least 11 mo, there was no increase in chromosomal aberrations or sister chromatid exchange in circulating lymphocytes compared to migraine patients not taking feverfew matched for age and sex. The Ames salmonella mutagenicity test was also performed on urine samples from 10 patients using feverfew and 10 matched nonusers, with no indication of mutagenicity (Anderson et al., 1988).

No problems have been reported in offspring of pregnant women who used feverfew, but feverfew has purportedly been associated with spontaneous abortion in cattle and uterine contractions in term human pregnancies (USP, 1998a).

## 8.5 Case Reports of Toxicity Due to Commercially Available Products

Adverse effects associated with feverfew use include dizziness, lightheadedness, nausea, heartburn, indigestion, bloating, gas, constipation, diarrhea, inflammation, and ulceration of the oral mucosa, weight gain, palpitations, heavier menstrual flow, contact dermatitis, and rash (USP, 1998a). Feverfew belongs to the Compositae family (Anonymous, 1994), and persons allergic to other members of this family, such as chamomile, ragweed, asters, chrysanthemums (Benner and Lee, 1973) and echinacea, could also be allergic to feverfew. Eighteen percent of 300 feverfew users questioned reported adverse effects, with mouth ulceration reported in 11.3% (Johnson et al., 1985). Feverfew-induced mouth ulceration is not a manifestation of contact dermatitis; it is a systemic reaction. In contrast, inflammation of the tongue and oral mucosa accompanied by lip swelling and loss of taste is probably due to direct contact with feverfew and is not associated with use of feverfew capsules or tablets (Awang, 1993).

In the study by Johnson and colleagues, in which 10 patients who had been taking fresh feverfew leaves were switched to placebo, patients experienced recurrence of migraine, tension headaches, joint pain and stiffness, nervousness, insomnia and disrupted sleep, and tiredness. The investigators dubbed these symptoms the "postfeverfew syndrome." Dr. Johnson had documented this syndrome in a previous publication when approx 10% of 164 patients who discontinued feverfew reported anxiety, poor sleep, and joint and muscle aches, pains, and stiffness (Johnson et al., 1985).

## 8.6 Drug Interactions

In vitro studies suggest that feverfew may inhibit platelet aggregation, leading to recommendations that patients avoid use of feverfew with anticoagulants and medications with antiplatelet activity (USP, 1998a). Platelets from 10 patients who had taken feverfew for at least 3½ years responded normally to aggregation induced by ADP and thrombin compared to platelets from four control patients who had stopped taking feverfew at least 6 mo earlier. In patients who had been taking feverfew for at least 4 yr, the threshold for platelet aggregation in response to 11α,9A-epoxymethanoprostaglandin $H_2$ (U46619) and serotonin was elevated (Biggs et al., 1982). Whether these results translate into the potential for drug interactions and bleeding diatheses remains to be documented.

## 8.7 Chemical Analysis

Thin-layer chromatography (TLC) has been used to identify parthenolide and other sesquiterpene lactones (Pickman et al., 1980). The high-performance liquid chromatography (HPLC) elution profile of parthenolide has also been illustrated (Barsby et al., 1993a; Hay et al., 1994). HPLC analysis of parthenolide (Awang et al., 1991; Dolman et al., 1992; Heptinstall et al., 1992) and other sesquiterpene lactones (Dolman et al., 1992) using a spectrophotometric detector has been described in detail, as has nuclear magnetic resonance (NMR) analysis of parthenolide content (Awang et al., 1991). Information on identification and chemical analysis can also be found in the *National Formulary* (USP, 1998b).

## 8.8 Regulation

In the United States, feverfew may be marketed as a dietary supplement, but is not approved as a drug. A USP advisory panel, although recognizing that feverfew has a long history of use and lack of documented adverse effects, does not recommend its use owing to the paucity of scientific evidence of safety and efficacy. The panel encourages further research, including at least one properly designed clinical trial (USP, 1998a).

In Canada, the Health Protection branch allows sale of tablets and capsules made from feverfew crude dried leaves for decreasing the frequency and severity of migraine headaches. The products should be standardized to contain not <0.2% parthenolide. In France, feverfew has traditional use in the treatment of heavy menstrual flow and prevention of migraine headache (USP, 1998a).

## References


Anderson D, Jenkinson PC, Dewdney RS, Blowere SD, Johnson ES, Kadam NP. Chromosomal aberrations and sister chromatid exchanges in lymphocytes and urine mutagenicity of migraine patients: a comparison of chronic feverfew users and age matched nonusers. Hum Toxicol 1988;7:145–52.

Anonymous. Feverfew. The Lawrence review of natural products. St. Louis, MO: Facts and Comparisons, 1994.

Awang DVC. Feverfew fever. A headache for the consumer. HerbalGram 1993;29:34–6,66.

Awang DVC, Dawson BA, Kindack DG, Heptinstall S. Parthenolide content of feverfew [*Tanacetum parthenium* (L.) Schultz-Bip.] assessed by HPLC and $^1$H-NMR spectroscopy. J Nat Prod 1991;54:1516–21.

Barsby RWJ, Knight DW, McFadzean I. A chloroform extract of the herb feverfew blocks voltage-dependent potassium currents recorded from single smooth muscle cells. J Pharm Pharmacol 1993a;45:641–5.

Barsby RWJ, Salan U, Knight DW, Hoult JRS. Feverfew and vascular smooth muscle: extracts from fresh and dried plants show opposing pharmacological profiles, dependent upon sesquiterpene lactone content. Planta Med 1993b;59:20–5.

Benner MH, Lee HJ. Anaphylactic reaction to chamomile tea. J Allergy Clin Immunol 1973;52:307–8.

Biggs MJ, Johnson ES, Persaud NP, Ratcliffe DM. Platelet aggregation in patients using feverfew for migraine. Lancet 1982;ii:776.

Collier HOJ, Butt NM, McDonald-Gibson WJ, Saeed SA. Extract of feverfew inhibits prostaglandin biosynthesis. Lancet 1980;ii:922–3.

DeWeerdt CJ, Bootsma HPR, Hendriks H. Herbal medicine in migraine prevention: randomized, double-blind, placebo-controlled crossover trial of a feverfew preparation. Phytomed 1996;3:225–30.

Dolman DM, Knight DW, Salan U, Toplis D. A quantitiative method for the estimation of parthenolide and other sesquiterpene lactones containing alpha-methylenebutyrolactone functions present in feverfew, *Tanacetum parthenium.* Phytochem Anal 1992;3:26–31.

Groenewegen WA, Heptinstall S. Amounts of feverfew in commercial perparations of the herb. Lancet 1986;i:44–5.

Groenewegen WA, Heptinstall S. A comparison of the effects of an extract of feverfew and parthenolide, a component of feverfew, on human platelet activity in vitro. J Pharm Pharmacol 1990;42:553–57.

Hay AJB, Hamburger M, Hostettmann K, Hoult JRS. Toxic inhibition of smooth muscle contractility by plant-derived sesquiterpenes caused by their chemically reactive α-methylenebutyrolactone functions. Br J Pharmacol 1994;112:9–12.

Heptinstall S, Awang DVC, Dawson BA, Kindack D, Knight DW, May J. Parthenolide content and bioactivity of feverfew (*Tanacetum parthenium* [L.] schultz-Bip.). Estimation of commercial and authenticated feverfew products. J Pharm Pharmacol 1992;44:391–5.

Johnson ES, Kadam NP, Hylands DM, Hylands PJ. Efficacy of feverfew as prophylactic treatment of migraine. Br Med J 1985;291:569–73.

Knight DW. Feverfew: chemistry and biological activity. Nat Prod Rep 1995;12:271–6.

Lee K, Huang E, Piantadosi C, Pagano JS, Geissman TA. Cytotoxicity of sesquiterpene lactones. Cancer Res 1971;31:1649–54.

Makheja AN, Bailey JM. The active principle in feverfew. Lancet 1981;ii:1054.

Marles RJ, Kaminski J, Arnason JT. A bioassay for the inhibition of serotonin release from bovine platelets. J Nat Prod 1992;55:1044–56.

Murch SJ, Simmons CB, Saxena PK. Melatonin in feverfew and other medicinal plants. Lancet 1997;350:1598–9.

Murphy JJ, Heptinstall S, Mitchell JRA. Randomized, double-blind placebo-controlled trial of feverfew in migraine prevention. Lancet 1988;ii:189–92.

O'Neill LAJ, Barrett ML, Lewis GP. Extracts of feverfew inhibit mitogen-induced human peripheral blood mononuclear cell proliferation and cytokine mediated responses: a cytotoxic effect. Br J Clin Pharmacol 1987;23:81–3.

Palevitch D, Earon G, Carasso R. Feverfew (*Tanacetum parthenium*) as a prophylactic treatment for migraine: a double-blind placebo-controlled study. Phytother Res 1997;11:508–11.

Pattrick M, Heptinstall S, Doherty M. Feverfew in rheumatoid arthritis: a double blind, placebo controlled study. Ann Rheum Dis 1989;48:547–9.

Pickman AK, Huang ES, Piantidosi C, Pagano JS, Geissman TA. Visualisation reagents for sesquiterpene lactones and polyacetylenes on TLC. J Chromatogr 1980; 189:187–98.

Tyler VE. The honest herbal. 3rd edit., Binghamton, NY: Pharmaceutical Products Press, 1993.

Tyler VE. Herbs of choice: the therapeutic use of phytomedicinals. Binghamton, NY: Pharmaceuticals Products Press, 1994.

United States Pharmacopeial Convention (USP). Feverfew. Botanical monograph series. Rockville, MD: United States Pharmacopeial Convention, 1998a.

United States Pharmacopoeia (USP). National Formulary. 18th edit., Suppl 9. Rockville, MD: United States Pharmacopeial Convention, 1998b.

# Chapter 9

# Garlic


## James Allman and Melanie Johns Cupp


*Allium sativum*, *Allii sativi bulbus*, knoblauch (Blumenthal, 1998)

## 9.1 History and Traditional Uses

Over the centuries, garlic has been used to ward off vampires, demons, witches, and evil beings; as an aphrodisiac to improve performance and desire; and as a cure-all for everything from athlete's foot to hemorrhoids and cancer (Tyler, 1993).

## 9.2 Current Promoted Uses

Garlic is promoted to lower cholesterol and blood pressure, delay atherosclerotic processes, prevent heart attack and stroke, improve circulation, and prevent cancer.

## 9.3 Products Available

Centrum® Herbals "Garlic" capsules, 300 mg
Herbscience® Garlic, 600 mg caplets
Kwai®, 600 μg of allicin/100 mg of dried garlic, 100 mg tablets (*see* detailed description below)
Kyolic® Aged Garlic Extract™, 600-mg caplets
Nature Made® Extra Strength Odor-controlled garlic, 500 mg
Nature Made® Garlic Oil, 500-mg softgel
Nature Made® Odorless Garlic, 500-mg tablets
Nature Made® High Potency Garlic Oil, 1500-mg softgels
Nature's Resource® Garlic Powder, 180-mg enteric coated tablets


From Forensic Science: *Toxicology and Clinical Pharmacology of Herbal Products*
Edited by: M. J. Cupp © Humana Press Inc., Totowa, New Jersey

Nature's Resource® Garlic Cloves, 580-mg capsules
One-a-Day® Garlic Oil macerate, 600-mg softgel
Sundown® Herbals Odor-Free Garlic, 400-mg tablets
Sundown® Herbals Odorless Garlic, 300 mg
Sun Source® Garlique®, 400-mg tablets

Average daily dosage: 4 g of fresh garlic (Blumenthal, 1997)
Equivalent daily dosages (4–12 mg of allicin or 2–5 mg of allicin) (Blumenthal, 1997)
- Fully dried powder, 400–1200 mg
- Fresh air-dried bulb, 2–5 g
- Garlic oil, 2–5 mg
- Dried bulb, 2–4 g TID
- Tincture (1:5 in 45% alcohol), 2–4 mL TID (Blumenthal, 1997)

Garlic contains various sulfur-containing compounds, all of which are derived from allicin, which is formed from alliin by the action of allinase, which is released when garlic is chopped (Srivastava and Tyagi, 1993). Allicin then produces diallyl sulfide, diallyl disulfide, diallyl trisulfide, ajoenes, methyl allyl trisulfides, vinyl dithiins, and other sulfur compounds, depending on how the garlic is prepared.

Different methods of processing garlic, resulting in products containing different sulfur-containing thiosulfinate derivatives, have been discussed (Srivastava and Tyagi, 1993). Cooking whole or coarsely chopped garlic destroys allinase, the enzyme necessary for production of allicin, ajoene, diallyl sulfide, diallyl disulfide, and vinyl dithiins; only cysteine sulfoxides such as alliin remain. Crushing or finely chopping garlic followed by boiling in an open container leads to volatilization and loss of many chemically unstable but potentially medicinal thiosulfinates. Steam distillation produces an oily mass of active compounds including diallyl, methyl allyl, dimethyl, and allyl 1-propenyl oligosulfides that originate from the thiosulfinates. Maceration of garlic in vegetable oil or soybean oil produces vinyl dithiins, ajoenes, and diallyl and methyl allyl trisulfides. This latter method is the one used to prepare commercially available garlic capsules. When garlic is allowed to ferment (cold aging), water-soluble *S*-allyl cysteine, *S*-allyl-mercaptocysteine, and other biologically active compounds are produced.

Kwai® brand coated garlic powder tablets contain dried garlic powder prepared by freeze-drying fresh garlic (Isaacsohn et al., 1998). The tablets are odorless because they contain alliin, but not allicin, the source of garlic's characteristic odor. After the tablets are ingested, the alliin is converted to allicin in the gastrointestinal tract by the enzyme allinase, which can come into contact with alliin once the coated tablets disintegrate and mix with intestinal water.

## 9.4 Pharmacologic/Toxicologic Effects

### 9.4.1 Cardiovascular Effects

Warshafsky et al. (1993) completed a meta-analysis using Medline (1966–1991) to collect all randomized, placebo-controlled trials that tested the effectiveness of oral garlic preparations in lowering cholesterol in humans. Inclusion criteria included trials in which at least 75% of participants had elevated cholesterol levels, defined as 5.17 mmol/L (200 mg/dL). Studies were excluded if they did not contain enough data to compute effect size. Of the 28 studies found, all but five were excluded. Four of the five studies claimed to be double-blinded. All five used parallel group design. Three of the studies used Kwai® powder tablets in doses of 600, 800, and 900 mg/d. One study used 1000 mg (4 mL) of Kyolic® aqueous extract per day and the other study used 700 mg of spray-dried powder per day. None of the studies included dietary restrictions on subjects participating. The authors concluded that total cholesterol levels decreased by a statistically significant ($p < 0.001$), yet clinically small, 9% compared to placebo, in patients given the equivalent of half a clove per day. Several more recent studies have confirmed the results of this meta-analysis.

Berthold et al. (1998) performed a double-blind, randomized, placebo-controlled, crossover trial to examine the effects of garlic oil on serum lipoproteins, cholesterol absorption, or cholesterol synthesis. The product used was an enteric coated preparation (Tegra®, Hermes, Arzneimittel GmbH, Munich Germany) of steam-distilled garlic oil. The daily dosage corresponded to 4–5 g of fresh garlic cloves, or 4000 U of allicin equivalents per day. Diallyl disulfide (>30%) and diallyl trisulfide (>25%) were assumed to be the active ingredients. Twenty-six patients with moderately high cholesterol (240–338 mg/dL) and triglyceride (<265 mg/dL) were recruited through the local newspaper. Subjects had not taken any lipid-lowering agents within the prior 8 wk; however, some subjects were taking antihypertensive medication, hormone replacement therapy, or thyroid hormones. Subjects were allowed to eat their "normal" diets throughout the study, but could not eat any additional garlic. Twenty-five subjects finished the 12-wk study, with one subject dropping out because of scheduling conflicts. Garlic oil did not affect any of the parameters studied.

Similar results have been obtained with garlic powder. Isaacsohn et al. (1998) conducted a randomized, double-blinded, placebo-controlled study that concluded that 900 mg/d of Kwai® garlic powder tablets (*see* Section 9.3) for 12 wk was ineffective in lowering cholesterol. The 50 subjects (28 garlic treatment, 22 placebo) recruited from a lipid clinic were also instructed on the National Cholesterol Education Program Step 1 Diet or other low-fat diet. Dietary compliance was measured using the Food Record Rating (FRR) Score.

Garlic did not produce statistically significant changes in serum lipoprotein or triglyceride levels. No significant changes in blood pressure were noted.

In another study using garlic powder, Jain and colleagues (1993) compared the effects of 300 mg of garlic powder three times a day to placebo on serum lipids, serum glucose, blood pressure, and other parameters in 42 subjects with hypercholesterolemia (total cholesterol of at least 220 mg/dL). Baseline measurements were taken to compare against readings at 6 and 12 wk of treatment. No significant treatment differences were noted at the end of wk 6, but by wk 12 total cholesterol was lowered by 6% with garlic tablets vs 1% with placebo ($p < 0.01$). The major reduction in total cholesterol was attributed to lowering low-density lipoprotein (LDL) cholesterol—11% in garlic treated patients vs 3% in placebo. No significant changes were noted for triglycerides, high-density lipoprotein (HDL) cholesterol, serum glucose, blood pressure, and body weight. Adverse effects included belching with a garlic taste, garlic odor, mild abdominal discomfort in two patients, a mild rash, and prolonged oozing from a razor cut.

This latter side effect may be explained by platelet inhibition by various garlic components. Boullin (1981) demonstrated the platelet inhibitory effect of four cloves of garlic (10 g) ingested by three subjects who had not taken aspirin for at least 14 d prior to testing. Aggregation and platelet shape changes were induced with 5-hydroxytryptamine and ADP. Samples taken after 1 h showed complete platelet inhibition and a small platelet change. The author attributed the platelet inhibition to methyl allyl trisulfide (MATS), which had been shown by other investigators (Ariga et al., 1981) to inhibit platelet aggregation in vitro.

The effects of ajoene, an allicin metabolite, on platelet aggregation have also been described (Srivastava and Tyagi, 1993). Ajoene was extracted from chopped garlic using ethanol. Blood was donated by from healthy donors who had not taken aspirin or any other drug affecting platelets for 2 wk prior to giving blood. Ajoene was added to the platelet sample, then stirred for 30 s at 37°C, followed by a waiting period of 4.5 min at room temperature before substances to induce aggregation (arachidonate, calcium, collagen, epinephrine, ADP) were added. The study included a platelet-rich plasma control treated with vehicle. The inhibition of platelet aggregation was found to be dose dependent and irreversible. Platelet inhibition was attributed to inhibition of thromboxane production, perhaps via cyclooxygenase inhibition.

Other investigators have shown that oily garlic extracts, which contain ajoene, are able to inhibit enzymes necessary for arachidonic acid conversion to thromboxane (Srivastava anad Tyagi, 1993). Makheja et al. (1979) demonstrated the effect of garlic oil on platelet thromboxane synthesis. Human and rabbit platelets were incubated with garlic oil, resulting in almost complete suppression of thromboxane production. These investigators also measured oxygen consumption to confirm that platelet cyclooxygenase was also inhibited, but activity of lipoxygenase did not appear to be decreased.

An in vitro study demonstrated that the concentrations of an aqueous extract of garlic required to inhibit ADP, epinephrine, and collagen-induced platelet aggregation were much less than those needed to inhibit thromboxane production (Srivastava, 1984). This finding suggests that inhibition of thromboxane synthesis is not the only mechanism by which garlic inhibits platelet aggregation.

Aqueous garlic extract contains adenosine, which inhibits platelets by activating adenylate cyclase and subsequently increasing intracellular cAMP, thus decreasing production of the arachidonic acid metabolite thromboxane, which causes platelet aggregation. Investigators have demonstrated that adenosine does not affect thromboxane production by affecting incorporation of arachidonic acid into the platelet membrane, by inhibiting cyclooxygenase or lipoxygenase enzymes, or by inhibiting release of arachidonic acid from the platelet membrane when stimulated. Allicin, in addition to adenosine, is another garlic component capable of decreasing thromboxane production without affecting the arachidonic acid cascade (Srivastava anad Tyagi, 1993). Thus, garlic's ability to inhibit platelet aggregation may be the result of multiple mechanisms effected by multiple garlic components present in varying amounts in aqueous vs oily garlic extracts.

Bordia et al. (1998) conducted a study to determine the effects of garlic on lipids, glucose, fibrinogen, and fibrinolytic activity in patients with past myocardial infarction (> 6 mo). All patients were taking nitrates and aspirin; the aspirin was discontinued 2 wk prior to inclusion to the study. Sixty patients were administered either two capsules twice daily of garlic oil (30 subjects) or placebo (30 patients). Each capsule contained the ethyl acetate extract from 1 g of peeled and crushed raw garlic. In addition, the investigators studied the in vitro effects of garlic oil, diallyl disulfide, and diallyl trisulfide on platelet aggregation and arachidonic acid metabolite formation. Compared to baseline, cholesterol levels decreased by 12.8% ($p < 0.01$), triglyceride levels decreased by 15.2% ($p < 0.01$), HDL levels increased by 22.3% ($p < 0.05$), and fibrinolytic activity increased by 55.1% ($p < 0.01$) after 3 mo of garlic treatment. Blood glucose and fibrinogen did not change compared to baseline. Placebo-treated patients did not exhibit a statistically significant change in any of these values. In vitro, garlic oil and the two garlic components tested inhibited both platelet aggregation and thromboxane synthesis. Diallyl trisulfide, a reversible platelet inhibitor, was more potent than diallyl disulfide in inhibiting thromboxane synthesis.

### 9.4.2. Gastrointestinal Effects

Garlic was effective against castor oil induced diarrhea, and relieved abdominal distension/discomfort, belching, and flatulence in 30 patients (Ross, 1998).

Small doses of garlic are purported to increase the tone of smooth muscle in the gastrointestinal tract, while large doses decrease such actions (Tyler, 1993). An ethanol–chloroform extract of fresh bulb antagonized acetylcholine and prostaglandin E induced rat fundus smooth muscle contraction at a concentration of 0.002 mg/mL; however, an ethanol extract of fresh garlic bulb caused rat fundus smooth muscle stimulation at a concentration of 0.016 mg/mL (Ross, 1998).

The gastrointestinal side effects of garlic extracts and commercially available products are described in Section 9.4.1.

### 9.4.3 Antimicrobial Activity

Therapy of cryptococcal meningitis with a combination of oral and parenteral garlic has been reported to produce a 69% cure rate. Garlic has also been claimed to suppress oropharyugeal or vaginal candidia colonization, clear candida cystistis in diabetics or patients with Foley catheters, cure dermatophytic infections, and treat systemic aspergillosis. Based on these reports, and the in vitro activity of garlic extracts against bacteria and fungi, Caporaso, Smith, and Eng (1983) studied the antifungal activity of human urine and serum from five volunteers who had consumed a 10–25 mL of fresh extract of garlic. The contents of a 1500 mg garlic extract capsule distributed by the Windmill Natural Vitamin Co. (Morton Grove, IL) was also assayed for antifungal activity. Several yeasts *(Candida sp., Cryptococcus sp.)* and mycelial fungi species *(Aspergillus sp., Mucor pusillus,* and *Rhizopus sp.)* were tested. All the yeast and mycelial fungi species except C. *glabrata* and R. *arrhizus* were susceptible to the garlic extract at a 1:100 dilution or greater. Similar results were obtained with urine samples from the volunteers. When serum the human volunteers was used, susceptibility dropped significantly. only serum samples taken at 30 and 60 min postingestion were active against the yeasts. The commercial preparation did not exhibit antifungal activity. Because an in vitro study suggests that allicin is the antifungal component of garlic (Barone and Tansey, 1977), the authors postulated that their results were due to instability of allicin at the relatively high pH of human serum ex vivo, binding of allicin to serum protein, inactivation of allicin in serum, or rapid distribution of allicin out of the vascular compartment into body tissues. Clinical use of oral garlic extracts for purposes of treating fungal infections appears to be limited because the gastrointestinal tolerance of the amount of garlic extract used in this study was poor, and larger amounts cause severe burning sensations in the esophagus and stomach, and vomiting. (Caporaso et al., 1983).

Limited data is available suggesting efficacy of topical garlic on fungal infections. Freshly cut garlic applied topically acted more quickly than tolnaftate against *Microsporum crisis* lesions on the arm of a young woman (Rich, 1982); ajoene 0.4% cream was used in the treatment of tines pedis in thirty-seven soldiers, resulting in a culture-negative cure in 7–14 d (Ledezma et al., 1996); and culture-confirmed sporotichosis was successfully treated using garlic juice (Tutakne et al., 1983). Well-designed studies are needed to confirm the safety and efficacy of topical application of garlic, especially in light of case reports of garlic burns (*See* 9.5 Case reports of toxicity).

### *9.4.4 Antineoplastic Effects*

Hu and colleagues completed a study (Hu et al., 1997) to evaluate garlic's ability to retard chemical carcinogenesis induced by benzo[a]pyrene (BP), a widespread environmental pollutant abundant in cigarette smoke and automobile exhaust. BP is believed to be a risk factor in human chemical carcinogenesis. BP is not carcinogenic *per se*; it requires metabolic activation to act as a carcinogen. BP's carcinogenic metabolites can be inactivated in vivo by conjugation with glutathione by the enzyme glutathione *S*-transferase (GST). Compounds that increase tissue GST levels would thus protect against carcinogenic effects of BP metabolites. The investigators found that the garlic organosulfides diallyl sulfide, diallyl disulfide, dipropyl sulfide, dipropyl disulfide, and diallyl trisulfide were capable of inducing GST expression in murine liver and forestomach, as well as of preventing forestomach neoplasia. This study confirmed the results of previous studies that organosulfides protect mice against BP-induced cancer.

Like BP, nitrosamines are ubiquitous environmental carcinogens. Takada and colleagues (1994) tested the effects of the garlic components diallyl sulfide (DAS), diallyl disulfide (DDS), diallyl trisulfide (DAT), allyl methyl sulfide (AMS), allyl methyl trisulfide (AMT), dipropyl sulfide (DPS), dipropyl disulfide (DPD), dimethyl disulfide (DMD), methyl propyl disulfide (MPD), and propylene sulfide (PS) on nitrosamine-induced hepatocarcinogenesis in rats. One hundred fifty rats were divided into 12 groups to evaluate the effects of these organosulfur compounds. Groups 1–5 were injected with diethylnitrosamine (DEN) 200 mg/kg of body wt to initiate hepatocarcinogenesis. After 2 wk on a basal diet, they received DAS (100 mg/kg; group 1), DDS (25 mg/kg; group 2), AMS (150 mg/kg; group 3) DPS (150 mg/kg; group 4), and DPD (150 mg/kg; group 5). At week three, they underwent partial hepatectomy (PH). Group 6 received DEN and underwent PH but were not given any organosulfides. Groups 7–11 received saline instead of DEN, but did receive the test compounds and underwent PH. Group 12 animals received placebos only and underwent PH. In a second experiment, 150 other rats were divided into 12 groups, and were treated in the same manner as the first group, except that groups 1–5 received 150 mg/kg of DAT, 100 mg/kg of AMT, 100 mg/kg of MPD, 50 mg/kg of PS, and 50 mg/kg of DMD, respectively. At wk 8, the rats were killed. In a third experiment, combination treatment with various organosulfides was examined in 105 rats given multiple test doses. Unexpectedly, the investigators discovered that DAS, DAT, AMS, AMT, and DPS promoted hepatocarcinogenesis. The authors proposed that this was a result of organosulfide administration during the promotion phase rather than prior to nitrosourea administration.

Lu and colleagues (1996) examined the effects of an aqueous extract of selenium-enriched garlic (garlic grown in selenium-rich soil) containing 40–45 μg selenium/mL, an aqueous extract of regular garlic containing <0.01 μg/mL of selenium, selenium-methylselenocysteine (a seleno-amino acid found in selenium-garlic), and sodium selenite (used for fertilizing selenium-garlic) on murine tumors (Lu et al., 1991). In vitro, both the extract of selenium-enriched garlic and selenium-methylselenocysteine resulted in growth inhibition, $G_1$ phase arrest, and DNA double-strand breaks in neoplastic murine mammary cells. Selenite produced single-strand breaks (an indicator of genotoxicity) and $S/G_2$-M phase arrest in addition to growth inhibition. In addition, dietary supplementation with selenium-enriched garlic extract provided protection against methylnitrosourea-induced mammary tumors. Regular garlic extract did not produce effects in vitro, nor did it protect against tumors when administered as a dietary supplement. The authors concluded that the beneficial effects observed could be attributed to selenium-methylselenocysteine.

### 9.4.5 Immunostimulant Effects

Lau and colleagues tested an aqueous garlic extract from Wakunaga Pharmaceutical Co. (Hisoshima, Japan), the protein fraction isolated from this same extract, and three additional extracts obtained from health food stores in Loma Linda, CA for ability to stimulate murine T-lymphocyte function and macrophage activity in vitro. Using a chemiluminescence assay and a lymphoblastogenesis assay, both Japanese extracts were shown to stimulate macrophage activity, and the protein fraction from the Japanese protein extract stimulated lymphocyte activity. Of the three extracts sold in American health food stores, only one stimulated macrophage activity. The authors concluded that the antineoplastic activity of garlic might be the result of immunostimulation. Although not addressed by the authors, the in vivo antifungal activity of garlic might also be explained by immunostimulation, especially in light of the in vitro study by Caporaso and colleagues discussed in Section 9.4.3 that did not support the clinical antifungal activity of garlic extract.

## 9.5 Case Reports of Toxicity

Chopped garlic and oil mixes left at room temperature can result in fatal botulism food poisoning, according to the FDA (Lecos, 1998). Such products need to be kept refrigerated, especially those that do not contain acidifying agents such as phosphoric or citric acid. *Clostridium botulinum* bacteria are dispersed throughout the environment, but are not dangerous in the presence of oxygen. The spores produce a deadly toxin in anaerobic, low acid conditions. The garlic oil in mixture provides the environment for the spores to produce their toxin, leading to botulism. At least 40 cases were reported in the late 1980s.

Garlic allergy can manifest as occupational asthma, contact dermatitis, urticaria, angioedema, rhinitis, and diarrhea. A 35-yr-old woman experienced several episodes of urticaria and angioedema associated with ingestion of raw or cooked garlic. Touching garlic also resulted in urticaria. Two garlic extracts as well as fresh garlic produced a 4+ reaction on skin prick tests, but no other food allergens produced positive results. The patient's symptoms were immunoglobulin E (IgE) mediated, but she also produced specific IgG, which confounded the results of IgE testing (Asero et al., 1998).

Twelve garlic workers with respiratory symptoms associated with garlic exposure underwent skin prick tests (SPTs) using garlic powder in saline, commercial garlic extract, and various other possible allergens; bronchial provocation tests with garlic powder; oral challenge with garlic dust; and specific IgE testing using the CAP (CAP System; Pharmacia, Uppsala, Sweden) methodology. Patients were classified into two groups depending on the results of the bronchial provocation tests. Seven patients had positive responses (rhinitis or asthma) to the inhalation challenge test, and were designated as Group 1. Six of these patients reacted to the garlic SPT, and five had specific garlic IgE. In addition, six patients had specific IgE to onion, three to leeks, and four to asparagus. In Group 2 (patients who did not respond to the inhalation challenge), one patient had a positive response to the garlic SPT, one to the onion SPT, and two to the leek SPT. None had garlic or onion IgE. Three patients in Group 1 reported that in the past, they had experienced urticaria, asthma, and angioedema, and anaphylaxis after garlic ingestion. Two of these patients were administered garlic orally in increasing doses up to 1600 mg. The patient who had reported anaphylaxis tolerated the full dose, while the patient who reported urticaria developed a 35% decrease in forced expiratory volume in 1 s ($FEV_1$) and angioedema of the eyelids at a dose of 500 mg. Using immunoblot and IgE immunoblot inhibition analysis, the investigators also attempted to elucidate the specific garlic component to which the patients reacted. Using pooled sera from Group 1, the investigators found that several garlic allergens crossreact with grass and *Chenopodiaceae* pollens (Anibarro et al., 1997).

Other cases of occupational allergy and asthma associated with garlic extract include an 11-yr-old boy who helped with garlic harvesting on his parents' farm and a 15-yr-old who helped collect and store garlic (Couturier and Bousquet, 1982); a 49-yr-old proprietor of a spice marketing and packing firm (Falleroni et al., 1981); a 30-yr-old electrician working in a spice processing plant (Lybarger et al., 1982); and a 16-yr-old who had helped his father load stored garlic into a van for several years (Armentia, 1996). Symptoms described included wheezing (Falleroni et al., 1981); cough, dyspnea, and chest tightness (Lybarger et al., 1982); rhinitis (Falleroni et al., 1981; Couturier and Bousquet, 1982; Armentia, 1996); and conjunctivitis (Couturier and Bousquet, 1982). Garlic allergy was confirmed using a wide variety of tests including scratch testing (Couturier and Bousquet, 1982); SPT (Falleroni et al., 1981; Lybarger et al., 1982; Armentia, 1996); IgE to garlic using radioallegosorbent test (RAST) (Lybarger et al., 1982), polystyrene tube solid phase radioimmunoassay (PTRIA) technique (Falleroni et al., 1981), CAP system (Armentia, 1996); oral challenge (Lybarger et al., 1982); bronchial provocation (Falleroni et al., 1981; Couturier and Bousquet, 1982; Lybarger, 1982; Arementia, 1996); and basophil degranulation (Couturier and Bousquet, 1982). Test methodologies are detailed in the references cited. Patients with occupational garlic allergy are often allergic to other foods as well as to airborne allergens, including peanuts, onion, ragweed pollen (Falleroni et al., 1981), asparagus, and chives (Lybarger et al., 1982).

Topically applied garlic can cause "garlic burns" as well as allergic garlic dermatitis. A 17-mo-old infant suffered partial thickness burns when a plaster made of garlic in petroleum jelly was applied to the skin for 8 h (Parish et al., 1987). Another infant, age 6 mo, suffered garlic burns when his father, disappointed that no antibiotics had been prescribed for a treatment of suspected aseptic meningitis, applied crushed garlic cloves by adhesive band to the wrists for 6 h (Garty, 1993). One week later, a round ulceration 1 cm in diameter surrounded by a slightly raised, erythematous border was noted on the left wrist. A similar, more superficial lesion was also seen on the right wrist. When questioned, the parents explained that these ulcerations were the residual blisters that had formed after garlic application. The author of this case report described this reaction as a second-degree chemical burn. An allergic mechanism was ruled out because the infant had not previously been exposed to garlic or onions. A patch test was not done for ethical reasons.

Although Garty hypothesized that the infants' delicate skin predisposed them to garlic burns, such reactions have also been reported in older children and adults. For example, a 6-yr-old child developed a necrotic ulcer on her foot after her grandmother applied crushed garlic under a bandage as a remedy for a minor sore (Canduela et al., 1995).

A 38-yr-old woman developed a garlic burn after applying a poultice made from fresh, uncooked garlic to her breast for treatment of a self-diagnosed *Candida* infection secondary to breastfeeding her 6-mo-old son (Roberge et al., 1997). Despite a burning sensation upon application, she left the poultice in place for 2 d. The infant continued to feed with no apparent adverse effects. Two days after removal of the poultice, she presented to the emergency room. Physical exam revealed that the area where the poultice had been applied appeared as a burn with skin loss, ulceration, crusting, hyperpigmentation, granulation tissue, serous discharge, minor bleeding, and erythema on the periphery. The area was tender. The patient was treated with 1% silver sulfadiazine cream.

Another adult suffered garlic burns after applying a compress of crushed garlic wrapped in cotton to her chest and abdomen for 18 h (Farrell and Staughton, 1996). The erythematous, blistering rash was in a dermatomal distribution on the right side of the patient's chest and upper abdomen, approximating the dermatomal distribution of thoracic segments 8 and 9. She reported that the pain had been present for a week and had a stabbing quality. She was initially diagnosed with herpes zoster and was prescribed acylcovir before admitting to use of topical garlic after further questioning. Biopsy revealed full thickness necrosis, many pyknotic nuclei, and focal separation of the necrotic epidermis from the dermis. The burns healed with scarring. The patient refused patch testing, and specific IgE RAST testing to garlic was negative.

The nonspecific appearance of garlic burns has been exploited. Three soldiers applied fresh ground garlic to their lower legs and antecubital fossa to produce an erythematous, vesicular rash in an effort to avoid military duty (Kaplan et al., 1990).

Eight patients who developed contact dermatitis after rubbing cut fresh garlic cloves on fungal skin infections responded to a topical fluorinated steroid but had negative garlic patch tests, suggesting irritation rather than allergy (Lee and Lam, 1991). Patch testing with 1% diallyl disulfide in petrolatum has also been recommended when allergy is suspected (Delaney and Donnelly, 1996).

*See* Sections 9.4.1 and 9.4.3 for additional adverse effects.

## 9.6 Drug Interactions

There are no documented drug interactions, but garlic's antiplatelet effect might be dangerous in patients taking warfarin or antiplatelet agents such as aspirin, clopidogrel, ticlopidine, or dipyridamole.

## 9.7 Pharmacokinetics/Toxicokinetics

### 9.7.1 Absorption

The bioavailability of the garlic component *S*-allyl-L-cysteine (SAC) was 64.1%, 76.6%, and 98.2% in rats after oral administration of 12.5 mg/kg, 25 mg/kg, and 50 mg/kg, respectively. Bioavailability was 103% in mice and 87.2% in dogs. SAC is rapidly absorbed from the gastrointestinal tract, with a peak plasma concentration occurring at 0.25 h in dogs, 0.5 h at doses of 12.5 mg/kg and 25 mg/kg in rats, and at 1 h in rats administered 50 mg/kg (Nagae et al., 1994).

### 9.7.2 Distribution

Egen-Schwind and colleagues (1992) found that 1,2-vinyl dithiin, a component of oily preparations of garlic, accumulates in fatty tissues, while 1,3-vinyl dithiin is more hydrophilic and is rapidly eliminated from serum, kidney, and fat tissue. The latter compound was detected in rat liver over the first 24 h after administration, while 1,2-vinyl dithiin was not. Both 1,3-vinyl dithiin and 1,2-vinyl dithiin were detected in the serum, kidney, and fat.

In rats, mice, and dogs, SAC is distributed mainly in the liver, kidney, and plasma (Nagae et al., 1994). In rats, SAC levels are highest in the kidney, and plasma and tissue levels peak 15–30 min after oral administration.

Garlic apparently distributes into human amniotic fluid and breast milk. Ten women were given placebo or garlic oil capsules 45 min prior to routine amniotic fluid sampling. Four of the five amniotic fluid samples from the women who had ingested garlic were judged by a blinded panel to have a stronger and more garlic-like odor than a paired amniotic fluid sample from a woman in the placebo group (Mennella et al., 1995). Ingestion of garlic for 3 d by nursing women decreased the infants' feeding time compared to infants of mothers who had taken placebo (Mennella and Beauchamp, 1993).

### 9.7.3 Metabolism/Elimination

De Rooij et al. (1996) conducted a study to evaluate the urinary excretion of *N*-acetyl-*S*-allyl-L-cysteine (allylmercapturic acid, ALMA). The importance of this study lies in the use of ALMA as a biomarker for occupational exposure to alkyl halides; if garlic produces detectable urine concentrations of ALMA, garlic consumption could interfere with toxicologic studies. Six human volunteers were administered 200 mg of garlic extract in tablet form (Kwai®). The volunteers ranged from 20 to 27 yr old and body weights ranged from 60 to 90 kg. Urine samples were collected prior to administration of the garlic and up to 24 h post-administration. Gas chromatography–mass spectrometry (GC–MS) was used to evaluate the excretion of ALMA.

γ-glutamyl-*S*-allyl-L-cysteine (GAC) is ALMA's most likely precursor. γ-glutamine is hydrolyzed from GAC by glutamine-transpeptidase, resulting in *S*-allyl-L-cysteine. This compound then undergoes acetylation via *N*-acetyl transferase to form ALMA. It is difficult to calculate to what extent GAC is excreted as ALMA in the urine because GAC content of garlic varies from product to product. By assuming that GAC represents 1% of the dry weight of garlic bulbs, and that the tablets represented 100% dry garlic, the researchers approximated that 10% of GAC is excreted as ALMA within the first 24 h of garlic ingestion. The average elimination half-life of ALMA was $6.0 \pm 1.3$ h (De Rooij et al., 1996).

*N*-acetyl-*S*-(2-carboxypropyl) cysteine, *N*-acetyl-*S*-allyl-L-cysteine (ALMA, allylmercapturic acid), and hexahydrohippuric acid were identified in urine of humans ingesting garlic or onions (Jandke and Spiteller, 1987). It is important to note that the study participants' urine contained *N*-acetyl-*S*-(2-carboxypropyl)-cysteine at baseline in minute amounts, even before garlic ingestion, but increased after ingestion of garlic or onions. As with the De Rooij study, the importance of these findings lies in the use of urinary excretion of mercapturic acids as a marker for industrial exposure to halogenated alkanes such as vinyl chloride.

Elimination of other garlic components has also been studied. Allicin is metabolized in rat liver homogenate more rapidly than the vinyl dithiins, the main consitutents of oily preparations of garlic. As discussed in Section 9.7.2 Distribution, 1,2-vinyldithiin is lipophilic and tends to accumulate in fat, while 1,3-vinyldithiin is less lipophilic and more quickly eliminated from the serum, fat, and kidney. Both vinyldithiins can be detected in the serum, fat, and kidney using GC–MS for at least 24 h after oral administration (Egen-Schwind et al., 1992).

*S*-Allylcysteine (SAC) is thought to undergo first-pass metabolism in rats based on nonlinear increases in AUC (area under the plama concentration vs time curve) after oral administration. SAC is likely metabolized to *N*-acetyl-SAC (ALMA) by acetyltransferase in the liver and kidney. The high concentration of SAC in rat kidney has been attributed to conversion of *N*-acetyl-SAC back into SAC by kidney acylase. Thirty to fifty percent of the SAC dose is excreted in the urine in rats as *N*-acetyl-SAC, and <1% of the dose is excreted as unchanged SAC in the urine and bile. In mice both SAC (16.5%) and the *N*-acetylated metabolite (7.2%) are excreted in the urine, while in dogs <1% of the dose was found in the urine as either SAC or *N*-acetyl-SAC. The half-life of SAC in rats ranges from 1.49 h with an intravenous dose of 12.5 mg/kg to 2.33 h with an oral dose of 50 mg/kg. In mice, the half-life of SAC is 0.77 h when given orally and 0.43 h for intravenous administration, and in dogs approx 10 h after either oral or intravenous administration (Nagae et al., 1994).

## 9.8 Analysis of Biofluids

Jandke and Spiteller (1987) performed GC–MS to analyze urine samples obtained after ingestion of garlic and onions. *N*-acetyl-*S*-(2-carboxypropyl) cysteine, *N*-acetyl-*S*-allyl-L-cysteine (ALMA, allylmercapturic acid), and hexahydrohippuric acid were identified. De Rooij and colleagues (1996) also used GC–MS to identify ALMA in human urine. Gas chromatographic sulfur selective analysis with a flame photometric detector as well as mass selective analysis was performed. Sulfur selective detection was approx 10 times less sensitive than GC–MS in selective ion monitoring (SIM) mode. The vinyl dithiins, found in oily garlic preparations, were detected in rat serum, kidney, fat, and liver using GC–MS (Egen-Schwind et al, 1992). Details of these analyses can be obtained from the cited references.

## 9.9 Regulatory Status

Garlic is approved in Germany as a nonprescription drug. The oil, extract, and oleo resin have been deemed generally recognized as safe (GRAS) as food substances by the FDA, and garlic is also regulated as a dietary supplement in the United States. In Canada garlic is approved as a food supplement; garlic is on the general sale list in the United Kingdom; in France it is accepted for the treatment of minor circulatory disorders; and in Sweden it is classified as a natural product (Blumenthal, 1997).

## References

Anibarro B, Fontela JL, De La Hoz F. Occupational asthma induced by garlic dust. J Allergy Clin Immunol 1997;100:734–8.

Ariga T, Oshiba S, Tamada T. Platelet aggregation inhibitor in garlic. Lancet 1981;i:150–1.

Armentia A. Can inhalation of garlic dust cause asthma? Allergy 1996;51:137–8.

Asero R, Mistrello G, Roncarolo D, Antoniotti PL, Falagiani P. A case of garlic allergy. J Allergy Clin Immunol 1998;101:427–8.

Barone FE, Tansey MR. Isolation, purification, identification, synthesis, and kinetics of activity of the anticandidal component of *Allium sativum* and a hypothesis for its mode of action. Mycologia 1977;69:793–825.

Berthold HK, Sudhop T, von Bergmann K. Effect of a garlic oil preparation on serum lipoproteins and cholesterol metabolism. A randomized controlled trial. JAMA 1998;279:1900–2.

Blumenthal, M. The complete German Commission E monographs. Therapeutic guide to herbal medicines. Garlic. Austin Texas: American Botanical Council, 1998.

Blumenthal, M. Popular herbs in the U.S. market. Garlic cloves. American Botanical Council. Austin, Texas, 1997.

Bordia A, Verma SK, Srivastava KC. Effect of garlic (*Allium sativum*) on blood lipids, blood sugar, fibrinogen and fibrinolytic activity in patients with coronary artery disease. Prostagland Leukotr Essen Fatty Acids 1998;58:257–63.

Boullin DJ. Garlic as a platelet inhibitor. Lancet 1981;i:776–7.

Canduela V, Mongil I, Carrascosa M, Docio S, Cagigas P. Garlic: always good for the health [letter]? Br J Dermatol 1995;132:161–2.

Caporaso N, Smith SM, Eng RHK. Antifungal activity in human urine and serum after ingestion of garlic (*Allium sativum*). Antimicrob Agents Chemother 1983;23:700–2.

Couturier P, Bousquet J. Occupational allergy secondary to inhalation of garlic dust. J Allergy Clin Immunol 1982;70:145.

Delaney TA, Donnelly AM. Garlic dermatitis. Austr J Dermatol 1996;37:109–10.

De Rooij BM, Boogaard PJ, Rijksen DA, Commandeur JNM, and Vermeulen NPE. Urinary excretion of *N*-acetyl-*S*-allyl-L-cysteine upon garlic consumption by human volunteers. Arch Toxicol. 1996;70:635–9.

Egen-Schwind C, Eckard R, Jekat FW, Winterhoff H. Pharmacokinetics of vinyldithiins, transformation products of allicin. Planta Med 1992;58:8–13.

Falleroni AE, Zeiss R, Levitz D. Occupational asthma secondary to inhalation of garlic dust. J Allergy Clin Immunol 1981;68:156–60.

Farrell AM, Staughton RCD. Garlic burns mimicking herpes zoster. Lancet 1996;317:1195.

Garty B. Garlic burns. Pediatrics 1993;91:658–9.

Hu X, Benson PJ, Srivastava SK, Xia H, Bleicher RJ, Zaren HA, et al. Induction of glutathione *S*-transferase as a bioassay for the evaluation of potency of inhibitors of benzoapyrene-induced cancer in a murine model. Int J Cancer 1997;73:897–901.

Isaacsohn JL, Moser M, Stein EA, Dudley K, Davey JA, Liskov E, Black HR. Garlic powder and plasma lipids and lipoproteins. A multicenter, randomized, placebo controlled trial. Arch Intern Med 1998;158:1189–94.

Jain AK, Vvargas R, Gotzkowsky S, McMahon FG. Can garlic reduce levels of serum lipids? A controlled clinical study. Am J Med 1993;94:632–5.

Jandke J, Spiteller G. Unusual conjugates in biological profiles originating from consumption of onions and garlic. J Chromatogr 1987;421:1–8.

Kaplan B, Schewach-Millet M, Yorav S. Facial dermatitis induced by application of garlic. Int J Dermatol 1990;29:75–6.

Lau BHS, Yamasaki T, Gridley DS. Garlic compounds modulate macrophage and T-lymphocyte functions. Mol Biother 1991;3:103–7.

Lecos C. Chopped garlic in oil mixes. URL: www.fda.gov. Accessed 1998 October 27.

Ledezma E, DeSousa L, Jorquera A, Sanchez J, Lander A, Rodriguez E. Jain MK, Apitz-Castro R. Efficacy of ajoene an organosulphur derived from garlic, in the short-term therapy of tinia pedis. Mycoses 1996;39:393–5.

Lee TY, Lam TH. Contact dermatitis due to topical treatment with garlic in Hong Kong. Contact Dermatit 1991;24:193–6.

Lu J, Pei H, Ip C, et al. Effect on an aqueous extract of selenium enriched garlic on in vitro markers and in vivo efficacy in cancer prevention. Carcinogenesis 1996;9:1903–7.

Lybarger JA, Gallagher JS, Pulver DW, Litwin A, Brooks S, Bernstein IL. Occupational asthma induced by inhalation and ingestion of garlic. J Allergy Clin Immunol 1982;69:448–54.

Makheja AN, Vanderhoek JY, Bailey JM. Inhibition of platelet aggregation and thromboxane synthesis by onion and garlic. Lancet 1979;i:781.

Mennella JA, Beauchamp GK. The effects of repeated exposure to garlic-flavored milk on the nursling's behavior. Pediatr Res 1993;34:805–8.

Mennella JA, Johnson A, Beauchamp GK. Garlic ingestion by pregnant women alters the odor of amniotic fluid. Chem Senses 1995;20:207–9.

Nagae S, Ushijima M, Hatono S, Imai J, Kasuga S, Matsuura H, et al. Pharmacokinetics of the garlic compound *S*-allylcysteine. Planta Med 1994;60:214–7.

Parish RA, McIntyre S, Heimbach DM. Garlic burns: a naturopathic remedy gone awry. Pediatr Emerg Care 1987;3:258–60.

Rich GE. Garlic an antibiotic? Med J Aust 1982;1:60.

Roberge RJ, Leckey R, Spence R, Krenzelok EJ. Garlic burns of the breast. Am J Emerg Med 1997;15:548–9.

Ross IA. Medicinal plants of the world. Chemical constituents, traditional and modern medicinal uses. Alluim Sativum. Totowa, NJ: Humana Press, 1998.

Srivastava KC. Effects of aqueous extracts of onion, garlic, and ginger on platelet aggregation and metabolism of arachidonic adin in the blood vascular system: in vitro study. Prostagland Leukotr Med 1984;13:227–35.

Srivastava KC, Tyagi OD. Effects of a garlic-derived principle (ajoene) on aggregation and arachidonic acid metabolism in human blood platelets. Prostagland Leukotr Essent Fatty Acids 1993;49:587–95.

Takada N, Matsuda T, Otoshi T, et. al. Enhancement by organosulfur compounds from garlic and onions of diethylnitroasamine-induced glutathione S-transferase positive foci in the rat liver. Cancer Res 1994;54:2895–9.

Tutakne MA, Satyanarayanan G, Bhardwaj JR, Sethi IC. Sporotrichosis treated with garlic juice. A case report. Indian J Dermatol 1983;28:41–5.

Tyler, VE. Garlic. In: The honest herbal. A sensible guide to the use of herbs and related remedies, 3rd edit., New York: Pharmaceutical Products Press, 1993.

Warshafsky S, Kamer, RS, Sivak SL. Effect of garlic on total serum cholesterol. Ann Intern Med 1993;119:599–605.

# Chapter 10

# Ginger

## Charity Metz and Melanie Johns Cupp

*Zingiber officinale* Roscoe, Zingerberis rhizoma, ingwerwurzelstok (Blumenthal, 1998), Jamaican ginger, African ginger, cochin ginger (Tyler, 1994), *Zingiber capitatum*, *Zingiber zerumbet* Smith (Anonymous, 1991), calicut, gengibre, gingembre, jenjibre, zenzero (USP, 1998a)

## 10.1 History and Traditional Uses

Ginger is a perennial plant with thick tuberous rhizomes from which an above ground stem rises about 3 ft (Leung, 1980). The plant produces an orchidlike flower (Anonymous, 1991) with petals that are greenish-yellow streaked with purple (USP, 1998a). Ginger is cultivated in areas of abundant rainfall (at least 80 in./yr) (USP, 1998a). Native to southern Asia, ginger is cultivated in tropical areas such as Jamaica, China, Nigeria, and Haiti (Leung, 1980).

Ginger was introduced to Jamaica and the West Indies by Spaniards in the 16th century, and exports from Jamaica to the rest of the world amount to >2 million pounds/yr (Tyler et al., 1981).

Ginger is an ingredient in more than half of all traditional Chinese medicines (Awang, 1992), and has been used since the 4th century BC (Tyler, 1981). Marco Polo documented its use in India in the late 13th century (Tyler, 1981). African and West Indies cultures have also used ginger medicinally (Awang, 1992), and the Greeks and Romans used it as a spice (Tyler, 1981). The Chinese utilized ginger for stomach aches, diarrhea, nausea, cholera, bleeding (Leung, 1980), asthma, heart conditions, respiratory disorders (USP, 1998a), toothache, and rheumatic complaints (Awang, 1992). In China, the root and stem are used to combat aphids and fungal spores (Anonymous, 1991).

From Forensic Science: *Toxicology and Clinical Pharmacology of Herbal Products*
Edited by: M. J. Cupp © Humana Press Inc., Totowa, New Jersey

Ginger has purported to have use as a carminative, diaphoretic, spasmolytic, expectorant, peripheral circulatory stimulant, astringent, appetite stimulant, antiinflammatory agent, diuretic, and digestive aid (USP, 1998a). It has also been used to treat migraines, fever, flu, amenorrhea (USP, 1998a), snake bites, and baldness (Leung, 1980).

## 10.2 Current Promoted Uses

In the United States, ginger is promoted to relieve and prevent nausea caused by motion sickness, morning sickness, and other etiologies.

## 10.3 Products Available

The best quality ginger comes from Jamaica and consists of whole ginger with the epidermis completely peeled from the rhizomes and dried in the sun for 5–6 d, although high-quality, partially scraped ginger used pharmaceutically also comes from Bengal and Australia (USP, 1998a). Extracts are prepared from the unpeeled root, as essential oil can be lost from peeled ginger (Leung, 1980).

Ginger is commercially available in the United States as the dried powdered root, syrup, tincture, capsules, tablets, tea, oral solution, powder for oral solution, as a spice, and in candy, ice cream, and beer (USP, 1998a).

Ginger root is available from several manufacturers as a tea, liquid extract, and as 50 mg, 250 mg, 400 mg, 470 mg, 500 mg, 535 mg, and 550 mg capsules. Examples include:

Alvita® Teas Ginger Root tea bag
Breezy Morning Teas Jamaican Ginger tea bag
Celestial Seasonings® Ginger Ease™ Herb tea bag
Aura Cacia Essential Oil Ginger
Abunda Life Chinese Ginger powder
Frontier Ginger — Hawaiian Root capsule
Nature's Herbs® Ginger Root, 535-mg capsule
Nature's Way® Ginger Root, 550-mg capsule
Nature's Plus® Liquid Ginger Extract, 4% volatile oils
Health Plus Ginger Root extract, 50-mg capsule
Nature's Answer® Ginger Root Low Alcohol (Liquid)
Nature's Answer® Ginger Root Alcohol Free (Liquid)
Nature's Herb® Ginger Root Extract (Liquid)
Nature's Way® Ginger Extract (Liquid)
Quanterra™ Stomach Relief, 250 mg dried ginger root powder (Zintona®) capsule

## 10.4 Pharmacologic/Toxicologic Effects

### 10.4.1 Gastrointestinal Effects

A study was conducted to evaluate the effect of ginger on the nystagmus response to vestibular or optokinetic stimuli, as measured by electronystagmographic (ENG) techniques (Holtmann et al., 1989). Study subjects were screened prior to study enrollment and were excluded if they responded abnormally to vestibular or optokinetic tests. Thirty-eight subjects, 20 women and 18 men between the ages of 22 and 34, were given 1 g of ginger (Zintona®), 100 mg dimenhydrinate, or placebo in a double-blind, crossover fashion 90 min prior to each test. Ginger had no effect on the ENG, in contrast to dimenhydrinate, which decreased nystagmus response to caloric, rotary, and optokinetic stimulations. Therefore, a central nervous system (CNS) effect was ruled out as ginger's antiemetic mechanism of action, and a direct gastrointestinal effect was proposed.

The antimotion sickness effect of ginger was also compared to that of dimenhydrinate (Dramamine®) in 18 male and 18 female college students who were self-rated as having extreme or very high susceptibility to motion sickness (Mowrey and Clayson, 1982). The subjects were given either two ginger capsules (940 mg), one dimenhydrinate capsule (100 mg), or two placebo capsules (powdered chickweed herb [*Stellaria media*]). Twenty to twenty-five minutes after consuming the capsule(s), subjects were led blindfolded to a previously concealed rotating chair. None of the dimenhydrinate or placebo subjects were able to remain in the chair a full 6 min, and three patients in the placebo group vomited. Half of the ginger subjects stayed the full 6 min. It was concluded that 940 mg of ginger was superior to 100 mg of dimenhydrinate in preventing motion sickness. It is important to note that none of the subjects in the dimenhydrinate group specifically asked to have the test terminated; the test was stopped by the investigator because of the magnitude of the subjects' self-reported "intensity of stomach feeling." Although the study subjects were blinded not only to the treatments used, but also to the purpose of the study, it is unclear if the investigator was also blinded.

Another placebo-controlled study tested the effectiveness of ginger in preventing postoperative nausea and vomiting (Arfeen et al., 1995). This randomized, double-blind study included 108 subjects slated for elective gynecologic laparoscopy. The number of subjects provided 80% power to detect a reduction in the incidence of nausea from 30% to 20%. All patients received 10 mg of diazepam orally and were randomized to receive two 500 mg ginger capsules, one 500 mg ginger capsule and one placebo capsule, or two placebo capsules 1 h prior to surgery. Nausea, when present, was rated on a scale of 1 to 3 (mild, moderate, severe). Although there was a trend favoring ginger, the difference was not statistically significant ($p = 0.36$). The investigators concluded that neither dose of ginger was effective in preventing postoperative nausea and vomiting. Blinding may have been problematic in this study because of the characteristic taste and smell of ginger, which was noted by one of the patients. Adverse effects were reported by five of the ginger patients and consisted of flatulence and a bloated feeling, heartburn (two patients), nausea, and burping. One patient in the placebo group complained of "feeling windy and having the urge to burp."

A second placebo-controlled study tested the efficacy of ginger in prevention of postoperative nausea and vomiting (Phillips et al., 1993). This randomized, double-blind study consisted of 120 subjects slated for elective gynecologic laparoscopy. The subjects were given either 1 g of ginger, 100 mg of metoclopramide, or a placebo (1 g of lactose) 1 h prior to surgery. The incidence of nausea and vomiting with metoclopramide was 27%, 21% with ginger, and 41% with placebo. Ginger was similar in effectiveness to metoclopramide in preventing postoperative nausea and vomiting ($p = 0.34$) and significantly more effective than lactose ($p = 0.006$).

A randomized, double-blind crossover study was conducted to determine the efficacy of ginger in hyperemesis gravidarum (Fisher-Rasmussen, 1990). Thirty pregnant women at <20 wk gestation previously admitted to the hospital for hyperemesis gravidarum participated in the study. The treatment included a 250 mg ginger capsule or a lactose capsule three times a day for the first 4 d. After a 2-d wash-out period, the subjects received the alternate treatment for 4 d. Ginger was significantly more efficacious in reducing symptoms of hyperemesis gravidarum than placebo ($p = 0.035$).

### *10.4.2 Anti-Inflammatory Activity*

Ginger components 6-gingerol, 6-dehydrogingerdione, 10-dehydrogingerdione, 6-gingerdione, and 10-gingerdione inhibit prostaglandin synthestase in vitro (Kiuchi et al., 1982). The latter four components were found to have greater potency as prostaglandin inhibitors than indomethacin. In an additional study of ginger's ability to affect arachidonic acid metabolism in human platelets and rat aorta, an aqueous extract of ginger was able to inhibit production of thromboxane and prostaglandins in a dose-dependent manner (Srivastava, 1984).

The antiinflammatory effects of ginger oil on arthritic rats were studied (Sharma et al., 1994). A 0.05-mL suspension of heat-killed *Mycobacterium tuberculosis* bacilli in liquid paraffin (5 mg/mL) was injected into the knees and paws to induce arthritis in treatment rats. Rats were randomized to receive 33 mg/kg of ingwerol (ginger oil obtained by steam distillation of dried ginger root), 33 mg/kg of eugenol (a component of clove oil purported to have antiinflammatory activity), or normal saline orally for 26 d, beginning just prior to the induction of arthritis. Compared to normal saline, both treatments were effective in decreasing both knee and paw swelling.

### *10.4.3 Use in Migraine*

A case reported the use of ginger for the prevention of migraines (Mustafa and Srivastava, 1990). A 42-yr-old woman suffered migraine with aura for 10 yr once or twice every 2 or 3 mo. Because the frequency and duration of migraine increased, the patient was prescribed 500–600 mg of powdered ginger to be taken at the onset of aura, then every 4 h for the next 3–4 d. The patient reported some relief within 30 min of the first dose. Then she added uncooked fresh ginger to her diet. In a 13-mo period, she reported only six migraines. These results should be confirmed in a double-blind, controlled trial.

### *10.4.4 Cardiovascular Effects*

In vitro studies of gingerol using canine cardiac tissue and rabbit skeletal muscle demonstrated $Ca^{2+}$-ATPase activation in the cardiac and skeletal sarcoplasmic reticulum (SR) (Kobayashi et al., 1987). Gingerol (3–30 $\mu M$) increased $Ca^{2+}$-ATPase pumping rate in a dose-dependent manner. A 100–fold dilution with fresh saline solution of 30 $\mu M$ gingerol completely reversed $Ca^{2+}$-ATPase activation. The investigators concluded that gingerol may be a useful pharmacologic tool in the study of regulatory mechanisms of the SR $Ca^{2+}$ pumping systems, and their effect on muscle contractility.

Another in vitro study examined the effect of 6-, 8-, and 10-gingerol on isolated left atria of guinea pigs (Shoji et al., 1982). The study found the gingerols had a dose-dependent positive inotropic effect that was evident at doses as low as $10^5$, $10^{-6}$, and $3 \times 10^{-5}$ g/mL for 6-, 8-, and 10-gingerol, respectively. Thus, 8-gingerol was the most potent gingerol in regard to cardiotonic activity.

In vitro, aqueous ginger extract has dose-dependent antithromboxane synthetase activity that correlates with its ability to inhibit aggregation of human platelets in response to ADP, collagen, and epinephrine (Srivastava, 1984). However, this may not be clinically significant; inhibition of platelet aggregation has been demonstrated in humans only after consumption of 5 g of raw ginger daily for 1 wk (Srivastava, 1989). A single 2-g dose of dried ginger did not affect platelet function (Lumb, 1994).

### 10.4.5 Mutagenicity

A study showed that 6-gingerol and 6-shogaol isolated from *Zingiber officinale* using column chromatography were mutagenic at 700 μM in the Hs30 strain of *Escherichia coli* (Nakamura and Yamamoto, 1983). 6-gingerol was noted to be a potent mutagen while 6-shogaol was $10^4$ less mutagenic. Another study documented the antimutagenicity of zingerone, another ginger component, in addition to the mutagenicity of gingerol and shogaol in *Samonella typhimurium* strains TA 100, TA 1535, TA 1538, and TA 98 (Nagabhushan et al., 1987). Gingerol and shogaol activated by rat liver enzymes at doses of 5–200 mcg/plate mutated strains TA 100 and TA 1535 while zingerone was non-mutagenic in all four strains. Zingerone also suppressed the mutagenicity of gingerol and shogaol in a dose dependent manner. Although all three compounds are similar in chemical structure, zingerone has a shorter side chain than the mutagenic compounds; thus the side chains may be responsible for the mutagenic activity of gingerol and shogaol.

### 10.4.6 Reproduction

In addition to its mutagenic activity, concern has been raised that the receptor binding of testosterone may be affected in the fetus because of ginger's inhibition of thromboxane synthetase (Backon, 1991). Commission E contraindicates ginger's use during pregnancy for morning sickness, although this contraindication has been disputed by some owing to the lack of reported problems despite its long history of use in pregnancy in traditional Chinese medicine (Blumenthal, 1998).

## 10.5 Case Reports of Toxicity Due to Commercially Available Products

Consumption of Jamaica ginger, an alcoholic ginger extract that was popular as a beverage in the rural southern United States during prohibition, resulted in a peripheral polyneuritis (Harris 1930). In reported cases, the first symptom to appear was sore calves for 1 or 2 d. After the soreness disappeared, walking became notably difficult for the case subjects. Subjects could not walk without the aid of a cane or crutches within a week. Bilateral weakness of the upper and lower extremities and foot drop, without sensory disturbance or pain, was a common physical finding. The skin on the feet was noted to be red and glossy, but not swollen. Deep tendon reflexes were inconsistent among patients; ankle jerks were not present in any subject, but some had normal knee reflexes. There were no cranial nerve deficits. Although the beverage contained 60–90% alcohol, alcoholic neuropathy was ruled out as an etiology of the syndrome because of the sporadic nature of Jamaica ginger consumption. Jamaica ginger was later found to have been adulterated with triorthocresyl phosphate (Valaer, 1930). This chemical had been added to the beverage presumably as a tasteless substitute for the oleo resin of ginger so that the product would be more palatable. Additional research with alcohol and true U.S.P. ginger fluid extract failed to produce paralysis. There have not been any cases of neuropathy associated with use of ginger in any form.

## 10.6 Drug Interactions

Although no drug interactions with ginger have been reported, caution should be used in patients taking anticoagulants and antiplatelet drugs because of its potential antiplatelet effect (USP, 1998a).

## 10.7 Chemical Analysis

Information on the chemical identification and analysis of ginger and its components can be found in the USP–NF (USP, 1998b). Gas chromatography–mass spectroscopy (GC–MS) has also been used to confirm the purity and identity of gingerol, shogaol, and zingerone (Connell and Sutherland, 1969).

## 10.8 Regulatory Status

In Austria and Switzerland, ginger is registered as an over-the-counter (OTC) drug indicated for the prevention of motion sickness, nausea, and in Austria, for vomiting in febrile pediatric patients. Australia's Therapeutic Goods Administration's *Listed Products* category includes ginger as an acceptable active ingredient. Likewise, in the United Kingdom ginger is on the General Sale List of the Medicines Control Agency. In Belgium, ginger rhizome is permitted as a traditional digestive aid, and the German Commission E approves ginger for dyspeptic complaints and the prevention of motion sickness (USP, 1998a). Ginger is listed as an official monograph in the United States Pharmacopoeia-National Formulary (USP, 1998b). Ginger is regulated as a dietary supplement in the United States. It is also considered "generally recognized as safe (GRAS) as a food substance" by the FDA (Tyler, 1994).

## References

Anonymous. The Lawrence review of natural products. St. Louis, MO: Facts and Comparisons, 1991.

Arfeen Z, Owen H, Plummer JL, Ilsley AH, Sorby-Adams RAC, Doecke CJ. A double-blind randomized controlled trial of ginger for the prevention of postoperative nausea and vomiting. Anaesth Intens Care 1995;23:449–52.

Awang DVC. Ginger. CPJ RPC 1992; (July):309–11.

Backon J. Ginger in preventing nausea and vomiting of pregnancy: a caveat due to its thromboxane synthetase activity and effect on testosterone binding [letter]. Eur J Obstet Gynecol Reprod Biol 1991;42:163–4.

Blumenthal M. The Complete German Commission E monographs: therapeutic guide to herbal medicines. Austin, TX: American Botanical Council, 1998.

Connell OW, Sutherland MD. A reexamination of gingerol, shogaol and zingerone, the pungent principles of ginger. Austr J Chem 1969;22:1033–43.

Fisher-Rasmussen W, Kjaer SK, Dahl C, Asping U. Ginger treatment of hyperemesis gravidarum. Eur J Obstet Gynecol Reprod Biol 1990;38:19–24.

Harris S. Jamaica ginger paralysis (a peripheral polyneuritis). South Med J 1930; 23:375–80.

Holtmann S, Clarke AH, Scherer H, Hohn M. The anti-motion sickness mechanism of ginger. A comparative study with placebo and dimenhydrinate. Acta Otolaryngol 1989;108:168–74.

Kiuchi F, Shibuya M, Sankawa U. Inhibitors of prostaglandin biosynthesis from ginger. Chem Pharmacol Bull 1982;30:754–7.

Kobayashi M, Shoji N, Ohizumi Y. Gingerol, a novel cardiotonic agent, activates $Ca^{2+}$pumping ATPase in skeletal and cardiac sarcoplasmic reticulum. Biochim Biophys Acta 1987;903:96–102.

Lumb AB. Effect of dried ginger on human platelet function. Thromb Haemost 1994;71:110–1.

Leung AY. Ginger. In: Encyclopedia of common natural ingredients used in food, drugs, and cosmetics. New York, John Wiley and Sons, 1980; pp. 1845.

Mowrey DB, Clayson DE. Motion sickness, ginger, and psychophysics. Lancet 1982;i:6557.

Mustafa T, Srivastava KC. Ginger (*Zingiber officinale*) in migraine headache. Journal of Ethnopharmacology 1990;29:267–73.

Nagabhushan M, Amonkar AJ, Bhide SV. Mutagenicity of gingerol and shogaol and antimutagenicity of zingerone in salmonella/microsome assay. Cancer Lett 1987;36:221–33.

Nakamura H, Yamamoto T. The active part of the [6]-gingerol molecule in mutagenesis. Mutat Res 1983;122:87–94.

Phillips S, Ruggier R, Hutchinson SE. *Zingiber officinale* (ginger)—an antiemetic for day case surgery. Anaesthesia 1993;48:715–7.

Shoji N, Iwasa A, Takemoto, Ishida Y. Cardiotonic principles of ginger (*Zingiber officinale* Roscoe). J Pharm Sci 1982;71:1174–5.

Srivastava KC. Effects of aqueous extracts of onion, garlic and ginger on platelet aggregation and metabolism of arachidonic acid in the blood vascular system: in vitro study. Prostagland Leukotr Med 1984;13:227–35.

Srivastava KC. Effect of onion and ginger consumption on platelet thromboxane production in humans. Prostagland Leukotr Essent Fatty Acids 1989;35:183–5.

Sharma JN, Srivastava KC, Gan EK. Suppressive effects of eugenol and ginger oil on arthritic rats. Pharmacology 1994;49:314–8.

Tyler VE. Digestive system problems. In: Herbs of Choice: the therapeutic use of phytomedicinals, Binghamton, NY: Pharmaceuticals Products Press, 1994.

Tyler VE, Brady LR, Robbers JE. Pharmacognosy, 8th edit., Philadelphia, PA: Lea and Febiger;1981, p. 156.

United States Pharmacopeial Convention (USP). Ginger. Botanical monograph series. Rockville, MD: United States Pharmacopeial Convention, 1998a.

United States Pharmacopoeia (USP). National Formulary. 18th edit., Suppl 9. Rockville, MD: United States Pharmacopeial Convention, 1998b.

Valaer P. The examination of cresyl-bearing extracts of ginger. Am J Pharm 1930;102:571–4.

# Chapter 11

# Saw Palmetto

*Amy Meadows and Melanie Johns Cupp*

*Serenoa repens* (Bartram) Small, *Sabal serrulata* (Michaux) Nichols, *Serenoa serrulatum* Schultes (USP, 1998)

## 11.1 History and Traditional Uses

Saw palmetto is a dwarf palm tree that grows in Texas, Florida, Georgia, and southern South Carolina (Chavez, 1998). The tree grows up to 6 ft tall and has wide leaves divided into fan-shaped lobes that are gray to blue-green in color. The plant produces purple-black berries from September to January (Nemecz, 1998).

The earliest known use of saw palmetto was in the 15th century BC in Egypt to treat urethral obstruction (Nemecz, 1998). The Native Americans also used saw palmetto to treat genitourinary conditions (Chavez, 1998). In the early 20th century it was used in conventional medicine as a mild diuretic and as a treatment for benign prostatic hypertrophy (BPH) and chronic cystitis (Tyler, 1993). Historically, saw palmetto has also been used to increase sperm production, increase breast size, and increase sexual vigor (Anonymous, 1994). Early settlers in the United States observed that animals which ate the berries grew fat and healthy, and by the 1870s saw palmetto was purported to improve general health, reproductive health, disposition, and body weight, and to stimulate appetite (Nemecz, 1998).

## 11.2 Current Promoted Uses

Saw palmetto is promoted as a treatment for BPH, to improve prostate health and urinary flow, and to improve reproductive and sexual functioning.

From Forensic Science: *Toxicology and Clinical Pharmacology of Herbal Products*
Edited by: M. J. Cupp © Humana Press Inc., Totowa, New Jersey

## 11.3 PRODUCTS AVAILABLE

Saw palmetto is commercially available alone and in combination products:

Nature's Way® Prostactive Saw Palmetto is a soft gelcap with 320 mg of saw palmetto per gelcap.
Nature's Way® Standardized Saw Palmetto Extract contains 160 mg of saw palmetto in a soft gelcap.
Nature's Way® Saw Palmetto contains 585 mg of saw palmetto in a capsule.
Nature's Fingerprint® Saw Palmetto contains 500 mg of saw palmetto in a capsule.
Sundown® Saw Palmetto contains 450 mg of saw palmetto per capsule.
Centrum® Saw Palmetto contains 160 mg of saw palmetto per soft gelcap.
Quanterra™ Prostate contains 160 mg of saw palmetto in a capsule.
Celestial Seasonings® Saw Palmetto contains 160 mg of saw palmetto in a brown soft gelcap.
One-A-Day® Prostate Health contains 320 mg of saw palmetto, zinc, and pumpkin seed oil in a soft gelcap.
Sundown® Saw Palmetto Complex contains 450 mg of saw palmetto, zinc, pygeum, and nettles in a gelcap.
Saw Palmetto Formula contains 500 mg of saw palmetto, zinc, pumpkin seed, prostate glandular powder, and pygeum bark in a tablet.
Spring Valley Saw Palmetto Extract contains 80 mg of saw palmetto and pumpkin seed oil in a soft gelcap.
Propalmex™ is a red and green soft gelcap that contains 160 mg of saw palmetto, zinc, and pumpkin seed oil extract.
Prostata® is a preparation containing saw palmetto, zinc picolinate, pyridoxine, L-alanine, glutamic acid, *Apis mellifica* pollen, silica, hydrangea extract, panax ginseng, and *Pygeum africanum.*

## 11.4 PHARMACOLOGIC/TOXICOLOGIC EFFECTS

### *11.4.1 Immunologic Effects*

Saw palmetto is purported to stimulate immune function (Blumenthal and Riggins, 1997).

### *11.4.2. Genitourinary/Endocrine Effects*

Saw palmetto's benefits in treatment of BPH are hypothesized to be due in part to antiandrogen effects (Wilt et al., 1998). Saw palmetto is a multisite inhibitor of androgen action. In an in vitro study (Briley et al., 1983), a liposterolic saw palmetto extract called Permixon® was shown to compete with

**Kava Root extract (30% kavalactones)**

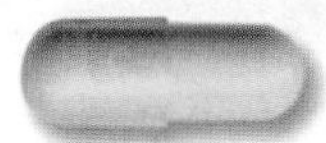

KavatrolTM 200 mg

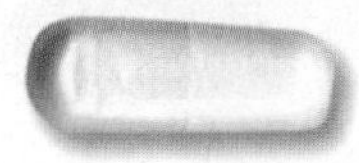

Nature's ResourceTM
Kava Kava 150 mg

**Cranberry Juice Concentrate**

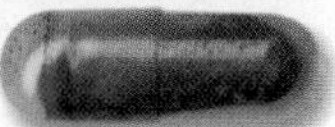

Nature's ResourceTM
Cranberry 405 mg

**Feverfew Leaf**

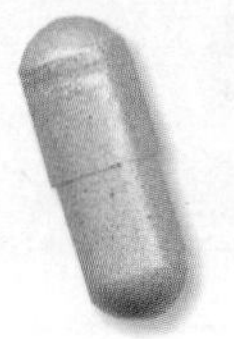

Nature's ResourceTM

Feverfew
380 mg

**Saw Palmetto Berry Extract**

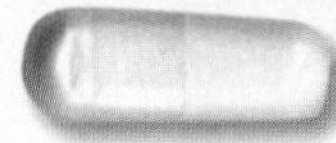

Nature's ResourceTM
Saw Palmetto

(at least 45% fatty acids and sterols)
80 mg

QuanterraTM
Prostate 160 mg

Propalmex®

Saw palmetto
(85-95% free fatty acids and phytosterols)
160 mg

Pumpkin seed oil extract
(85-95% free fatty acids)
40 mg

Zinc (as zinc gluconate)
7.5 mg

**St. John's Wort Extract (0.3% hypericin)**

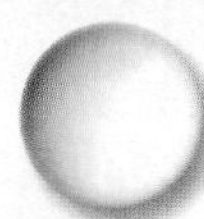

KiraTM (LI 160) 300 mg
(from upper parts of flowers and leaves)

Celestial Seasonings®
St. John's Wort 300 mg

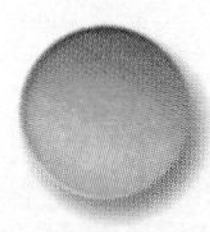

MovannaTM (WS-5572)
(from flowers and leaves)
300 mg

QuanterraTM
Emotional Balance
(LI 160 WS) 300 mg
(aerial part, dried extract)

AlterraTM 450 mg
(extended-release tablet)

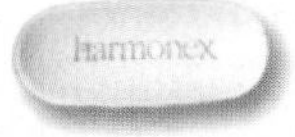


HarmonexTM
St. John's wort extract
(flower) 450 mg

Siberian ginseng extract (root)
(0.8% eleutherosides) 90 mg

**Ginkgo Biloba Leaf Extract**

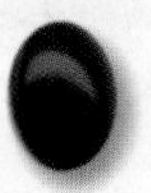

QuanaterraTM
Mental Sharpness
(EGb 761®) 60 mg

GinkobaTM 40 mg

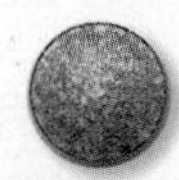

GinkaiTM

(LI 1370) 50 mg
(25% ginkgo flavonoids and 6% terpenoids)

## Valerian Root

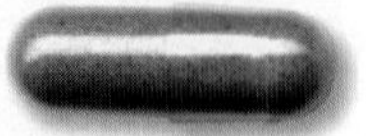

Nature's Resource™
Valerian
530 mg

## Garlic

Garlique®
Garlic powder (bulb)
(not less than 5000 mcg allicin yield)
400 mg

Kwai®
dried garlic clove powder (600 mcg allicin)
100 mg

Kyolic™
aged garlic extract
600 mg

## Dong Quai Root

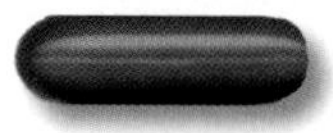

GNC Herbal Plus®
Concentrated Dong Quai
1000 mg

## Ginger Root

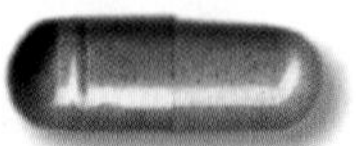

Nature's Way® Herbal Formula
Ginger Root
550 mg

## Panax Ginseng Extract

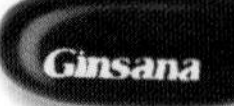


Ginsana®
(G115®) (root)
100 mg

Your Life® Ginseng
(7% ginsenosides)
100 mg

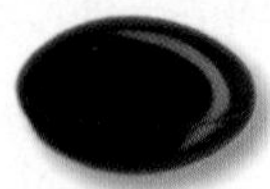

Nature Made®
Ginseng 250 mg

## Echinacea

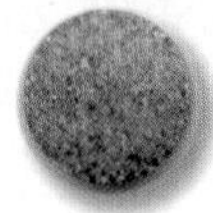

Echinex™

Extract of Echinacea purpurea root and herb (4% phenolic compounds) 250 mg

Extract of Siberian ginseng root (0.8% eleutherosides) 100 mg

Extract of ginger root (5% gingerols) 100 mg

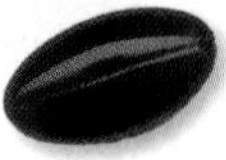

Nature Made®

Echinacea entire plant extract 125 mg

*E. purpurea, E. angustifolia* and/or *E. pallida*
(4% polyphenols and 2% echinacosides)

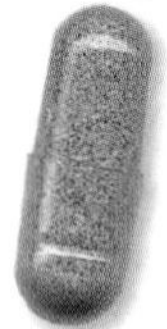

Nature's Resource™

*Echinacea purpurea* herb
350 mg

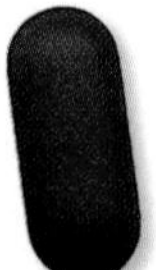

Your Life®
Echinacea extract 125 mg
*Echinacea angustifolia* & *Echinacea purpurea*
(4% phenolic compounds)

a radiolabeled synthetic androgen for the cytosolic androgenic receptor of rat prostate tissue. Another in vitro study found that saw palmetto lipid extract inhibits 5-α reductase, the enzyme responsible for the conversion of testosterone to its active metabolite dihydrotestosterone (DHT); inhibits 3–ketosteroid reductase, the enzyme responsible for DHT metabolism to other active androgens; and blocks androgen receptors (Sultan et al., 1984).

Saw palmetto may also improve BPH signs and symptoms by inhibiting estrogen receptors in the prostate (Wilt et al., 1998). Saw palmetto extract in a dose of 160 mg or placebo three times daily was administered to 35 elderly men, and prostatic tissue was collected (Di Silverio et al., 1992). The investigators found that some component of the saw palmetto extract inhibits nuclear estrogen receptors in the prostates of BPH patients.

Clinically, 160 mg of Permixon® twice daily was superior to placebo in a double-blind trial in 110 men with BPH (Champault et al., 1984). A statistically significant ($p < 0.001$) benefit compared to placebo was seen in nocturia, flow rate, post-void residual, self-rating, physician rating, and dysuria. Compared to baseline, both placebo and saw palmetto were beneficial in improving nocturia ($p < 0.001$), but only saw palmetto improved flow rate and post-void residual compared to baseline ($p < 0.001$). Headache was the only adverse effect.

A double-blind study (Carraro et al., 1996) compared Proscar® (finasteride, a prescription 5-α reductase inhibitor), 5 mg daily, with Permixon®, 160 mg twice daily for 6 mo. Both finasteride and saw palmetto improved International Prostate Symptom Score and quality of life compared to baseline, with no statistical difference between the two treatments. Finasteride improved peak urinary flow rate more than saw palmetto ($p = 0.035$), and residual volume was decreased more with finasteride than with saw palmetto ($p = 0.017$). Finasteride decreased prostate volume more than saw palmetto ($p < 0.001$), and only finasteride decreased prostate specific antigen (PSA) compared to baseline ($p < 0.001$). Although only one patient in each treatment group withdrew because of sexual problems, the finasteride patients experienced a statistically significant deterioration in the sexual function score compared with baseline ($p < 0.01$). Twice as many patients withdrew from the saw palmetto group because of side effects (28 vs 14), but there were no statistically significant differences noted between the two groups in regard to any adverse effect. Hypertension was the most common adverse effect, occurring in 3.1% of the saw palmetto patients and 2.2% of the finasteride patients. Other adverse effects included decreased libido, abdominal pain, impotence, back pain, diarrhea, flulike illness, urinary retention, headache, nausea, constipation, and dysuria. A drawback of this study is that no placebo group was included; more data on the efficacy of these two drugs compared to placebo are needed.

The findings of Carraro and colleagues discussed above suggest that Permixon® does not affect PSA. These results were confirmed by an in vitro study in which Permixon® 10 mcg/mL (calculated plasma concentration achieved with therapeutic doses), did not interfere with secretion of PSA (Bayne et al., 1999). These results imply that PSA can continue to be used for prostate cancer screening in men taking saw palmetto.

A meta-analysis (Wilt et al., 1998) of randomized trials comparing saw palmetto to placebo or other therapy was recently published. The authors concluded that despite methodology problems, saw palmetto appears to improve urologic symptoms and urinary flow to an extent similar to that of finasteride, but with fewer adverse effects.

In regard to other endocrine effects, one Web site (www.hometownrx.com/Doc/Herbs/Sawpalm.html) claims there is preliminary evidence that saw palmetto can aid those with "thyroid deficiency."

### *11.4.3 Anti-Inflammatory Effects*

Anti-inflammatory effects have been hypothesized to improve BPH symptoms (Wilt et al., 1998). An acidic, lipophilic saw palmetto extract (Talso®) was shown in vitro to inhibit both the cyclooxygenase and 5-lipoxygenase pathways, preventing the formation of inflammatory producing prostaglandins and leukotrienes (Breu et al., 1992).

## *11.5 Case Reports of Toxicity Due to Commercially Available Products*

A case of toxicity associated with the use of Prostata®, a preparation containing saw palmetto, zinc picolinate, pyridoxine, L-alanine, glutamic acid, *Apis mellifica* pollen, silica, hydrangea extract, panax ginseng, and *Pygeum africanum*, was reported in the *Annals of Internal Medicine* (Hamid et al., 1997). A 65-yr-old man developed acute and protracted cholestatic hepatitis after taking Prostata®. The man stopped taking the product after 2 wk of use because he developed jaundice and severe pruritus. On physical exam, the patient's abdomen was not tender and his liver and spleen were not palpable. Lab results were as follows: bilirubin 8.2 mg/dL, aspartate aminotransferase 1238 IU/L, alanine aminotransferase 1364 IU/L, alkaline phosphatase 179 IU/L, γ-glutamyl transferase 391 IU/L, hematocrit 41%, leukocyte count $3.3 \times 10^3/mm^3$, platelet count 153,000 cells/$mm^3$, serum protein 6.3 g/dL, albumin 3.6 g/dL, carcinoembryonic antigen (CEA) <2 mg/μL. Serologic testing was negative for hepatitis A virus IgM, hepatitis B surface antigen, cytomegalovirus IgM, and hepatitis C virus antibodies. The patient was negative for antinuclear antibodies and antismooth muscle antibodies, but positive for antimitochondrial antibodies. Liver enzyme levels remained abnormal for more than 3 mo. Liver biopsy was done after 2 mo and showed parenchymal infiltrate of neutrophils and lymphocytes that involved the portal tracts, early bridging, and mild periportal fibrosis. There was no evidence of bile duct damage, cirrhosis, or granulomas. The authors postulated that the patient's cholestasis was an extension of saw palmetto's estrogenic or anti-androgen effect.

## *11.6 Pharmacokinetics/Toxicokinetics*

Limited pharmacokinetic data are available because saw palmetto is a mixture of various compounds (Plosker and Brogden, 1996).

### *11.6.1 Absorption*

A mean peak plasma drug concentration of 2.6 mg/L of the "second component" with a high-performance liquid chromatography (HPLC) retention time of 26.4 min was measured in 12 healthy young men after a single oral dose of 320 mg of saw palmetto. The time to peak concentration occurred 1.5 h after administration (De Bernardi Di Valserra et al., 1994). A 640-mg rectal dose of saw palmetto extract produced a peak of 2.6 μg/mL occurring 3 h after the dose (De Bernardi Di Valserra and Tripodi, 1994).

### *11.6.2 Distribution*

Rat studies indicate that prostate concentrations are higher than those achieved in other genitourinary tissues or in the liver (Plosker and Brogden, 1996).

### *11.6.3 Metabolism/Excretion*

The elimination half-life of the "second component" discussed previously was 1.9 h and the mean area under the concentration vs time curve (AUC) was 8.2 mg/L × h after a single oral dose of 320 mg (De Bernardi Di Valserra et al., 1994). The AUC of the "second component" produced by a 640-mg rectal dose of saw palmetto extract was 10 mg/L × h, and plasma levels were detectable up to 8 h post-dose (De Bernardi Di Valserra and Tripodi, 1994).

## *11.7 Analysis of Biofluids*

HPLC has been used to interpret plasma levels of the "second component" of saw palmetto (De Bernardi Di Valserra and Tripodi, 1994; De Bernardi Di Valserra et al., 1994).

## 11.8 Chemical Analysis

Identification and chemical analysis of saw palmetto is described in the *National Formulary* (USP, 1998).

## 11.9 Regulatory Status

The German Commission E lists saw palmetto as an approved herb. The berry is the only part of the plant approved for use. The approved uses include urination problems associated with BPH stages I and II and urination problems associated with prostate adenoma. This evaluation is based on reasonable proof of safety and efficacy (Blumenthal, 1998).

Saw palmetto is considered a dietary supplement by the FDA (Tyler, 1993). Saw palmetto was previously included in the NF (National Formulary) and the USP (United States Pharmacopeia), but was deleted in 1950 and 1916, respectively. Saw palmetto was deleted because no active ingredient could be found to account for its use (Nemecz, 1998). Saw palmetto was again included in the NF as an official monograph in 1998 (Anonymous, 1998).

## References

Anonymous. Saw palmetto. The Lawrence review of natural products. St. Louis, MO: Facts and comparisons, 1994.

Bayne CW, Donnelly F, Ross M, Habib FK. Serenoa repens (Permixon): a 5alpha-reductase types I and II inhibitor—new evidence in a coculture model of BPH. Prostate 1999;40:232–41.

Blumenthal M. The complete German Commission E monographs. Therapeutic guide to herbal medicine. Austin, TX: American Botanical Council, 1998.

Blumenthal M, Riggins CW. Popular herbs in the US market. Therapeutic monographs. Saw palmetto berry. Austin, TX: American Botanical Council, 1997 .

Breu W, Hagenlocher M, Redl K, Tittel G, Stadler F, Wagner H. Antiphlogistic activity of an extract from *Sabal serrulata* fruits prepared with supercritical carbon dioxide. In-vitro inhibition of cyclooxygenase and 5–lipoxygenase metabolism. Arzneim Forsch 1992;42:547–51.

Briley M, Carilla E. Fauran F. Permixon, a new treatment for benign prostatic hyperplasia, acts directly at the cytosolic androgen receptor in rat prostate [abstract]. Br J Pharmacol 1983;79:327P.

Carraro J, Raynaud J, Koch G, Chisholm GD, Di Silverio F, Teillac P, et al. Comparison of phytotherapy (Permixon®) with finasteride in the treatment of benign prostatic hyperplasia; a randomized international study of 1,098 patients. Prostate 1996;29:231–40.

Champault G, Patel JC, Bonnard AM. A double-blind trial of an extract of the plant *Serenoa repens* in benign prostatic hyperplasia. Br J Clin Pharmacol 1984;18:461–2.

Chavez ML. Saw palmetto. Hosp Pharmacy 1998;33:1335–61.
De Bernardi Di Valerra M, Tripodi AS, Contos S, Germogli R. *Serenoa repens* capsules: a bioequivalence study. Acta Toxicol Ther 1994;15:21–39.
De Bernardi di Valserra M, Tripodi AS. Rectal bioavailability and pharmacokinetics of *Serenoa repens* new formulation in healthy volunteers. Arch Med Intern 1994; 46:77–86.
Di Silverio F, D'Eramo G, Lubrano C, Flammia GP, Sciarra A, Palma E, et al. Evidence that *Serenoa repens* extract displays an antiestrogenic activity in prostatic tissue of benign prostatic hypertrophy patients. Eur Urol 1992;21:309–14.
Hamid S, Rojter S, Vierling J. Protracted cholestatic hepatitis after the use of Prostata. Ann Intern Med 1997;127:169–79.
Nemecz G. Saw palmetto. US Pharm 1998 (Jan);23:97–8, 100–2.
Plosker GL, Brogden RN. *Serenoa repens* (Permixon®). A review of its pharmacology and therapeutic efficacy in benign prostatic hyperplasia. Drug Aging 1996;9:379–95.
Sultan C, Terraza A, Devillier C, Carilla E, Briley M, Loire C, Descomps B. Inhibition of androgen metabolism and binding by a liposterolic extract of "*Serenoa repens* B" in human foreskin fibroblasts. J Steroid Biochem 1984;20:515–9.
Tyler VE. The honest herbal, 3rd edit., Binghamton, NY: Pharmaceutical Products Press, 1993.
United States Pharmacopoeia (USP). National Formulary, 18th edit., Suppl 9, Rockville, MD: United States Pharmacopeial Convention, 1998.
Wilt TJ, Ishani A, Stark G, MacDonald R, Lau J, Mulrow C. Saw palmetto extracts for treatment of benign prostatic hyperplasia. JAMA 1998;280:1604–9.

# *Chapter 12*

# Panax *Ginseng*

*Angela Morgan and Melanie Johns Cupp*

Korean ginseng, Asian ginseng, Oriental ginseng, Chinese ginseng (Muller and Clauson, 1998), Japanese ginseng, American ginseng (Awang, 1991)

Note that the term "ginseng" can refer to the species of the genus *Panax*, as well as to *Eleutherococcus senticosus* (Siberian or Russian ginseng) (Awang, 1991). Unless otherwise noted, the information in this monograph refers specifically to species of the genus *Panax*. Depending on the particular botanical reference, there are three to six different species of *Panax ginseng*, and three with purported medicinal benefits: panax ginseng (Chinese or Korean ginseng), *Panax pseudo-ginseng* (Japanese ginseng), and *Panax quinquefolium* (American ginseng) (Awang, 1991a). In this chapter, the term "panax ginseng" will be used to refer to these species, and "Siberian ginseng" will be used to refer to *Eleutherococcus senticosus*. The chemical composition of Siberian ginseng differs from that of panax ginseng (Awang, 1991a); thus, the distinction between the two is important in a discussion of therapeutic and adverse effects.

## *12.1 History and Traditional Uses*

Panax ginseng is a perennial herb that starts flowering in its fourth year (Leung, 1980). It grows in the United States, Canada, and the mountainous forests of eastern Asia (Tyler et al., 1981). The translucent, yellowish-brown roots are harvested when plants reach between 3 and 6 yr of age (Tyler et al., 1981). This herb has been used in the Orient for 5000 yr as a tonic (Chong and Oberholzer, 1988). According to traditional Chinese medicine's "philosphy of opposites," American ginseng (*Panax quinquefolis* L.) is a "cool" or "yin" tonic

From Forensic Science: *Toxicology and Clinical Pharmacology of Herbal Products*
Edited by: M. J. Cupp © Humana Press Inc., Totowa, New Jersey

used to treat "hot" symptoms such as stress, insomnia, palpitations, and headache, while Asian ginseng (*Panax ginseng* L.) is "hot" or "yang" and is used to treat "cold" diseases (Awang, 1998). In the Orient, ginseng is considered a cure-all. This stems from the "Doctrine of Signatures" because the root is said to resemble a man's appearance and is therefore useful to treat all of man's ailments (Anonymous, 1990). Throughout history the root has been used as a treatment for asthenia, atherosclerosis, blood and bleeding disorders, colitis, and relief of symptoms associated with aging, cancer, and senility (Anonymous, 1990). Ginseng is also widely believed to be an aphrodisiac (Tyler, 1993).

## 12.2 Current Promoted Uses

Ginseng is promoted as a tonic capable of invigorating the user physically, mentally, and sexually. It is also said to possess antistress activity, or to serve as an "adaptogen." Claims that ginseng can improve athletic performance, enhance longevity, or treat toxic hepatitis are not supported by human trials.

## 12.3 Products Available

Two commercial forms of the herb are available. "White" ginseng consists of the dried root and "red" ginseng is prepared by steaming the fresh, unpeeled root before drying (Blumenthal, 1997). Many different formulations of the herb are available including capsules, gelcaps, powders, tinctures, teas, slices to eat in salads, and whole root to chew. There are also a wide variety of products that claim to contain ginseng such as ginseng cigarettes, toothpaste, cosmetics, soaps, beverages (including beer), candy, baby food, gum, candy bars, and coffee. Prices vary widely based on the quantity and quality of the ginseng root used (Kennedy, 1995). Tinctures are more expensive but last for years. Powder capsules are cheaper but have a shelf-life of only 1 yr (Schiedermayer, 1998). Panax ginseng price ranges from $28 to more than $200 per pound depending on the quality (Tyler, 1997). One of the problems in the manufacture of ginseng is the lack of quality control and standardization (Muller and Clauson, 1998). Although the amount of ginsenosides, the purported active ingredients, ranges widely among brands and often differs from the content stated on the label, testing by *Consumer Reports* revealed that the amount of ginsenosides in Ginsana®, the ginseng market leader in the United States, is well standardized (Anonymous, 1998). (*See* Section 12.9 for discussion of factors affecting ginsenoside content.) The manufacturer (Pharmaton, Ridgefield, CT) claims that each Ginsana® capsule contains 100 mg of standardized, concentrated ginseng (Janetzky and Morreale, 1997). A study (Cui et al., 1996) of the Swedish Ginsana® product revealed consistency in ginsenoside content between batches.

Ginsana® is available in the United States in softgel capsules and chewy squares. The capsules are green because chlorophyll is added. Other brands of ginseng are most commonly available in capsule or tablet form and are usually brown. Dosage strengths normally range between 50 mg and 300 mg of panax ginseng extract per capsule or tablet. Also, several combination products are available. For example, Ginkogin® is a combination of panax ginseng, ginkgo biloba, and garlic. There are other types of ginseng on the market including Siberian, Brazilian, and Indian ginseng. These are not of the genus *Panax* and do not contain ginsenosides (Tyler, 1997).

## *12.4 Pharmacologic/Toxicologic Effects*

### *12.4.1 Endocrine Effects*

Panax ginseng may exert hypoglycemic effects possibly by accelerating hepatic lipogenesis and increasing glycogen storage (Yokozawa et al., 1975; Oshima et al., 1985; Sotaniemi et al., 1995). In a study of 36 newly diagnosed type II diabetics, ginseng at a dose of 200 mg daily exerted a statistically significant benefit on glycosylated hemoglobin ($HbA_{1c}$) compared to 100 mg of ginseng daily or placebo after 8 wk of therapy, and patients receiving 100 mg of ginseng had smaller mean fasting blood glucose levels than patients taking 200 mg of ginseng or placebo (Sotaniemi et al., 1995). The actual difference among the mean $HbA_{1c}$ in the three groups was small; the 200-mg ginseng group had a mean glycosylated hemoglobin of 6% vs 6.5% for the 100-mg ginseng and placebo groups. Likewise, the actual difference among mean fasting blood glucose in the three groups was small; the mean fasting blood glucose was 7.7 mmol/L for the 100-mg ginseng group, 7.4 mmol/L for the 200-mg ginseng group, and 8.3 mmol/L for the placebo group at the end of the study. The observed differences might be attributed to differences in body weight among the three groups. The small study sample limits the generalizability of these results.

All the ginsenosids (saponins) so tested have shown anti-fatigue actions in mice (Kaku et al., 1975). This may reflect the purported "adaptogenic" action of ginseng, which can be defined as an increase in resistance to stresses and is thought to be secondary to normalization of body processes through regulation of the production of various hormones (Awang, 1998).

Ginseng appears to have a modulating effect on the hypothalamic–pituitary–adrenal axis by inducing secretion of adrenocorticotropic hormone (ACTH) from the anterior pituitary to increase plasma cortisol (Hiai et al., 1979; Fulder, 1981), perhaps accounting for improvement in 11 quality of life measurements in a large double-blind study using ginseng extract G115 (Caso Marasco et al., 1996).

Although many products containing ginseng are marketed specifically for postmenopausal women, a recent review concluded that there is insufficient evidence that ginseng is effective for treatment of menopausal symptoms (Schiedermayer, 1998). In vitro, Siberian ginseng extract, but not panax ginseng extract, binds to estrogen receptors. Both extracts have affinity for progestin, glucocorticoid, and mineralocorticoid receptors (Pearce et al., 1982).

### *12.4.2 Neurologic Effects*

Commercially available panax ginseng products have been reported to have stimulant effects on the central nervous system in humans (Seigel, 1979) (*See* section 12.5). In animal models, ginseng extracts have been shown to have CNS stimulant effects (Takagi et al., 1972). Ginsenoside Rg1 inhibits neuronal apoptosis in vitro (Li et al., 1997), and ginsenoside Rb1 reverses short-term memory loss in rats (Awang, 1998). It has been suggested that ginseng may hold promise for the treatment of dementia in humans (Awang, 1998; Li et al., 1997).

### *12.4.3 Cardiovascular Effects*

In animal studies, ginsenoside Rb1 decreases blood pressure, perhaps due to relaxation of smooth muscle (Kaku et al., 1975). In humans, small studies suggest ginseng may decrease systolic blood pressure at a dose of 4.5 g/d (Han et al., 1998), and enhance the efficacy of digoxin in class IV heart failure (Ding et al., 1995). In contrast, ginsenoside Rg1 has been purported to have hypertensive effects (Awang, 1998).

An in vitro study using a crude extract of ginseng saponins and rabbit corpus cavernosal smooth muscle suggests that some component of ginseng may be a nitric oxide donor, capable of causing relaxation of smooth muscle in the corpus carvernosum (Kim et al., 1998). This finding might provide a scientific basis for claims that ginseng enhances sexual potency, and for the results of a study that showed increased penile rigidity and girth compared to placebo or trazodone in paitients with erectile dysfunction (Choi et al., 1995).

Red ginseng powder may be useful in hyperlipidemia; it was shown to decrease triglycerides as well as increase high-density lipoprotein (HDL) in a pilot study (Yamamoto et al., 1983). A previous rat study lends validity to ginseng's ability to decrease triglyceride levels (Yokozawa et al., 1975), but a study in diabetic patients showed no effect on total cholesterol, low-density lipoprotein (LDL), HDL, or triglyceride levels (Sotaniemi et al., 1995).

### *12.4.4 Hematologic Effects*

Panax ginseng may inhibit platelet aggregation by regulating the levels of cGMP and thromboxane $A_2$ (Park et al., 1995).

### 12.4.5 Immunologic Effects

Red ginseng stimulates accumulation of neutrophils in a dose-dependent manner following intraperitoneal injections in mice (Toda et al., 1990). Data show panax ginseng extracts are also able to stimulate an immune response in humans. Chemotaxis of polymorphonuclear cells was increased compared to placebo. Both the phagocytosis index and fraction were enhanced in the ginseng groups and intracellular killing was increased compared to the placebo group. Total lymphocytes and helper T cells were increased as well (Scaglione et al., 1990). There have been other reports of increases in cell-mediated immunity as well as natural killer cell activity (Singh et al., 1984).

### 12.4.6 Antineoplastic Effects

Data from in vitro studies, animal models, case-control studies, and cohort studies suggest ginseng may prevent or ameliorate various cancers. These studies have been reviewed in detail elsewhere (Xiaoguang et al., 1998; Ahn 1997; Yun 1996). Prospective, placebo-controlled studies of ginseng's ability to prevent or treat cancer are lacking.

## 12.5 Case Reports of Toxicity Due to Commercially Available Products

In 1979 the term "ginseng abuse syndrome" (GAS) was coined as the result of a study (Siegel, 1979) of 133 people who had been using a variety of ginseng preparations for at least 1 mo. Most study subjects experienced CNS excitation and arousal. Fourteen patients experienced GAS, defined as hypertension, nervousness, sleeplessness, skin eruptions, and morning diarrhea. Five of these subjects also exhibited edema. The effects of ginseng on mood appeared to be dose dependent; four patients experienced depersonalization and confusion at doses of 15 g, and depression was reported following doses >15 g. Twenty-two subjects in all experienced hypertension. All of the patients experiencing GAS or hypertension were also using caffeinated beverages. Six other subjects also experienced GAS but were considered "atypical" because they were either using Siberian ginseng instead of panax ginseng, or were injecting ginseng, and thus were not included in the study results. One subject experienced anaphylaxis followed by confusion and hallucinations after injection of 2 mL of ginseng extract. The average daily dose of the 14 patients experiencing GAS was 3 g of ginseng root, and most users reported titrating the dose to minimize nervousness and tremor. One subject experienced hypotension, weakness, and tremor when ginseng use was abruptly discontinued. The author compared ginseng's effects to those of high doses of corticosteroids. GAS seemed to be found predominantly during the first year of use, possibly because by the 18-mo follow-up visit, ginseng use had declined to an average of 1.7 g daily, and by the 24-mo visit, half of the GAS patients had discontinued ginseng use, and 21% of the remaining subjects had stopped using it. Eight subjects were still experiencing diarrhea and nervousness at 2 yr follow-up. Because this study was not controlled, the existence of GAS has been questioned (Tyler, 1993).

Hypertension, shortness of breath, dizziness, inability to concentrate, a loud palpable fourth heart sound, "thrusting" apical pulse, and hypertensive changes on fundal examination were reported in a 39-yr-old man who had taken various ginseng products for 3 yr (Hammond and Whitworth, 1981). His blood pressure measured 140/100 mm Hg on three occasions over 6 wk, and when referred for management of his hypertension it was 154/106 mm Hg. He was advised to discontinue the ginseng products, and 5 d later was normotensive at 140/85 mm Hg. At 3 mo follow-up, he remained normotensive and his other symptoms had resolved. No attempt was made to confirm the identity or composition of the ginseng products.

An episode of Stevens-Johnson syndrome was reported in a 27-yr-old man following ginseng administration (two pills a day for 3 d). Infiltration of the dermis by mononuclear cells was noted. The patient recovered completely within 30 d (Dega et al., 1996).

An association between ginseng and mastalgia has been reported. A 70-yr-old woman developed swollen, tender breasts with diffuse nodularity after using a panax ginseng powder (Gin Seng) for 3 wk. Symptoms ceased following discontinuation of the herb and reappeared with two additional rechallenges. Prolactin levels were within normal limits (Palmer et al., 1978).

A 72-yr-old woman experienced vaginal bleeding after taking 200 mg daily of a Swiss-Austrian geriatric formulation of ginseng (Geriatric Pharmaton, Bernardgrass, Austria) for an unspecified time (Greenspan, 1983). In a similar case, a 62-yr-old woman had undergone a total hysterectomy 14 yr previously and had been taking Rumanian ginseng alternating with Gerovital® every 2 wk for 1 yr (Punnonen and Lukola, 1980). The patient derived a marked estrogenic effect from the product based on microscopy of vaginal smears as well as the gross appearance of the vaginal and cervical epithelium. The patient was dechallenged from the products for 5 wk, rechallenged with Gerovital for 2 wk, then rechallenged with ginseng for 2 wk. Estrone, estradiol, and estriol levels were essentially unchanged over this time period, but the estrogenic effects on the vaginal smear coincided with ginseng use. Using gas chromatography, the investigators found no estrogen in the tablets the patient had been taking. They did discover that a crude methanolic extract of the ginseng product competed with estradiol for the estrogen and progesterone binding sites in human myometrial cytosol.

A 44-yr-old woman who had experienced menopause at age 42 experienced three episodes of spotting associated with use of Fang Fang ginseng face cream (Shanghai, China). Interestingly, these episodes of bleeding were associated with a decrease in follicle-stimulating hormone (FSH) levels and a disordered proliferative pattern on endometrial biopsy. The woman discontinued use of the cream and experienced no further bleeding (Hopkins et al., 1988).

Whether the products used in these reports of vaginal bleeding and mastalgia contained panax ginseng or Siberian ginseng (*Eleutherococcus senticosus*) was not investigated. Whether panax or Siberian ginseng causes estrogenic effects requires further study.

Maternal ingestion of 650 mg of Siberian ginseng (Jamieson Natural Sources, Toronto) twice daily was associated with androgenization in a neonate (Koren et al., 1990). The product had been taken for the previous 18 mo, including the pregnancy. During pregnancy, the mother noted increased and thicker hair growth on her head, face, and pubic area, and had experienced repeated premature uterine contractions during late pregnancy. At birth, the Caucasian child weighed 3.3 kg, had thick black pubic hair, hair over the entire forehead, and swollen red nipples. The woman continued to take the ginseng product for 2 wk after the baby's birth, during which time she breast-fed the baby. She was advised to discontinue the product when the baby was 2 wk old, and his pubic and forehead hair began to fall out. By 7½ wk of age, hair was scant, but his testes were enlarged. Weight gain was 1.1 kg during the first 3½ wk of life, and 1.4 kg during the next 3½ wk. At age 7½ wk, his weight (5.8 kg), length (60.6 cm), and head circumference (41.5 cm) were at or above the 97th percentile. At that time, testosterone, 17-hydroxyprogesterone, and cortisol levels were normal. Subsequent information did not confirm the product's androgenic effects. A sample of the raw material used in manufacturing the preparation used by this patient was identified as *Periploca sepium* (Chinese silk vine), not Siberian ginseng. No androgenic effects were noted in rats administered the manufacturer's sample (Waller et al., 1992). *Periploca sepium* ("jia-pi") was reported previously to be mislabeled as Siberian ginseng ("wu-jia-pi"), perhaps due to similarities in the Chinese terms for these herbs (Awang, 1991b).

## 12.6 Drug Interactions

A probable interaction between warfarin and a panax ginseng product has been reported (Janetzky and Morreale, 1997). A 47-yr-old man with a St. Jude-type mechanical aortic valve had been controlled on warfarin with an international normalized ratio (INR) of 3.1 (goal 2.5–3.5). He experienced a subtherapeutic INR of 1.5 following 2 wk of ginseng administration (Ginsana® three times daily). Other medications included 30 mg of diltiazem three times daily, nitroglycerin as needed, and 500 mg of salsalate three times daily as needed. He had been on all of these medications for at least 3 yr before the abrupt change in his INR. Discontinuation of ginseng resulted in an increase in INR to 3.3 within 2 wk.

Manic-like symptoms were reported in a patient treated with phenelzine and ginseng. The symptoms disappeared with cessation of the herbal therapy (Jones and Runikis, 1987). Users should also exercise caution if ginseng is taken in combination with caffeinated beverages; as discussed in Section 12.5, hypertension and nervousness have been reported when the two are combined (Siegel, 1979).

Although Siberian ginseng is not of the same genus as panax ginseng, it may be confused with and substituted for panax ginseng, and thus a discussion of drug interactions with Siberian ginseng is warranted. Siberian ginseng has been reported to inhibit the metabolism of hexobarbital in mice by 66% (Mendon et al., 1984). Siberian ginseng ingestion was associated with elevated digoxin levels in a 74-yr-old man whose digoxin levels had been maintained between 0.9 and 2.2 ng/L (normal, 0.6–2.6 ng/L) for more than 10 yr. He was asymptomatic for digoxin toxicity despite a level of 5.2 ng/L. EKG, potassium level, and serum creatinine level were normal. The level decreased upon dechallenge, and increased upon rechallenge. The product was analyzed for digoxin or digitoxin contamination, but none was found. The product was not analyzed to determine if it did in fact contain Siberian ginseng. It was hypothesized that some component of Siberian ginseng might impair digoxin elimination or interfere with the digoxin assay. The type of digoxin assay used in this case was not specified (McRae, 1996).

## 12.7 Pharmacokinetics/Toxicokinetics

The structures and nomenclature of the chemical constituents of panax ginseng have been discussed elsewhere (Phillipson and Anderson, 1984). *See also*, Section 12.9.

### *12.7.1 Absorption*

β-Sitosterol is a steroid sapogenin that has been isolated from ginseng. Approximately 50–60% of a dose of β-sitosterol is absorbed from the gastrointestinal tract in rats (Schon and Engelhardt, 1960). After oral administration of radiolabeled ginsenoside Rg1, blood radioactivity peaked at 2.1 h. Bioavailability was 49% (Liu and Xiao, 1992).

### *12.7.2 Distribution*

Studies of the distribution of [$^3$H]ginsenoside Rg1 following intravenous injection have been performed in mice (Liu and Xiao, 1992). Tissue radioactivity was greatest in the kidney, followed by the adrenal gland, liver, lungs, spleen, pancreas, heart, testes, and brain. Plasma protein binding was 24%, and tissue protein binding was 48% in the liver, 22% in testes, and 8% in the brain.

### *12.7.3 Metabolism/Elimination*

The blood radioactivity decreased in a triphasic manner after intravenous injection of [$^3$H]ginsenoside Rg1 to mice (Liu and Xiao, 1992). Other Chinese studies have characterized the biotransformation of ginsenoside 20(*S*)-Rg2, one of the main constituents of ginseng roots and leaves. Its metabolism is complex and involves multiple hydrolysis reactions in the gastrointestinal tract. Metabolites of 20(*S*)-Rg2 include 20(*S*)-Rh1 and 20(*S*)-protopanaxatriol. Details of the biotransformation of 20(*S*)-Rg2 and chemical structures of the ginsenosides are available in the cited reference (Liu and Xiao, 1992).

Corroborating two rat studies (Odani et al., 1983a,b) suggesting that only trace amounts of ginsenosides are excreted in the urine, low levels of ginsenoside aglycones were identified using gas chromatography–mass spectroscopy (GC–MS) to analyze urine samples of 65 athletes claiming to have ingested ginseng within the 10 d prior to urine collection (Cui et al., 1996). An aglycone (molecule from which the sugar moiety has been removed) of ginsenosides, 20(*S*)-protopanaxatriol, was found at concentrations between 2 and 35 ng/mL in approx 90% of the urine samples studied. Another aglycone, 20(*S*)-protopanaxadiol, was barely detectable despite the fact that the ginsenosides from which it is derived were the major ginsenosides found in the commercially available Swedish ginseng products analyzed by the investigators. This indicates that these two ginsenosides have different pharmacokinetics. Because the actual amount of ginseng ingested and the time since ingestion were unknown, little else can be inferred from these data.

## *12.8 Analysis of Biofluids*

Colorimetry, thin-layer chromatography (TLC), gas–liquid chromatography (GLC), droplet counter current chromatography (DDC), and high-performance liquid chromatography (HPLC) are not sensitive enough to quantify ginsenosides in biofluids, tissues, and organs, but radioimmunoassay is both highly sensitive and specific (Sankawa et al., 1982).

Use of radioimmunoassay to determine ginsenoside Rg1 in the biological fluids, tissues, and organs of animals fed ginseng has been described (Sankawa et al., 1982). GC–MS methods have also been used in determination of ginsenosides in human urine (Cui et al., 1996).

## 12.9 Chemical Analysis

There are over 30 ginsenosides found in *Panax sp.*, but "total ginsenosides" content is usually based on HPLC analysis of 6–8 major ginsenosides, including $Rb_1$, $Rb_2$, Rc, Rd, Re, Rf, $Rg_1$, and $Rg_2$. The ginsenoside content of American and Asian ginseng differs. $Rb_2$ and $Rg_2$ are low in Asian ginseng. American ginseng lacks Rf and $Rg_2$, and is low in $Rb_2$ and $Rg_1$. $Rb_1$, Rc, Rd, and Re are the predominant ginsenosides in American ginseng. Rb1 concentrations are commonly ten times those of $Rg_1$, and may exceed twenty (Awang, 1998). The concentration of ginsenosides in American ginseng is affected by harvest date, humidity, and drying temperature (Reynolds, 1998,b).

Panax ginseng identification using TLC, and determination of ginsenside Rb1 and Rg1 content using liquid chromatography has been described in the *National Formulary* (USP, 1998). HPLC using a UV detector is another method for identification of ginsenosides (Soldati and Stitcher, 1980; Sankawa et al., 1982; Sollorz, 1985; Ma et al., 1995). This method may be more reliable than mixed melting point determination, elemental analysis, and TLC owing to the high molecular weight of the compounds (Wagner et al., 1985). GC and GC–MS have also been used to analyze ginsenoside content of Swedish ginseng preparations (Cui et al., 1996).

## 12.10 Regulatory Status

The German Commission E approves panax ginseng as a nonprescription drug for use as a "tonic for invigoration and fortification in times of fatigue and debility, for declining capacity for work and concentration, and also for use during convalescence (Blumenthal, 1998). In the United States, ginseng is regulated as a dietary supplement.

## References

Ahn YO. Diet and stomach cancer in Korea. Int J Cancer 1997;Suppl 10:7–9.

Anonymous. Ginseng. Lawrence review of natural products. St. Louis, MO: Facts and Comparisons;1990.

Anonymous. Ginsana: Tonic or dud? Consumer Reports on Health 1998;10(7):2.

Awang DVC. The anti-stress potential of North American ginseng. J Herbs Spices Med Plants 1998;6:87–91

Awang DVS. Maternal use of ginseng and neonatal androgenization [letter]. JAMA 1991a;265:1828.

Awang DVS. Maternal use of ginseng and neonatal androgenization [letter]. JAMA 1991b/266:363.

Blumenthal M. Popular herbs in the U.S. market. Austin, TX: American Botanical Council, 1997.

Blumenthal M. Ginseng root. The complete German Commission E monographs. Austin, TX: American Botanical Council;1998.

Caso Maraso A, Vargas Ruiz R, Salas Villagomez A, Begona Infante C. Double-blind study of a multivitamin complex supplemented with ginseng extract. Drugs Exp Clin Res 1996;22:323–9.

Choi HK, Seong DH, Rha KH. Clinical efficacy of Korean red ginseng for erectile dysfunction. Int J Impot Res 1995;7:181–6.

Chong S, Oberholzer V. Ginseng – is there a use in clinical medicine? Postgrad Med J 1988;64:841–6.

Cui J, Garle M, Bjorkhem I, Eneroth P. Determination of aglycones of ginsenosides in ginseng preparations sold in Sweden and in urine samples from Swedish Athletes. Scand J Clin Lab Invest 1996;56:151–60.

Dega H, Laporte J, Frances C, Herson S, Chosidow O. Ginseng as a cause for Stevens–Johnson syndrome? Lancet 1996;347:1344.

Ding DZ, Shen TK, Cui YZ. [Effects of red ginseng on the congestive heart failure and its mechanism]. Chung Kuo Chung Hsi I Chieh Ho Tsa Chih 1995;15:325–7.

Fulder S. Ginseng and the hypothalamic–pituitary control of stress. Am J Chin Med 1981;9:112–18.

Greenspan EM. Ginseng and vaginal bleeding. JAMA 1983;249:2018.

Hammond TG, Whitworth JA. Adverse reactions to ginseng [letter]. Med J Aust 1981;1:492.

Han KH, Choe SC, Kim HS, Sohn DW, Nam KY, Oh BH, et al. Effect of red ginseng on blood pressure in patients with essential hypertension and white coat hypertension. Am J Chin Med 1998;26:199–209.

Hiai S, Yokoyama H, Oura H. Features of ginseng saponin-induced corticosterone secretion. Endocrinol Japon 1979;26:737–40.

Hopkins MP, Androff L, Benninghoff AS. Ginseng face cream and unexplained vaginal bleeding. Am J Obstet Gynecol 1988;159:1121–2.

Janetzky K, Morreale A. Probable interaction between warfarin and ginseng. Am J Health Syst Pharm 1997;54:692–93.

Jones B, Runikis A. Interaction of ginseng with phenelzine. J Clin Psychopharmacol 1987;7:201–2.

Kaku T, Miyata T, Uruno, T, Sako, I, Kinoshita A. Chemico-pharmacological studies on saponins of panax ginseng. Arzneim Forsch 1975;25:539–47.

Kennedy B. Herb of the month: ginseng. Total Health 1995;17:48.

Kim HJ, Woo DS, Lee G, Kim JJ. The relaxation effects of ginseng saponin in rabbit corporal smooth muscle: is it a nitric oxide donor? Br J Urol 1998;82:744–8.

Koren G, Randor S, Martin S, Danneman D. Maternal use of ginseng and neonatal androgenization [letter]. JAMA 1990;264:2866.

Leung A. Encyclopedia of common natural ingredients used in food, drugs, and cosmetics. New York: John Wiley and Sons, 1980.

Li J, Zhang X, Zhang J. Study of the anti-apoptotic mechanism of ginsenoside Rg1 in cultured neurons. Acta Pharmaceut Sinica 1997;32:406–10.

Liu C, Xiao P. Recent advances on ginseng research in China. J Ethnopharmacol 1992;36:27–38.

Ma YC, Zhu J, Sun L, Sain S, Kont K, Plaut-Carcasson YY. A comparative evaluation of ginsenosides in commercial ginseng products and tissue culture samples using HPLC. J Herbs Spices Med Plants 1995;3(4):41–50.

McRae S. Elevated serum digoxin levels in a pateint taking digoxin and siberian ginseng. Can Med Assoc J 1996;155:293–5.

Mendon PJ, Ferguson PW, Watson CF. Effects of *Eleutherococcus senticus* extracts on hexobarbital metabolism in vivo and in vitro. J Ethnopharmacol 1984;10:235–41.

Muller J, Clauson K. Top herbal products encountered in drug information requests (part 1). Drug Benefit Trends 1998;10:43–50.

Odani T, Tanizawa H, Takino Y. Studies on the absorption, distribution, excretion, and metabolism of ginseng saponins. II. The absorption, distribution, excretion of ginsenoside-Rg1 in the rat. Chem Pharamcol Bull 1983a;31:292–8.

Odani T, Tanizawa H, Takino Y. Studies on the absorption, distribution, excretion, and metabolism of ginseng saponins. III. The absorption, distribution, excretion of ginsenoside-Rb1 in the rat. Chem Pharamcol Bull 1983b;31:1059–66.

Oshima Y, Konno C, Hikino H. Isolation and hypoglycemic activity of panaxans I, J, K, and L, glycans of panax ginseng roots. J Ethnopharmacol 1985;14:255–9.

Palmer BV, Montgomery ACV, Monteiro JCMP. Gin Seng and mastalgia. Br Med J 1978;1:1284.

Park H, Rheem M, Park K, Nam K, Park KH. Effect of nonsaponin fraction from panax ginseng on cGMP and thromboxane A2 in human platelet aggregation. J Ethnopharmacol 1995;49:157–62.

Pearce PT, Zois I, Wynne KN, Funder JW. Panax ginseng and *Eleutherococcus senticosus* extracts — in vitro studies on binding to steroid receptors. Endocrinol Jpn 1982;29:567–73.

Phillipson JD, Anderson LA. Ginseng-quality, safety and efficacy? Pharm J 1984;232:161–5.

Punnonen R, Lukola A. Oestrogen-like effect of gingseng. Br Med J 1980;281:1110.

Reynolds LB. Effects of drying on chemical and physical characteristics of American ginseng (*Panax quinquefolius* L.) J Herbs Spices Med Plants 1998;6(2):9–21.

Reynolds LB. Effects of harvest date on some chemical and physical characteristics of American ginseng (*Panax quinquefolius* L.) J Herbs Spices Med Plants 1998;6(2):63–9.

Sankawa U, Sung C, Han B, Akiyama T, Kawashima K. Radioimmunoassay for the determination of ginseng saponin, ginsenoside RG1. Chem Pharmacol Bull 1982;30:1907.

Scaglione F, Ferra F, Dugnan S, Falchi M, Santoro G, Fraschi F. Immunomodulatory effects of two extracts of panax ginseng. Drugs Exp Clin Res 1990;16:537–42.

Schiedermayer D. Little evidence for ginseng as treatment for menopausal symptoms. Altern Med Alert 1998;1:77–8.

Schon N, Engelhardt P. Tierexperimentelle untersuchungen zur frage der resorption von β-sitosterin. Arzneim Forsch 1960;10:491–6.

Siegel R. Ginseng abuse syndrome. Problems with the panacea. JAMA 1979;241:1614–5.

Singh V, Agarwal S, Gupta B. Immunomodulatory activity of panax ginseng extract. Planta Med 1984;50:462–5.

Soldati F, Sticher O. HPLC separation and quantitative determination of ginsenosides from *Panax ginseng*, *Panax quinquefolius* and from ginseng drug preparations. Planta Med 1980;38:348–57.

Sollorz G. Quality evaluation of ginseng roots. Quantitative HPLC determination in ginsenosides. Deutch Apoth Ztg 1985;125:2052–55.

Sotaniemi E, Haapakoski E, Rautio A. Ginseng therapy in non-insulin-dependent diabetic patients. Diabetes Care 1995;18:1373–5.

Takagi K, Saito H, Nabata H. Pharmacological studies of panax ginseng root: estimation of pharmacological actions of panax ginseng root. Jpn J Pharmacol 1972;22:245–59.

Toda S, Kimura M, Ohnishi M. Induction of neutrophil accumulation by red ginseng. J Ethnopharmacol 1990;30:315–8.

Tyler V. Ginseng: king of zing? Prevention 1997;49:69.

Tyler V. The honest herbal,. 3rd edit., Binghamton, NY: Pharmaceutical Products Press, 1993.

Tyler VE, Brady LR, Robbers JE. Pharmacognosy, 8th edit., Philadelphia: Lea and Febiger, 1981.

United States Pharmacopeial Convention. National Formulary, 18th edit., Suppl. 9. Rockville, MD: United States Pharmacopeial Convention, 1998.

Wagner H, Hikino H, Farnsworth N. Economic and medicinal plant research, vol. 1. Orlando: Academic Press, 1985.

Waller DP, Martin AM, Farnsworth NR, Awang DVC. Lack of androgenicity of Siberian ginseng. JAMA 1992;267:692–3.

Xiaoguang C, Hongyan L, Xiaohong L, Zhaodi F, Yan L, Lihua T, Rui H. Cancer chemopreventive and therapeutic activities of red ginseng. J Ethnopharmacol 1998;60:71–8.

Yamamoto M, Uemura T, Nakama S, Uemiya M, Kumagai A. Serum HDL-cholesterol-increasing and fatty liver-improving actions of panax ginseng in high cholesterol diet-fed rats with clinical effect on hyperlipidemia in man. Am J Chin Med 1983;11:96–101.

Yokozawa T, Seno H, Oura H. Effect of ginseng extract on lipid and sugar metabolism. Chem Pharmacol Bull 1975;23:3095–3100.

Yun TK. Experimental and epidemiological evidence of the cancer-preventive effects of *Panax ginseng* C.A. Meyer. Nutr Rev 1996;54(11 Pt 2):S71–81.

# Chapter 13

# Cranberry

*Angela J. Lawson and Melanie Johns Cupp*

## 13.1 History and Traditional Uses

Cranberry (*Vaccinium macrocarpon*) is a small evergreen shrub that grows in mountains, forests and damp bogs from Alaska to Tennessee. Native Americans introduced the Europeans to cranberry as a food, dye, and medicine (Tyler, 1993). In the 1920s canned cranberry sauce was introduced, and in the 1940s cranberry juice became commercially available. Cranberry has been used to prevent and treat urinary tract infections since the 19th century (Siciliano, 1996).

## 13.2 Current Promoted Uses

Cranberry juice has been widely used for the prevention, treatment, and symptomatic relief of urinary tract infections (Sobota, 1984). Also, cranberry juice has been given to patients to help reduce urinary odors in incontinence (Kraemer, 1964; DuGan and Cardaciotto, 1966; Anonymous, 1994). Another potential benefit of the use of cranberry is a decrease in the rates formation of kidney stones (Sternlieb, 1963; Zinsser et al., 1968; Light et al., 1973).

## 13.3 Products Available

Cranberry is available in a variety of forms such as fresh or frozen cranberries, cranberry juice cocktail, other cranberry drinks, cranberry sauce, and powder in hard or soft gelatin capsules (Hughes and Lawson, 1989; Siciliano, 1996). Cranberries are approx 88% water and contain flavonoids, anthrocyanins (odain), cetechin, triterpinoids, β-hydroxybutyric acid, citric acid, malic acid,

From Forensic Science: *Toxicology and Clinical Pharmacology of Herbal Products*
Edited by: M. J. Cupp © Humana Press Inc., Totowa, New Jersey

glucuronic acid, quinic acid, benzoic acid, ellagic acid, and vitamin C (Siciliano, 1996). Fresh or frozen cranberries are a good source of cranberry because they contain pure fruit; however, because of their high acidity and extremely sour taste, they are less readily used in clinical practice (Tyler, 1993). Pure cranberry juice is tart like lemon juice because of the high citric and quinic acid content (Siciliano, 1996). Cranberry juice cocktail is more palatable but is only 25–33 % juice and contains corn syrup as a sweetener (Hughes and Lawson, 1989; Siciliano, 1996), while other cranberry juice drinks contain as little as 10% juice (Siciliano, 1996). These sweetened beverages are relatively high in calories (approx 140 kcal per 8 oz serving) (Siciliano, 1996) and could cause weight gain in a patient consuming the juice for medicinal purposes (Hughes and Lawson, 1989). Another drawback to sweetened beverages is that theoretically the sugar could act as a source of food for uropathogens (Hughes and Lawson, 1989). Cranberry sauce consisting of sweetened or gelled berries at a concentration half that of cranberry juice cocktail is also readily available to consumers (Siciliano, 1996). Cranberry capsules are a sugar-free source of cranberry. Hard gelatin capsules contain more crude fiber and organic acids than cranberry juice cocktail, while the soft gelatin capsules contain soybean oil and contain only 8% of the total organic acids found in fresh cranberries (Hughes and Lawson, 1989). Twelve capsules of cranberry powder are equivalent to 6 fl. oz of cranberry juice cocktail (Hughes and Lawson, 1989).

In the various studies and consumer references, many dosages and dosing regimens have been reported for the use of cranberry in prevention of renal calculi, prevention of urinary odor and prevention and treatment of urinary tract infections.

Dosages used or recommended in clinical studies and case reports:

Prevention of urinary tract infection: 8 oz. of cranberry juice four times a day for several days, then twice daily (Sternlieb, 1963); 300 mL/d as cranberry juice cocktail (Avorn, 1994)
Treatment of urinary tract infection: 6 oz. cranberry juice of daily for 21 d (Papas et al., 1966); cranberry juice 6 oz. twice daily (Moen, 1962)
Reduction of urinary odors: 16 oz. of cranberry juice daily (Kraemer, 1964); 3 oz. of cranberry juice daily, then increased by 1 oz. each week to a maximum of 6 oz. daily (DuGan and Cardaciotto, 1966)
Prevention of urinary stones: 1 quart of cranberry juice cocktail daily (Zinsser et al., 1968); 8 oz. of cranberry juice four times a day for several days, then 8 oz. twice daily (Sternlieb, 1963)

Dosages in lay references:

Prevention of urinary tract infection: 3 oz. daily as a cocktail (Tyler, 1993)
Treatment of urinary tract infection: 12–32 oz. daily as a cocktail (Tyler, 1993)

Various brand name products of cranberry available:

Nature's Resource® contains 405 mg of standardized cranberry juice concentrate per capsule. The recommended dose is two to four capsules three times a day with water at meals. The label also recommends drinking a full glass of water when taking the capsules and drinking 6–8 oz. of liquids per day.

Spring Valley® contains 475 mg of cranberry fruit per capsule. The recommended dose is two to four capsules three times a day preferably with meals.

Cranberry Fruit Sundown® Herbals contain 425 mg of cranberry fruit per capsule. The recommended is two to four capsules up to three times a day as needed.

Celestial Seasonings® Cranberry contains 400 mg of cranberry extract standardized to >35% organic acids. The recommended dose is one capsule every day as needed with a full glass of water.

Ocean Spray® Cranberry Juice Cocktail is 27% cranberry juice. It contains filtered water, high fructose corn syrup, cranberry juice concentrate, and ascorbic acid.

## 13.4 Pharmacologic/Toxicologic Effects

### 13.4.1 Antimicrobial Activity

Controversy exists on the pharmacologic mechanism of cranberry. In the mid-19th century German researchers discovered hippuric acid in the urine of people who ate cranberries (Siciliano, 1996). From the 1920s through the 1970s, many researchers thought that hippuric acid produced a bacteriostatic effect by acidifying the urine (Blatherwick and Long 1923; Bodel et al., 1959; Avorn et al., 1994). The ability of cranberry to prevent renal calculi has also been attributed to its ability to decrease urine pH and inhibit bacterial growth (Sternlieb, 1963; Zinsser et al., 1968; Walsh, 1992). Not all studies documented a change in urinary pH with cranberry administration, so a parallel line of thinking suggested that hippuric acid, which was structurally similar to mandelic acid, inhibited bacterial multiplication (Bodel et al., 1959). It was found that the concentration of hippuric acid in the urine rarely reached a concentration necessary for bacteriostatic effects (Bodel et al., 1959). Because hippuric acid is a weak acid, it exists in equilibrium with its conjugate base, and requires a urine pH of at least 5.0 to produce the minimum bacteriostatic hippuric acid concentration. Thus, these researchers felt that both urine pH and hippuric acid concentration were important for the bacteriostatic effect of cranberry. More recently, however, studies have shown that the mechanism of action of cranberry is the inhibition of bacterial adherence to mucosal surfaces (Sobota, 1984; Schmidt and Sobota, 1988; Zafriri et al., 1989; Ofek et al., 1991; Avorn et al., 1994). One study proposed that there are two substances in cranberry juice cocktail, fructose and a glycoprotein, responsible for inhibiting adherence of *Escherichia coli* to mucosal cells (Zafriri et al., 1989).

*Escherichia coli* is responsible for 85% of urinary tract infections (Schultz, 1984). Virtually all *E. coli* express type 1 fimbrae, and most uropathogenic *E. coli* express P fimbriae which are responsible for mediating the adherence of the bacteria to uroepithelial cells (Zafriri et al., 1989). Fructose is responsible for inhibiting the adherence of type 1 fimbriated *E. coli* while a polymeric compound inhibits P fimbriated *E. coli* (Zafriri et al., 1989). Recently, a study (Howell and Vorsa, 1998) identified this polymeric compound as condensed tannins (proanthocyanidins) based on the ability of proanthocyanidins purified from cranberries to inhibit the ability of P-fimbriated *E. coli* to attach to isolated uroepithelial cells at concentrations of 10–50 μg/mL. Blueberries, another member of the *Vaccinium* genus, may be a more palatable source of proanthicyanidins.

Epidemiologic data (Foxman et al., 1995) and data from a double-blind, placebo-controlled trial (Avorn et al., 1994) support the use of cranberry juice to prevent urinary tract infections, although in the latter study differences in baseline characteristics between study groups may have influenced the results. Cranberry extract in capsule form was more effective than placebo in preventing recurrent urinary tract infections in a small study (Walker et al., 1997).

Another potential benefit to the use of cranberry is its antiviral effect. One study (Konowalchuk and Speirs, 1978) evaluated the ability of various commercial juices and beverages to inactivate poliovirus type I (Sabin) in vitro. Cranberry juice had some antiviral activity that was noted to be enhanced at pH > 7 (Konowalchuk and Speirs, 1978). The antiviral effect of commercial juices is thought to be due to polyphenols, including tannins, which form complexes with viruses (Konowalchuk and Speirs, 1978).

### *13.4.2 Gastrointestinal Effects*

The ingestion of large amounts of cranberry (>3–4 L/d) may result in diarrhea and other gastrointestinal symptoms (Anonymous, 1994).

### *13.4.3 Renal Effects*

Ammoniacal fermentation, or alkalinization and decomposition of urine, is responsible for the foul odor of urine (Kraemer, 1964). The results of one study (Kraemer, 1964) found that a single dose of 16 oz of cranberry juice lowered the urine pH of six men with chronic urinary tract disorders, and decreased ammoniacal odor and turbidity. The urine pH of five of six men free of urinary tract infections was also lowered with this dose. In another study (DuGan and Cardaciotto, 1966), hospital personnel noted a decrease in urine odor in the geriatric wards of a nursing home, but a change in urine pH or change in ammonia levels in the air could not be detected. Other subjective comments by nursing home personnel included a decrease in complaints among patients who had experienced burning upon urination, and more frequent voiding.

Another potential effect of the use of cranberry is in the management of calculus formation because of the association between alkalinization of the urine and stone formation (Sternlieb, 1963; Zinsser et al., 1968; Light et al., 1973; Walsh, 1992). A specially prepared sweetened cranberry juice consisting of 80% juice was administered to 41 people who were randomly assigned to ingest 150, 180, 210, or 240 mL of the juice with each meal for 1 wk (Kinney and Blount, 1979). Each subject served as his or her own control. Urine pH was measured by the subjects at each voiding, and a urine sample was collected daily after the evening meal. Mean urine pH was decreased to a statistically significant extent with cranberry juice ingestion compared to baseline. The decrease was not dose related. Cranberry juice had some effect in lowering daily fluctuations in urine pH, but this effect again was not dose related. The effect of cranberry juice on urine pH persisted throughout the experimental period (i.e., the kidney did not compensate for changes in pH). Side effects included weight gain and increased frequency of bowel movements.

In another study of cranberry's effect on urinary pH (Schultz, 1984), two 6-oz servings of cranberry juice daily for 20 d were able to lower urinary pH more than orange juice in eight multiple sclerosis patients, but were unable to lower pH consistently to below 5.5.

## 13.5 Chemical Analysis

Extracts of pure proanthocyanidins have been prepared using reverse-phase and adsorption chromatography, and their identity confirmed with $^{13}C$ nuclear magnetic resonance imaging, ultraviolet spectroscopy, and chemical reagent tests (Howell and Vorsa, 1998).

## 13.6 Regulatory Status

In the United States, cranberry is considered a dietary supplement and food (Blumenthal, 1997).

## References

Anonymous. Cranberry. Lawrence review of natural products. St. Louis, MO: Facts and Comparisons, 1994.

Avorn J, Monane M, Gurwitz JH, Glynn RJ, Choodnovskiy I, Lipstiz L. Reduction of bacteriuria and pyruia after ingestion of cranberry juice. JAMA 1994;271:751–4.

Blatherwick NR, Long ML. Studies of urinary acidity. II. The increased acidity produced by eating prunes and cranberries. J Biol Chem 1923;57:815–8.

Blumenthal M. Popular herbs in the U.S. market. Austin, TX: American Botanical Council, 1997.

Bodel PT, Cotran R, Kass EH. Cranberry juice and the antibacterial action of hippuric acid. J Lab Clin Med 1959;54:881–8.

DuGan CR, Cardaciotto PS. Reduction of ammoniacal urinary odors by the sustained feeding of cranberry juice. J Psychiatr Nurs 1966;8:467–70.

Foxman B, Geiger AM, Palin K, Gillespie B, and Koopman JS. First-time urinary tract infection and sexual behavior. Epidemiology 1995;6:162–8.

Howell AB, Vorsa N. Inhibition of the adherence of P-fimbriated *Escherichia coli* to uroepithelial-cell surfaces by proanthocyanidin extracts from cranberries. N Engl J Med 1998;339:1085–6.

Hughes BG, Lawson LD. Nutritional content of cranberry products [letter]. Am J Hosp Pharm 1989;46:1129.

Kinney AB, Blount M. Effect of cranberry juice on urinary pH. Nurs Res 1979;28: 287–90.

Konowalchuk J, Speirs JI. Antiviral effect of commercial juices and beverages. Appl Environ Microbiol 1978;35:1219–20.

Kraemer RJ. Cranberry juice and the reduction of ammoniacal odor of urine. Southwest Med 1964;45:211–2.

Light I, Gursel E, Zinnser HH. Urinary ionized calcium in urolithiasis. Effect of cranberry juice. Urology 1973;1:67–70.

Moen DV. Observations on the effectiveness of cranberry juice in urinary infections. Wisc Med J 1962;61:282–3.

Ofek I, Goldhar J, Zafriri D, Lis H, Adar R, Sharon N. Anti-*Escherichia coli* adhesion activity of cranberry and blueberry juices [letter]. N Engl J Med 1991;324:1599.

Papas PN, Brusch CA, Ceresia GC. Cranberry juice in the treatment of urinary tract infections. Southwest Med J 1966;47:17–20.

Schmidt DR, Sobota AE. An examination of the anti-adherence activity of cranberry juice on urinary and nonurinary bacterial isolates. Microbios 1988;55:173–81.

Schultz A. Efficacy of cranberry juice and ascorbic acid in acidifying the urine in multiple sclerosis subjects. J Comm Health Nurs 1984;1:159–69.

Siciliano A. Cranberry. Herbal Gram 1996;38:51–4.

Sobota AE. Inhibition of bacterial adherence by cranberry juice: potential use for the treatment of urinary tract infections. J Urol 1984;131:1013–6.

Sternlieb P. Cranberry juice in renal disease. N Engl J Med 1963;268:57.

Tyler, VE. The honest herbal, 3rd edit., Binghamton, NY: Pharmaceutical Products Press, 1993.

Walker EB, Barney DP, Mickelsen JN, Walton RJ, and Mickelsen RA Jr. Cranberry concentrate: UTI prophylaxis [letter]. J Fam Pract 1997;45:167–8.

Walsh B. Urostomy and urinary pH. J ET Nurs 1992;9:110–3.

Zafriri D, Ofek I, Adar R, Pocino M, Sharon N. Inhibitory activity of cranberry juice on adherence of type I and type P fimbriated *Escherichia coli* to eucaryotic cells. Antimicrob Agents Chemother 1989;33:92–8.

Zinsser HH, Seneca H, Light I, Mayer G, Karp F, McGeoy G, Tarrasoli H. Management of infected stones with acidifying agents. NY State J Med 1968;68:3001–9.

# Chapter 14

# Borage

## Melanie Johns Cupp

*Borago officinalis* (L.), common borage, bee bread, common bugloss, starflower, ox's tongue, cool tankard (Anonymous, 1992)

## 14.1 History and Traditional Uses

Borage is found throughout North America and Europe. The plant reaches a height of 2 ft, and is covered with coarse hairs. It has oval leaves and bright blue, star-shaped flowers with black anthers that bloom from May to September (Anonymous, 1992).

Borage has a salty flavor and smells like cucumbers. The leaves can be preserved in vinegar or eaten raw or cooked like spinach (Tyler, 1993). It has also been used in salads (Anonymous, 1992). Borage syrup, candy, jam, and jelly recipes are available, and some people make borage tea (Tyler, 1993).

Writers from the first century AD noted that borage leaves and flowers steeped in wine dispelled melancholy (Tyler, 1993). This use continued into the Middle Ages (Anonymous, 1992), although any beneficial effect on mood was probably due to the wine (Tyler, 1993). As early as the second century AD, borage was used to treat sore throat when mixed with honey, and is still recommended by herbalists for this purpose (Tyler, 1993). An infusion of the leaves and stems was once used as a diuretic, diaphoretic, and emollient (Tyler et al., 1981). Other traditional uses include relief of symptoms of rheumatism, colds, and bronchitis. It is also purported to increase breast milk production (Anonymous, 1992). A poultice of fresh leaves has been used to treat inflammation (Tyler et al., 1981).

From Forensic Science: *Toxicology and Clinical Pharmacology of Herbal Products*
Edited by: M. J. Cupp © Humana Press Inc., Totowa, New Jersey

## 14.2 Current Promoted Uses

Borage oil is promoted as a source of essential fatty acids. Marketers claim deficiency of essential fatty acids triggers fluctuations in blood glucose that lead to hunger and weight gain. Other promoted uses include treatment of rheumatoid arthritis, diabetic neuropathy, dermatitis, and hypertension.

## 14.3 Products Available

Borage leaf and whole herb can be purchased by the ounce. Borage seed oil softgel, 1000 mg (240 mg of γ-linolenic acid plus linoleic acid and 10 IU of vitamin E [*d*-α-tocopherol]), 1300-mg borage oil capsules (300 mg of γ-linolenic acid, 494 mg of linoleic acid, 221 mg of oleic acid), borage oil hard gelatin capsules (67 mg of γ-linolenic acid and 170 mg of linoleic acid), and 500-mg borage oil capsules are available. The oil is also available in bulk.

## 14.4 Pharmacologic/Toxicologic Effects

Borage contains tannins, mucilage, malic acid, potassium nitrate, mineral salts (Tyler, 1993), and approx 20–25% γ-linolenic acid (GLA), an ω-6 polyunsaturated essential fatty acid (Leventhal et al., 1993; Tyler, 1993). These ingredients are purported to have constipating and astringent properties (tannins), diuretic effects (malic acid and potassium nitrate), and expectorant action (mucilage) (Tyler, 1993).

### 14.4.1 Anti-Inflammatory Effects

Arachidonic acid (AA), present in cell membrane phospholipids, is the precursor to eicosanoids such as leukotrienes and prostaglandins that cause inflammation. GLA displaces AA and promotes formation of eicosanoids that are associated with less inflammatory activity than those produced from AA (Palombo et al., 1997); thus, GLA is hypothesized to decrease formation of inflammatory AA eicosanoid metabolites (Leventhal et al., 1993). GLA is converted in vivo to dihomo-γ-linolenic acid (DGLA), the immediate precursor to prostaglandin $E_1$ ($PGE_1$), which has antiinflammatory and immunoregulatory activity. DGLA has been shown to suppress interleukin-1 (IL-1) mediated synovial cell proliferation in vitro by increasing $PGE_1$ formation (Leventhal et al., 1993). DGLA is not converted to inflammatory leukotrienes by 5-lipoxygenase; it is converted to 15-hydroxy-dihomo-γ-linolenic acid (15-hydroxyeicosatrienoic acid; 15-HETrE), which suppresses 5-lipoxygenase activity and inflammatory leukotriene $B_4$ production (Chilton-Lopez et al., 1996). GLA also suppresses inflammatory $PGE_2$ production (Leventhal et al., 1993).

Dietary GLA lowered AA and increased DGLA in alveolar macrophages, liver Kupffer cells, and liver endothelial cells in rats (Palombo et al., 1997). DGLA accumulation was also seen in murine peritoneal macrophage phospholipids (Chapkin and Carmichael, 1990) and in rat platelets (Engler et al., 1991) after dietary borage oil supplementation. Borage oil added to the diet of Atlantic salmon has also been demonstrated to alter the fatty acid composition of hepatocyte phospholipids. Borage oil increased the percentage of $n-6$ polyunsaturated fatty acids, decreased the percentage of $n-3$ polyunsaturated fatty acids, and increased fatty acid desaturation and elongation (Tocher et al., 1997a). Similar results were noted in a study using another type of fish (turbot), with a concomitant increase in $PGE_1$ (Tocher et al., 1997b). Turbot heart phospholipids demonstrated an increase in GLA and DGLA, and a decrease in AA, while $PGE_1$ content was increased in heart, kidney, and gill (Bell et al., 1995). These changes in phospholipid fatty acid composition have also been demonstrated in humans. GLA-enriched borage oil, 480 mg or 1500 mg, significantly ($p < 0.05$) increased DGLA in polymorphonuclear neutrophil (PMN) phospholipids and decreased PMN production of leukotriene $B_4$ (Ziboh and Fletcher, 1992).

The anti-inflammatory effects of borage seed oil have been demonstrated in animal models. A diet enriched with borage seed oil (23% GLA) was compared to one with safflower oil (<1% GLA) with regard to effects on acute inflammation induced by monosodium urate crystals, subacute or chronic inflammation caused by Freund's adjuvant in a subcutaneous air pouch, or adjuvant-induced arthritis (Tate et al., 1989). Borage seed oil, but not safflower oil, decreased inflammation in all models. In addition, the ratio of DGLA to AA was five times that in the livers of animals fed safflower oil.

In humans, T-lymphocyte proliferation, which is involved in the pathophysiology of rheumatoid arthritis (RA), was reduced with the administration of 2.4g GLA as borage seed oil, and was associated with increased GLA and DGLA concentrations in plasma cells and monocytes (Rossetti et al., 1997). In an open, uncontrolled study (Pullman-Moar et al., 1990), nine borage seed oil capsules daily were administered for 12 wk to seven patients with active RA, and to seven "normal" patients. DGLA increased in monocytes, and there was a decrease in the production of the inflammatory mediators $PGE_2$, leukotriene $B_4$, and leukotriene $C_4$ by stimulated monocytes. In addition, the DGLA content of the phospholipid bilayer of plasma cells, mononuclear cells, and platelets increased. Six of seven RA patients improved clinically.

A larger controlled study has also demonstrated the benefits of borage seed oil in RA. A 24-wk, randomized, double-blind study (Leventhal et al., 1993) compared four borage seed oil capsules three times daily with cottonseed oil capsule placebo RA patients (Leventhal et al., 1993). Each capsule contained 0.6 mL of oil and 13.6 IU of vitamin E. The borage seed oil contained 23% GLA, 62% linoleic acid, 8% oleic acid, and 7% other fatty acids, providing a total of 1.4 g GLA (Boracelle capsules with oil of borage, Bio Oil Research Ltd., Nantwich, Cheshire, England). The cottonseed oil placebo capsules contained 54% linoleic acid, 18% oleic acid, 24% palmitic acid, and 4% other fatty acids (Bio Oil Research Ltd). Thirty-seven adult patients with RA diagnoses according to the revised criteria of the American Rheumatism Association were enrolled in the study. Patients had been taking stable doses of nonsteroidal antiinflammatory drugs (NSAIDs) and/or 10 mg of prednisone or equivalent for at least a month, and were maintained on these doses throughout the study. Patients were excluded if they had taken other antirheumatic drugs within 3 mo of study enrollment. Patients were permitted to take medications for other medical conditions. Disease was assessed every 6 wk according to: (1) physician's global assessment on a scale from 0 to 4, (2) patient's global assessment on a scale from 0 to 4, (3) number of tender or painful joints upon pressure or passive motion (0–68), (4) number of joints with swelling (0–66), (5) joint pain or tenderness score (0–3), (6) joint swelling score (0–3), (7) duration of morning stiffness in minutes, (8) ability to perform occupational and domestic activities, and (9) grip strength. Complete blood count, including differential and platelet count, blood chemistries, urinalysis, and rheumatoid factor were checked at wk 0 and 24, and erythrocyte sedimentation rate (SED rate) was measured at wk 12 and 24. Important improvement was defined as a 25% improvement in continuous variables, and an improvement of two levels for scaled variables. Meaningful improvement was defined as important improvement of at least four of the following: tender joint count or score, swollen joint count or score, physician global assessment, patient global assessment, morning stiffness, or SED rate. Baseline and clinical data were similar between the two groups; however, more patients in the placebo group had required hydroxychloroquine in the past. Patients treated with GLA showed significant improvement from baseline in the joint tenderness score, joint swelling score, and platelet count, while the placebo group did not improve. Compared to placebo, GLA patients had significantly better joint tenderness counts and scores, joint swelling scores, global assessment by physician, pain by scaled assessment, and reduced platelet count. If only those patients who completed the study are considered (five patients in each group dropped out), baseline data between the placebo and GLA groups did not differ except that GLA patients had more morning stiffness and higher joint tenderness scores. Placebo patients who completed the study did not improve in any variable. The GLA patients who completed the study showed significant improvement from baseline in number of tender joints, joint tenderness score, number of swollen joints, swollen joint score, global assessment by physician, visual analog pain assessment, morning stiffness, and platelet count. Compared to placebo, GLA was significantly ($p < 0.05$) better than placebo in improving tender joint count, joint tenderness score, number of swollen joints, joint swelling score, global assessment by physician, and pain assessed by visual analog and by scaled assessment. Although seven GLA patients had meaningful improvement (important improvement in at least four measures), seven had no meaningful improvement, and none went into remission. No GLA patient showed deterioration. One placebo patient had meaningful improvement, eight had no meaningful improvement, and four deteriorated. Adverse effects included soft stools (two GLA and one placebo patient), flatulence (one GLA patient), belching (one GLA patient), and rash (one placebo patient). Although further study is needed, it appears that borge oil providing 1.4 g of GLA per day is a moderately effective adjunctive therapy in the treatment of RA. Lower doses of GLA (480–540 mg/d) have not shown the objective benefits demonstrated in this study.

### *14.4.2 Dermatologic Effects*

Seborrheic dermatitis is associated with aberrant serum levels of essential fatty acids and the presence of *Malassezia furfur*. Borage oil containing 25% GLA used topically has been effective in the treatment of seborrheic dermatitis in children, but it does not affect the growth of *Malassezia furfur* (Tollesson et al., 1997).

Dietary borage oil may have a beneficial effect on inflammatory skin disorders. Guinea pigs fed borage oil as part of their diet had elevated levels of DGLA and its metabolite 15-HETrE in epidermal phospholipids. Although there was no change in epidermal prostaglandins, 15-HETrE is thought to have antiinflammatory effects (Miller et al., 1990).

Human dermatologic conditions such as eczema and atopic dermatitis may benefit from borage oil. Compared to 3% safflower oil cream or placebo cream, cream containing 3% borage oil significantly decreased skin roughness and transepidermal water loss, and increased skin moisture in volunteers with dry skin or surfactant-induced scaly skin (Nissen et al., 1995). In another study, topical borage oil had no effect on visible signs of irritation, cutaneous blood flow, or transepidermal water loss in either normal or surfactant (sodium lauryl sulfate)-irritated skin (Loden and Andersson, 1996). Atopic dermatitis may benefit from oral administration of borage oil, but more study is needed to confirm efficacy and to identify which patient characteristics predict response (Bahmer and Schafer, 1992; Borrek et al., 1997).

### 14.4.3 Respiratory Effects

An uncontrolled study (Christophe et al., 1994) in patients with cystic fibrosis demonstrated an increase in vital capacity after 4 wk of supplementation with 1500 mg of borage oil (330 mg of GLA) daily. AA content of serum phospholipids was increased, although they would be expected to decrease based on results of other studies. AA, DGLA, and linoleic acid content of cholesterol esters also increased.

### 14.4.4 Carcinogenicity

Although other members of the Boraginaceae family contain hepatocarcinogenic pyrrolizidine alkaloids, there are no reports of similar compounds in common borage (Anonymous, 1992).

### 14.4.5 Hematologic Effects

GLA at a dose of 5.23 g provided as borage oil for 42 d in male volunteers increased platelet phospholipid DGLA (Barre and Holub, 1992), but borage oil at doses of 3 g/d has been shown not to affect human platelet aggregation (Bard et al., 1997).

### 14.4.6 Effects in Diabetic Neuropathy

Dietary supplementation with 1% borage oil and other GLA-containing oils ameliorated diminished motor and sensory nerve conduction velocity in diabetic rats, but efficacy did not correlate with GLA content of the various oils (Dines et al., 1996).

### 14.4.7 Cardiovascular Effects

Dietary borage oil decreased blood pressure in both spontaneously hypertensive and normotensive rats via an unknown mechanism. Cholesterol levels and activity of β-hydroxy-3-methylglutaryl coenzyme A (HMG-CoA) reductase were increased (Engler et al., 1992).

A diet supplemented with GLA and eicosapentaenoic acids improved oxygen delivery by decreasing vascular resistance and increasing cardiac index in endotoxin-induced lung injury in pigs. This mechanism is thought to involve attenuation of endotoxin-induced thromboxane $B_2$ synthesis (Murray et al., 1995). A study (Mancuso et al., 1997) in endotoxic rats demonstrated that in addition to attenuation of thromboxane B2 production, production of leukotriene $B_4$, leukotriene $C_4/D_4$, and $PGF_{1\alpha}$, as well as neutrophil accumulation, was attenuated. Lung phospholipid concentrations of AA were decreased and DGLA was increased.

Cardiovascular effects have also been demonstrated in humans. Borage oil at a dose of 4.5 mL/d for 4 wk in nine normotensive volunteers augmented arterial baroreflex control of vascular resistance as measured by plasma norepinephrine levels and vasoconstrictor response to a 40 mm Hg drop in lower body pressure (Mills et al., 1990).

Borage oil administered to male volunteers for 28 d attenuated the blood pressure, heart rate, and skin temperature response to the Stroop color–word conflict test, and improved task performance (Mills et al., 1989).

## 14.5 Case Reports of Toxicity

A 72-yr-old woman developed nausea, vomiting, diarrhea, "flickering" in her eyes, and palpitations after drinking what she believed to be borage leaf tea. Blood pressure was 120/75 mm Hg, and heart rate was irregular at 52 beats/min. She was taking no other medications. EKG revealed atrial fibrillation with a slow ventricular rate with pauses of up to 1.5 s, intermittent type I and type II block, and ST segment depression. Other aspects of the physical exam and laboratory investigations were unremarkable, except a digoxin level of 3.93 ng/mL and a digitoxin level of 133.5 ng/mL. Apparently, the patient had mistaken foxglove, which contains digitalis glycosides, for borage. The patient improved with symptomatic treatment. Although this patient's toxicity was not due to borage, this case demonstrates the need for clarification of the identity of herbal remedies used by patients for self-medication (Brustbauer and Wenisch, 1997).

## 14.6 Pharmacokinetics/Toxicokinetics

GLA is metabolized to DGLA in neutrophils by the addition of two carbons. DGLA is metabolized to 15-hydroxyeicosatrienoic acid (Chilton-Lopez et al., 1996) by 5-lipoxygenase (Miller et al., 1990).

## 14.7 Chemical Analysis

Capillary gas chromatography has been used to analyze GLA content of evening primrose oil (Gibson et al., 1992). GLA in borage seed oil has been separated using silver-ion high-performance liquid chromatography (HPLC) with on-line atmospheric pressure chemical ionization-mass spectrometric (APCI-MS) detection (Laasko and Voutilainen, 1996).

## 14.8 Regulatory Status

Borage oil is regulated as a dietary supplement in the United States. Borage is not approved by the German Commission E because of the possibility of hepatocarcinogenic/hepatotoxic pyrrolizidine alkaloids and undocumented effectiveness (Blumenthal, 1998).

## REFERENCES


Anonymous. Borage. The Lawrence review of natural products. St. Louis, MO: Facts and Comparisons, 1992.

Bahmer FA, Schafer J. [Treatment of atopic dermatitis with borage seed oil (Glandol)—a time series analytic study]. Kinderarztl Prax 1992;60:199–202.

Bard JM, Luc G, Jude B, Bordet JC, Lacroix B, Bonte JP, et al. A therapeutic dosage (3 g/d) of borage oil supplementation has no effect on platelet aggregation in healthy volunteers. Fundam Clin Pharmacol 1997;11:143–4.

Barre DE, Holub BJ. The effect of borage oil consumption on the composition of individual phospholipids in human platelets. Lipids 1992;27:315–20.

Bell JG, Tocher DR, MacDonald FM, Sargent JR. Diets rich in eicosapentaenoic acid and gamma-linolenic acid affect phospholipid fatty acid composition and production of prostaglandins E1, E2, and E3 in turbot (*Scophthalmus maximus*), a species deficient in delta 5 fatty acid desaturase. Prostagland Leukotr Essent Fatty Acids 1995;53: 279–86.

Blumenthal M. The complete German Commission E monographs. Therapeutic guide to herbal medicines. Austin, TX: American Botanical Council, 1998.

Borrek S, Hildebrandt A, Forster J. [Gamma-linolenic-acid-rich borage seed oil capsules in children with atopic dermatitis. A placebo-controlled double-blind study]. Klin Padiatr 1997;209:100–4.

Brustbauer R, Wenisch C. [Bradycardiac atrial fibrillation after drinking herbal tea]. Dtsch Med Wochenschr 1997;122:930–2.

Chapkin RS, Carmichael SL. Effects of dietary $n-3$ and $n-6$ polyunsaturated fatty acids on macrophage phospholipid classes and subclasses. Lipids 1990;25:827–34.

Chilton-Lopez T, Surette ME, Swan DD, Fonteh AN, Johnson MM, Chilton FH. Metabolism of gamma linolenic acid in human neutrophils. J Immunol 1996;156:2941–7.

Christophe A, Robberecht E, Franckx H, DeBsets F, van de Pas M. Effect of administration of gamma-linolenic acid on the fatty acid composition of serum phospholipids and cholesteryl esters in patients with cystic fibrosis. Ann Nutr Metab 1994;38:40–7.

Dines KC, Cotter MA, Cameron NE. Effectiveness of natural oils as sources of gamma-linolenic acid to correct peripheral nerve conduction velocity abnormalities in diabetic rats: modulation by thromboxane A2 inhibition. Prostagland Leukotr Essent Fatty Acids 1996;55:159–65.

Engler MM, Karanian JW, Salem N Jr. Ethanol inhalation and dietary $n-6$, $n-3$, and $n-9$ fatty acids in the rat: effect on platelet and aortic fatty acid composition. Alcohol Clin Exp Res 1991;15:483–8.

Engler MM, Engler MB, Erickson SK, Paul SM. Dietary gamma-linolenic acid lowers blood pressure and alters aortic reactivity and cholesterol metabolism in hypertension. J Hypertens 1992;10:1197–204.

Gibson RA, Lines DR, Neumann MA. Gamma linolenic acid (GLA) content of encapsulated evening primrose oil products. Lipids 1992;27:82–4.

Laakso P, Voutilainen P. Analysis of triacylglycerols by silver-ion high-performance liquid chromatography-atmospheric pressure chemical ionization spectrometry. Lipids 1996;31:1311–22.

Leventhal LJ, Boyce EG, Zurier RB. Treatment of rheumatoid arthritis with gammalinolenic acid. Ann Intern Med 1993;119:867–73.

Loden M, Andersson AC. Effect of topically applied lipids on surfactant-irritated skin. Br J Dermatol 1996;134:215–20.

Mancuso P, Whelan J, DeMichele SJ, Snider CC, Guszcza JA, Karlstad MD. Dietary fish oil and borage oil suppress intrapulmonary proinflammatory eicosanoid biosynthesis and attenuate pulmonary neutrophil accumulation in endotoxic rats. Clin Care Med 1997;25:1198–206.

Miller CC, Ziboh VA, Wong T, Fletcher MP. Dietary supplementation with oils rich in (*n* – 3) and (*n* – 6) fatty acids influences in vivo levels of epidermal lipoxygenase products in guinea pigs. J Nutr 1990;120:36–44.

Mills DE, Mah M, Ward RP, Morris BL, Floras JS. Alteration of baroreflex control of forearm vascular resistance by dietary fatty acids. Am J Physiol 1990;259 (6 Pt 2): R116–71.

Murray MJ, Kumar M, Gregory TJ, Banks PL, Tazelaar HD, De Michele SJ. Select dietary fatty acids attenuate cardiopulmonary dysfunction during acute lung injury in pigs. Am J Physiol 1995;269 (6 Pt 2):H2090–9.

Nissen HP, Biltz H, Muggli R. Borage oil. Cosmet Toiletr 1995;110:71–3, 76.

Palombo JD, De Michele SJ, Lydon E, Bistrian BR. Cyclic vs continuous enteral feeding with omega-3 and gamma-linolenic fatty acids: effects on modulation of phospholipid fatty acids in rat lung and liver immune cells. JPEN 1997;21:123–32.

Pullman-Moar S, Laposata M, Lem D, Holman RT, Leventhal LJ, DeMarcoD, Zurier RB. Alteration of the cellular fatty acid profile and the production of eicosanoids in human monocytes by gamma-linolenic acid. Arthrit Rheum 1990;33:1526–33.

Rossetti RG, Seiler CM, DeLuca P, Laposata M, Zurier RB. Oral administration of unsaturated fatty acids: effects on human peripheral blood T lymphocyte proliferation. J Leukoc Biol 1997;62:438–43.

Tate G, Mandell BF, Laposata M, Ohlinger D, Baker DG, Schumacher HR, Zurier RB. Suppression of acute and chronic inflammation by dietary gamma linolenic acid. J Rheumatol 1989;16:729–34.

Tocher DR, Bell JG, Dick JR, Sargent JR. Fatty acyl desaturation in isolated hepatocytes form Atlantic salmon (*Salmo salar*): stimulation of dietary borage oil containing gamma-linolenic acid. Lipids 1997a;32:1237–47.

Tocher DR, Bell JG, Ferndale BM, Sargent JR. Effects of dietary gamma-linolenic acid-rich borage oil combined with murine fish oils on tissue phospholipid fatty acid composition and production of prostaglandins E and F of the 1-, 2-, and 3-series in a marine fish deficient in delta 5 fatty acyl desaturase. Prostagland Leukotr Essent Fatty Acids 1997b;57:125–34.

Tollesson A, Frithz A, Stenlund K. Lalassezia furfur in infantile seborrheic dermatitis. Pediatr Dermatol 1997;14:423–5.

Tyler VE. The honest herbal, Binghamton, NY: Pharmaceutical Products Press, 1993.

Tyler VE, Brady LR, Robbers JE. Pharmacognosy, 8th edit., Philadelphia: Lea and Febiger, 1981.

Ziboh VA, Fletcher MP. Dose–response effects of dietary gamma-linolenic acid-enriched oils on human polymorphonuclear-neutrophil biosynthesis of leukotriene B4. Am J Clin Nutr 1992;55:39–45.

# *Chapter 15*

# Calamus

*Melanie Johns Cupp*

*Acorus calamus*, rat root, sweet flag, sweet myrtle, sweet root, sweet sedge (Anonymous, 1996), vekhand (Samudralwar and Garg 1996 ), sweet cane, sweet grass, sweet segg, cinnamon-sedge, beewort, myrtle-flag, myrtle-grass, myrtle-sedge, sweet rush (Harding, 1972)

## *15.1 History and Traditional Uses*

Calamus is a perennial iris-like plant that grows in moist habitats near swamps, ponds, and streams in North America, Europe, and Asia (Tyler, 1993), reaching heights of 6 ft (Anonymous, 1996). Calamus is described in the Indian Ayurvedic literature (Samudralwar and Garg, 1996) and has been known since biblical times (Tyler, 1993). It has been used for centuries to treat gastrointestinal distress including colic in children (Tyler, 1993), and as a sedative (Anonymous, 1996). A rhizome infusion is used to treat fevers and dyspepsia, while chewing the rhizome is recommended to clear the voice (Tyler, 1993), relieve dyspepsia, aid digestion (Harding, 1972), and remove tobacco odor from the breath (Anonymous, 1996). The powdered rhizome is used as a cooking spice (Tyler, 1993), and calamus oil, which is responsible for the plant's odor and taste (Anonymous, 1996), is used in pharmaceuticals and foods in India (Balachandran et al., 1991; Sivaswamy et al., 1991). In the United States, calamus was once used to flavor tooth powders, beer, bitters, and various tonics (Tyler, 1993), while in rural Pakistan it is commonly used even today as a medicine in children (Riazuddin et al., 1987).

From Forensic Science: *Toxicology and Clinical Pharmacology of Herbal Products*
Edited by: M. J. Cupp © Humana Press Inc., Totowa, New Jersey

## 15.2 Current Promoted Uses

Calamus is not promoted commercially in the United States.

## 15.3 Products Available

Calamus products are not widely available in the United States.

## 15.4 Pharmacologic/Toxicologic Effects

### 15.4.1 Carcinogenicity

There are four varieties of *Acorus calamus* based on content of isoasarone (β-asarone; *cis*-isoasarone), which has been shown to cause duodenal tumors in rats (Tyler, 1993). Type I is found in North America and contains practically no isoasarone (Anonymous, 1996). Type II is found in Europe and the oil contains <10% isoasarone, while the oils of types III and IV contain up to 96% isoasarone.

### 15.4.2 Mutagenicity/Genotoxicity

Calamus oil was strongly mutagenic in *Salmonella typhimurium* in one study (Sivaswamy et al., 1991), but had exhibited no mutagenic activity in a previous study (Riazuddin et al., 1987).

Calamus oil in a dose of 0.005 mL fed daily in powdered chow for 35 d was found to be genotoxic in Swiss mice (Balachandran et al., 1991). These effects were attributed to β-asarone, which was previously demonstrated to cause chromosomal aberrations and an increase in the rate of sister chromatid exchanges in human lymphocytes.

### 15.4.3 Antimicrobial Activity

In vitro, both isomers of asarone were shown to inhibit motility of *Toxocara canis* larvae and to have larvicidal activity, depending on duration of exposure (Sugimoto, 1995).

### 15.4.4 Central Nervous System Effects

The psychoactive effects of *Ascora calamus* in humans are not well documented, but there is limited evidence that the plant is used as an ingredient in intoxicating Indian ritual snuffs (de Smet, 1985), and the crude plant potentiates barbiturate and ethanol-induced sedation in mice (Anonymous, 1996). *Cis*-isoasarone is thought to be the component of calamus responsible for these sedative properties.

Calamus oil administered intraperitoneally at doses of 10–100 mg/kg in rats, mice, dogs, cats, and monkeys decreased spontaneous movements, muscle tone, and response to tactile and auditory stimuli in a dose-dependent fashion (Dhalla and Bhattacharya, 1968). Motor activity decreased by 95% at the highest dose compared to controls, and the animals became docile. This sedation was characteristic of that induced by chlorpromazine or reserpine. No deaths occurred at any dose. The onset of action was 10–20 min, and the effects lasted from 2 to 48 h depending upon the dose and animal to which it was administered. Repeated vomiting occurred in dogs, cats, and monkeys during the first 4 h after administration. The specific neurotransmitters involved in calamus oil-induced sedation are thought to be serotonin (Dhalla and Bhattacharya, 1968) or norepinephrine (Menon and Dandiya, 1967; Dhalla and Bhattacharya, 1968). Monoamine oxidase inhibition occurs in vitro, but at doses exceeding those necessary for sedation in animal models (Dhalla and Bhattacharya, 1968).

In mice, an alcohol extract of calamus roots and rhizomes at doses of 10–50 mg/kg administered intraperitoneally exhibited sedative properties as evidenced by decreased amphetamine-induced and spontaneous motor activity, but was less potent than chlorpromazine in this regard (Panchal et al., 1989). The alcohol extract did not protect frogs from strychnine-induced convulsions at doses up to 20 mg/kg administered intraperitoneally.

### *15.4.5 Musculoskeletal Effects*

(*See also* Section 15.4.4)

A water-soluble dried powder of an alcohol extract of the roots and rhizomes of *Ascora calamus* was shown to inhibit caffeine citrate-induced contractions of frog rectus muscle, but was unable to inhibit muscle contractions induced by acetylcholine (Panchal et al., 1989). Such spasmolytic effects have also been demonstrated with the volatile oil in smooth muscle in other animal models, including isolated rat intestine and uterus, isolated rabbit intestine and aorta, and isolated cat trachea (Maj et al., 1966). Calamus oil was also shown to protect guinea pigs from death due to histamine inhalation, and to improve perfusion in rat hind legs (Maj et al., 1966). In contrast to the sedative effects of calamus, isoasarone is not thought to be the component responsible for spasmolytic activity; isoasarone-free oil from the type I plant had a pronounced spasmolytic effect, while oil from the type IV plant (isoasarone-rich) has no spasmolytic effect (Anonymous, 1996).

### *15.4.6 Cardiovascular Effects*

In vitro, negative ino- and chronotropic effects have been demonstrated at doses of 1, 10, and 100 mg/mL (Panchal et al., 1989).

### 15.4.7 $LD_{50}$

The $LD_{50}$ of asarone in mice was 417.6 mg/kg given enterally, and 310 mg/kg given intraperitoneally (Belova et al., 1985).

### 15.4.8 Reproductive Effects

Calamus oil vapor was able to induce sterility in male houseflies (Mathur and Saxena, 1975). Calamus oil vapor prevented housefly hatching and molting at a 100 ppm dilution (Saxena and Rohdendorf, 1974).

### 15.4.9 Local Anesthetic Effects

Calamus extract at concentrations of 0.5% and 1% of exhibited no local anesthetic activity in guinea pigs and rabbits (Panchal et al., 1989).

## 15.5 Case Reports of Toxicity

Other than contact dermatitis (Mitchell and Rook, 1979), human toxicity has not been reported.

## 15.6 Chemical Analysis

Gas chromatographic (GC) analysis of asarone has been described (Sugimoto et al., 1995).

## 15.7 Regulatory Status

The use of calamus as a flavoring agent in dentifrices, beverages, and medicines in the United States was banned because of concerns over its carcinogenicity (Tyler, 1993; Anonymous, 1996). Despite this ban, calamus can still be found in some herb shops in the United States.

## References

Anonymous. Calamus. The review of natural products. St. Louis, MO: Facts and Comparisons, 1996.

Balachandran B, Sivaswamy SN, Sivaramakrishnan VM. Genotoxic effects of some foods and food components in Swiss mice. Indian J Med Res 1991;94:378–83.

Belova LF, Alibekov SD, Baginskaia AI, Sokolov SI, Pokrovshaia GV. Asarone and its biological properties. Farmakol Toksikol 1985;48:17–20

de Smet PA. A multidisciplinary overview of intoxicating snuff rituals in the western hemisphere. J Ethnopharmacol 1985;13:3–49

Dhalla NS, Bhattacharya IC. Further studies on neuropharmacological actions of acorus oil. Arch Int Pharmacodyn Ther 1968;172:352.

Harding AR. Ginseng and other medicinal plants. Columbus, OH: AR Harding, 1972.

Maj J, Malec D, Lastowski Z. pharamcological properties of the native calamus (*Acorus calamus* L). 3. Spasmolytic effect of etheric oil. Acta Pol Pharm 1966;23:477–82.

Mathur AC, Saxena BP. Induction of sterility in male houseflies by vapors of *Acorus calamus* L. oil. Naturwissenschaften 1975;62:576–7.

Menon MK, Dandiya PC. The mechanism of the tranquilizing action of asarone from *Acorus calamus* Linn. J Pharm Pharmacol 1967;19:170–5.

Mitchell J, Rook A. Botanical dematology. Vancouver: Greengrass, 1979.

Panchal GM, Venkatakrishna-Bhatt H, Doctor RB, Vajpayee S. Pharmacology of *Acorus calamus* L. Indian J Exp Biol 1989;27:561–7.

Riazuddin S, Malik MM, Nasim A. Mutagenicity testing of some medicinal herbs. Environ Mol Mutagen 1987;10:141–8.

Samudralwar DL, Garg AN. Minor and trace elemental determination in the Indian herbal and other medicinal preparations. Biol Trace Elem Res 1996;54:113–21.

Saxena BP Rohdendorf Be. Morphological changes in *Thermobia domestica* uunder the influence of *Acorus calamus* oil vapors. Experientia 1974;30:1298–300.

Sivaswamy SN, Balachandran B, Balanehru S, Sivaramakrishnan VM. Mutagenic activity of south Indian food items. Indian J Exp Biol 1991;29:730–7.

Sugimoto N, Goto Y, Akao N, Kiuchi F, Kondo K, Tsuda Y. Mobility inhibition and nematocidal activity of asarone and related phenylpropanoids on second-stage larvae of *Toxocara*. Biol Pharmaceut Bull 1995;18:605–9.

Tyler VE. The honest herbal, 3rd edit., Binghamton, NY: Pharmaceutical Products Press, 1993.

# Chapter 16

# Chaparral

*Kim Melgarejo and Melanie Johns Cupp*

*Larrea tridentata* Coville, synonymous with *L. divaricata* Cav. and *L. mexicana* Moric (Tyler, 1993), *L. glutinosa* Englem, creosote bush, greaseweed, hediondilla (Anonymous, 1993); *L. nitida*, *L. ameghinoi*, *L. cuneifolia* (Leonforte, 1986)

## 16.1 History and Traditional Uses

Chaparral is a broad term that describes any thicket of wild shrubs and dwarf trees, but chaparral, the herb, is known more specifically by the names listed above (Tyler, 1993). Chaparral is able to survive the arid deserts of the United States and Mexico. The shrub is a branched bush that grows to 9 ft in height. Its bilobed leaves have a resinous feel and strong smell (Anonymous, 1993). This olive-green bush was used medicinally by Native Americans. Chaparral purportedly possesses analgesic, expectorant, emetic, diuretic, and antiinflammatory properties, and has been used in the treatment of arthritis, colds, tuberculosis, and cancer. It has also been used as a hair tonic, and as an antidote for LSD flashbacks (Tyler, 1993). Tea made from boiled leaves has been used to treat sexually transmitted diseases and intestinal cramps, and to stimulate urination. The leaves were soaked in water to produce an extract used as a bath for rheumatism and chickenpox. The dried powdered leaves were used as a dusting powder for sores, and were mixed with badger oil to make an ointment used on burns to aid new skin formation (Waller and Gisvold, 1945).

Nordihydroguaiaretic acid (NDGA), purportedly the active constituent of chaparral, was first isolated in 1945 (Waller and Gisvold, 1945). NDGA was used as a food antioxidant from 1945 to 1967, in products such as lards, oils, candies, baking mixes, frozen foods, vitamins, and pharmaceuticals at levels of 0.01–0.02% (Smart et al., 1969).

From Forensic Science: *Toxicology and Clinical Pharmacology of Herbal Products*
Edited by: M. J. Cupp © Humana Press Inc., Totowa, New Jersey

## 16.2 Current Promoted Uses

Based on the finding that NDGA is an antioxidant, chaparral has been promoted as an anticancer agent (Tyler, 1993). In a recent review (Sheikh, 1997) of chaparral-associated hepatotoxicity, patients reported using chaparral as a general cleansing tonic, internal skin cleanser, blood thinner, arthritis remedy, antiasthmatic, nutritional supplement, and weight loss product.

## 16.3 Products Available

Chaparral can be found in health food stores and on various sites on the World Wide Web. Products available include leaves, stems, and bark in bulk to be used in brewing tea. The tea is made by steeping the dried leaves and stems in hot water. Approximately 7–8 g of leaves are used per quart of water (Smart et al., 1969). Capsules and tablets have also been formulated in various dosages. Products can be found containing chaparral as the only active ingredient, or in combination with other herbs. Dosages used by patients in a case series detailing chaparral-associated hepatotoxicity and other adverse effects (Sheikh, 1997) included 100-mg, 400-mg, 450-mg, and 480-mg capsules and 64.8-mg and 100-mg tablets.

There are several on-line sources for chaparral and chaparral-containing products advertising chaparral capsules, cut herb, herb powder, tincture, concentrated liquid for compresses, and various combination products for colds, flu, arthritis, detoxification, immune system enhancement, and adrenal protection.

## 16.4 Pharmacologic/Toxicologic Effects

### *16.4.1 Antineoplastic Activity*

Antineoplastic activity was first noted in 1959 when the National Cancer Institute (NCI) received correspondence from laypersons claiming that cancer patients were benefiting from the consumption of chaparral tea. In subsequent studies, the NCI determined that NDGA was effective against cancer cells in vitro, but not in mice (Anonymous, 1993). It was theorized that the antineoplastic activity of NDGA was dependent upon the difference between the primary method of production of energy in cancer cells vs normal cells; cancer cells were thought to more frequently utilize anaerobic glycolysis (Smart et al., 1969), a process that can be inhibited by NDGA. Specifically, NDGA is a reducing substance that maintains NAD in its reduced state (i.e., NADH). Without NAD, the conversion of glyceraldehyde 3-phosphate to 1,3-diphosphoglyceric acid is blocked, and so is the anaerobic synthesis of ATP (i.e., glycolysis). NDGA does not irreversibly inhibit the reaction, and NDGA's effect can be reversed in vitro by addition of NAD or pyruvate (Burk and Woods, 1963). This reversibility may explain NDGA's lack of antineoplastic effect in mice, or perhaps it is because, as in rats, it is metabolized in the gut to an oxidizing agent (Grice et al., 1968). Interestingly, there is evidence that NDGA has some antineoplastic activity in mice when combined with the antioxidant ascorbic acid (Smart et al., 1969). More recently, NDGA has been shown to interrupt mitochondrial respiration as well as anaerobic glycolysis processes via interruption of the $NAD^+/NADH$ balance (Pavani et al., 1994).

Case reports suggest chaparral may have some antineoplastic effects in humans. An elderly male had a 3–4 mm brown, slightly raised mole on his right cheek near the nasolabial fold that darkened and enlarged over 1–2 yr. The lesion was excised. He was told that it was malignant, but that it had been completely removed. It recurred within a year, requiring a second excision, then recurred and required a third excision. It recurred a fourth time, but the patient did not seek medical care until the lesion reached a size of 3 × 4 cm with small satellite lesions and a tender 5 × 7 cm mass in the right submandibular area. During the 6–9 mo prior to seeking medical attention, the patient had become pale, weak, lethargic, and slightly cachectic. A wedge biopsy of the facial lesion and a needle biopsy of the neck mass revealed malignant melanoma and necrotic debris, respectively. Because he was 85 yr old, the patient decided to forego the recommended surgical excision and radical neck dissection. One month later, the patient began drinking chaparral tea prepared by steeping 7–8 g of dried leaves and stems per quart of hot water. He drank two or three cups of the tea daily. He rarely missed a dose, and took no other medications. Three months later, his children noted that the facial lesion had decreased to the size of a dime, the neck mass had disappeared, and he looked better and had begun to regain lost weight. Eleven months after his initial diagnosis, he returned to the clinic. Physical exam revealed that the cheek lesion had decreased to 2 × 3 mm, and the satellite lesions and neck mass had disappeared. He had gained approx 25 lbs and looked healthier. The stems and leaves that the patient had been using to make the tea were positively identified by the University of Utah Department of Botany as *Larrea divaricata* Cav. The leaves and stems were analyzed by the College of Pharmacy and found to contain 7–8% NDGA dry weight. The patient's method of tea preparation extracted approx 40% of the NDGA, yielding a total daily dose of 200–250 mg of NDGA (Smart et al., 1969).

Additional cases of tumor regression associated with chaparral tea use were observed by physicians at the University of Utah and included two patients with melanoma, one with metastatic choriocarcinoma, and one with widespread lymphosarcoma. Of the melanoma patients, one experienced 95% regression with excision of the remaining tumor, but the other developed a new lesion after a 4-mo remission. The lymphosarcoma patient experienced a 75% regression in tumor size after only 2 d of chaparral use, after which he discontinued the tea. The choriocarcinoma patient responded to the tea for 2 mo despite poor response to other therapies, then relapsed (Anonymous, 1993). The benefit seen in these case reports may represent spontaneous regression, or in some cases may be attributable to other treatments administered.

### *16.4.2 Hepatotoxicity*

Several cases of hepatotoxicity associated with chaparral use have been described (*see* Section 16.5). The mechanism of chaparral-associated hepatotoxicity is unknown. It is not known if chaparral is an intrinsic hepatotoxin (i.e., toxic to everyone if the dose is sufficient) or an idiosyncratic hepatotoxin (i.e., toxic only to those who have certain genetically aberrant metabolic pathways or immune system defects). Proposed mechanisms of chaparral-associated hepatotoxicity include (1) inhibition of cyclooxygenase or cytochrome P-450, (2) an immune-mediated reaction, (3) formation of a toxic metabolite, (4) impairment of liver function by phytoestrogens found in chaparral, and (5) cholestatic mechanisms causing impairment of bile formation or excretion. There is likely overlap between the two categories and the various mechanisms. In addition, toxicity may be influenced by age, weight, nutritional status, exposure to other drugs and chemicals, cumulative dose, and preparation (i.e., tea, dried plant parts, etc.) (Sheikh et al., 1997).

Phytoestrogens are hypothesized to cause hepatotoxicity via mechanisms similar to hormonal estrogens. Chaparral contains lignans that are similar to known estrogenic substances. High-performance liquid chromatography (HPLC) revealed that chaparral tablets and capsules contain more of these estrogenic lignans than the tea, reflecting the observation that hepatotoxicity is associated more commonly with consumption of tablets and capsules than with the tea (Obermeyer et al., 1995).

Enzyme inhibition is also a proposed mechanism of chaparral-induced hepatotoxicity (Sheikh et al., 1997). NDGA inhibits cytochrome P-450 activity in rat epidermal and hepatic microsomes (Agarwal, 1991).

### *16.4.3 Effects on the Arachidonic Acid Cascade*

In a study by Salari and colleagues (1984), NDGA proved to be a potent and selective inhibitor of 5-lipoxygenase ($ID_{50} < 3 \times 10^{-7}\ M$). Specifically, it reduces the active ferric form of lipoxygenase to the inactive ferrous form (Kemal et al., 1987). NDGA is also an indirect inhibitor of phospholipase $A_2$; by virtue of its antioxidant effect, it prevents oxidative modification of cell membrane phospholipids (Robison et al., 1990).

### *16.4.4 Nephrotoxicity*

Chaparral has also been associated with cystic renal disease in rats (Grice et al., 1968; Goodman et al., 1970; Evan et al., 1979) and humans (Smith et al., 1994; *see* Section 16.5). Toxicity studies revealed that cystic nephropathy could be reliably induced in rats fed a 2% by wt concentration of NDGA for 6 wk (Evan et al., 1979). Renal toxicity may stem from the accumulation of the *o*-quinone metabolite. NDGA is converted to this metabolite in the rat ileum and cecum, absorbed into the bloodstream, and excreted by the kidney, where it is reabsorbed by the epithelial cells of the proximal convoluted tubules. In the rat, tubular changes are thus confined to the tubules in the outer cortex (i.e., the proximal convoluted tubules) (Grice et al., 1968).

Unlike NDGA, which is an antioxidant, its metabolite is an oxidizing agent. Accumulation of the *o*-quinone metabolite is hypothesized to increase the fragility of lysosomal membranes by lipid peroxidation, causing autolysis, desquamation of necrotic proximal tubular epithelial cells, and accumulation of cellular debris leading to blockage of the tubules. Cysts develop as the kidney attempts to replace the damaged tubular epithelium (Goodman et al., 1979).

Examination of kidneys from rats fed NDGA for 6 wk or longer revealed multiple dark, raised cystic structures over the entire kidney surface. On cut section, the cysts were seen to extend to the inner medulla. The size of the cysts varied from pinpoint to 4 mm, depending on duration of exposure. They were lined with flattened or cuboidal tubular epithelial cells that were sometimes distended with granular material. These cells were occasionally found to have been shed into the cyst cavity. The presence of a basement membrane and the structure of the cells lining the cysts supports the contention that the cysts are of tubular origin. Large cysts often contained remnants of smaller cysts, and they compressed adjacent tubules. The cysts contained casts which in turn contained cells in varying stages of degeneration. These cellular debris were located at the periphery of the casts, leaving a central pool of acellular material. This acellular material stained yellow-brown with hematoxylin-phloxin-saffron (HPS), blue-green with toluidine blue, blue-green to dark blue with Schmorl's method, and pale blue or bright orange-red with Alcian blue-safranin. It was strongly periodic acid-Schiff (PAS)-positive in the small casts, but negative or slightly positive in the large casts. Cellular components were (PAS)-negative, stained purple-blue with Alcian blue, blue-green with Schmorl's, and positive with the Fontana–Masson method for argentaffin (Goodman et al., 1970).

Focal necrosis of the proximal tubules was evident, with pale (i.e., lighter staining) cells that contained greatly enlarged lysosomes containing granular material and remnants of other cell organelles on electron microscopy. In some cases, the lysosomal membrane was interrupted. The nucleus and other organelles of these pale cells were similar to those of adjacent normal proximal tubular cells, indicating that they were probably proximal tubular cells that had lost their brush borders. The basement membrane of the proximal tubules was thickened and convoluted. An inflammatory interstitial reaction was also evident, with infiltration of lymphoid cells, fibroblast proliferation, and histiocytes (Goodman et al., 1970).

Ether-extracted freeze-dried kidney tissue contained the *o*-quinone metabolite of NDGA, seen as red-brown granules. It was also seen as yellow-brown material in histiocytes, degenerating proximal tubular epithelium, small acellular casts, and occasionally in the cells lining the cysts and in the lumen of the proximal convoluted tubules. No free NDGA was found in the rat kidneys (Goodman et al., 1970).

### 16.4.5 Carcinogenicity

Chaparral tea has been associated with cystic renal cell carcinoma. *See* Section 16.5.

### 16.4.6 Dermatologic Effects

*See* Section 16.5.

### 16.4.7 Antihyperglycemic Effects

NDGA has been shown to lower plasma glucose in two mouse models of type II diabetes. Insulin levels were unchanged. It appears that NDGA is able to improve insulin action (Luo et al., 1998).

## 16.5 Case Reports of Toxicity Due to Commercially Available Products

Several reports of chaparral-associated hepatitis have been published. In 1997, Sheikh and colleagues reviewed 13 reports of hepatotoxicity associated with chaparral ingestion reported to the FDA between 1992 and 1994. A patient with asymptomatic elevation of liver function tests (LFTs) was mentioned in this report, but the product taken by the patient contained pyrrolozidine alkaloids, which are known hepatotoxins, so this patient was considered separately from the other 13. Of the 13 patients, 11 were female. One had a history of drug abuse, two had a history of alcohol use, one was taking conjugated estrogen, one was taking both diltiazem and occasional acetaminophen, and one had a history of lovastatin use, all of which have been associated with hepatotoxicity. These patients became symptomatic only after using chaparral. One patient also had a remote history of hepatitis C, but her LFTs were normal until after she began taking chaparral. Clinical presentation varied. Chief complaints in most patients included fatigue, right upper quadrant pain, dark urine, light stools, nausea, and diarrhea. A few patients also reported anorexia, weight loss, fever, and itching. Most patients had acute hepatitis characterized by jaundice, increases in serum levels of alkaline phosphatase, alanine aminotransferase, aspartate aminotransferase, total bilirubin, γ-glutamyltransferase, and lactate dehydrogenase. Liver biopsy was performed on three patients, revealing acute cholangitis with cholestasis, acute cholangitis with cholestasis and cirrhosis, and subacute cholangitis with cholestasis and cirrhosis. Five of seven patients who underwent abdominal ultrasound had evidence of a thickened gallbladder. Three of these patients had gallstones as revealed on ultrasound or computed tomography (CT). An exploratory laparotomy was performed in one patient, revealing ascites and a nodular liver. T-tube cholangiography showed nonfilling of the gallbladder, but no evidence of biliary disease. Endoscopic retrograde cholangiopancreatography (ERCP) revealed narrowed intrahepatic bile ducts in one of the two patients in whom it was performed. The authors of the review concluded that cumulative dose, but not duration of use, appears to be a risk factor for chaparral-induced hepatotoxicity. In addition, they state that hepatotoxic drugs or viruses might predispose patients to chaparral-associated hepatotoxicity. Four of these 13 cases (Anonymous, 1992; Alderman et al., 1994; Gordon et al., 1995) were previously reported in the medical literature, and are described in the following paragraphs.

Two of the cases included in the review by Sheikh and colleagues were first reported by the Centers for Disease Control (CDC) in 1992 (Anonymous, 1992). A 42-yr-old man was evaluated for jaundice and icteric sclera after consuming three 500-mg capsules of chaparral per day for the previous 6 wk. Past medical history included no unusual dietary practices, no alcohol for the past 3 yr, and no exposure to hepatotoxins. On physical exam, the liver was palpated 3 cm below the right costal margin. Upper abdominal ultrasound was normal. Lab findings were negative for hepatitis A, B, and C, cytomegalovirus (CMV), and Epstein–Barr virus (EBV). Serum chemistry revealed total bilirubin of 16.6 mg/dL (normal is 0–0.3 mg/dL), alkaline phosphatase of 133 U/L (normal is is 0–135 U/L), γ-glutamyltranspeptidase (GGT) of 158 U/L (normal is 0–32 U/L), aspartate aminotransferase (AST) of 1077 U/L (normal is 0–48 U/L), and lactate dehydrogenase (LDH) of 405 U/L (normal is 0–225 U/L). He was diagnosed as having hepatic dysfunction secondary to chaparral ingestion. Twenty-six days after discontinuing the herb, his LFTs had returned to normal (Anonymous, 1992).

Another patient sought medical advice after having experienced right upper quadrant pain and jaundice for 4 wk. This 41-yr-old woman had consumed 150 tablets (64.8 mg four times daily) of chaparral for a skin condition over 11 wk prior to onset of symptoms (Anonymous, 1992; Sheikh et al., 1997). Physical exam revealed marked jaundice but no hepatomegaly. Abdominal ultrasound and barium enema were normal. Laboratory results ruled out hepatitis A and B. Liver function tests revealed normal alkaline phosphatase, total bilirubin of 30 mg/dL, AST of 3560 U/L, alanine aminotransferase (ALT) of 2790 U/L (normal is 0–53 U/L), GGT of 138 U/L, and LDH of 868 U/L. She became asymptomatic approx 4 mo after the initial physician visit (Anonymous, 1992).

In a similar case also included in the Sheikh et al. review, a 45-yr-old woman presented with painless jaundice, anorexia, fatigue, nausea, vomiting, and pruritus after consuming 160 mg/d of chaparral for 10 wk (Alderman et al., 1994; Sheikh et al., 1997). Past medical history included alcohol abuse for 4 yr. She began taking chaparral at the advice of her alcohol addiction counselor, who claimed it would help prevent cravings for alcohol. The patient denied a history of intravenous drug use, exposure to blood products, use of oral contraceptives, or infectious contact. Medications and herbs taken included 0.2 mg/d of clonidine; a multivitamin containing 400 IU of vitamin E, 1000 mg of vitamin C, 25 mg of magnesium, and 10,000 IU of vitamin A; lecithin 15 g/d; and three capsules daily containing 150 mg of passionflower, 100 mg of hops, and 25 mg of valerian. Although valerian has been associated with hepatotoxicity when taken in conjunction with scullcap (*see* Chapter 19), it has not been linked with hepatotoxicity when taken alone. The only other potential hepatotoxin she had taken was lovastatin, which was discontinued 2½ mo before beginning chaparral. Physical exam revealed a 14-cm liver with a smooth, nontender border. Despite being normal approx 1 mo prior, LFTs were markedly elevated: ALT was 1611 IU (normal is 0–65 IU), AST was 957 IU (normal is 0–50 IU), alkaline phosphatase (ALP) was 265 IU (normal is 35–130 U/L), GGT was 993 IU (normal is 0–65 IU), and total bilirubin was 11.6 mg/dL (normal is <1.4 mg/dL). Over the next 3 wk, jaundice, anorexia, fatigue, pruritus, and LFTs worsened. Hepatitis B and C, CMV, and EBV were ruled out, and autoantibody titers were normal. Albumin decreased to 2.6 g/dL, and prothrombin time (PT) and partial thromboplastin time (PTT) increased to 13.6 s (normal is 11–13 s) and 37.2 s (normal is 20–30 s). ERCP showed sparse, smooth, but severely narrowed intrahepatic and extrahepatic bile ducts. The cause of duct narrowing could not be determined, but could be due to epithelial injury or intrahepatic cholestasis. CT and ultrasound were normal, ruling out obstruction from a tumor or sclerosing cholangitis as causes of cholestasis. Liver biopsy revealed acute inflammation with neutrophil and lymphoplasmocytic infiltration, diffuse hepatic disarray and necrosis, focal acute pericholangitis, some ductal dilatation, and proliferation of the bile ductules in portal and periportal areas.

Laparoscopic liver biopsy 2 wk later revealed progressive changes with a predominantly mononuclear infiltrate, and further collapse of the reticular framework. Mallory bodies were not seen on either biopsy, ruling out alcoholic hepatitis. The diagnosis was drug-induced cholestatic hepatitis. A steroid taper was initiated, with almost complete resolution on biopsy 1 mo later. The steroid was continued for 7 more weeks, with normalization of symptoms and laboratory tests (Alderman et al., 1994).

In a case involving positive rechallenge with chaparral, a 71–yr-old white man developed biopsy-proven hepatitis 3 mo after ingesting a tablet form of chaparral leaf daily. His symptoms began with a flulike illness, followed by ascites and jaundice 2 wk later. Past medical history included daily wine consumption, but no exposure to infectious causes of hepatitis. Pertinent laboratory results included AST of 404 IU/L (normal is < 40 IU/L), ALT of 385 U/L (normal is < 40 IU/L), ALP of 149 U/L (normal is < 110 IU/L), bilirubin of 304 μmol/L (normal is < 20 μmol/L), and PT of 13 s. Moderate ascites was seen on CT. His symptoms and laboratory test abnormalities resolved over the next 2 mo after he discontinued using chaparral and alcohol, but recurred later with chaparral rechallenge. One month after reinstituting chaparral, he felt ill, complained of right upper abdominal pain, and exhibited jaundice and ascites. Physical exam also revealed icteric sclera and full abdominal flanks. The AST was 767 IU/L, ALT was 759 IU/L, ALP was 304 IU/L, GGT was 178 IU/L, bilirubin was 169 μmol/L, and PT was 16 s. Infectious hepatitis was ruled out based on serology results. Liver span was 8 cm. Transjugular liver biopsy showed diffuse mild to moderate hepatocellular necrosis with inflammation, portal tract expansion, mild cholestasis, and mild fibrous septation. After he stopped intake of chaparral a second time, LFTs and other laboratory tests normalized over the next 3 mo. Liver biopsy revealed mild fibrous septation with some resolution of necrosis and inflammation. The patient remained well with normal LFTs over the next 4 yr (Batchelor et al., 1995).

In a case reported by these same clinicians, a 43-yr-old woman developed hepatitis after ingestion of chaparral leaf tablets several times a day. Six weeks after beginning chaparral for relief of chronic tension headaches, she developed nausea and a flulike illness, followed by jaundice 2 wk later. The patient denied any risk factors for exposure to infectious hepatitis. Aspirin was her only medication. Physical exam was negative for hepatosplenomegaly, ascites, or stigmata of chronic liver disease. Laboratory results included AST of 1612 U/L, ALP of 129 U/L, and bilirubin of 166 μmol/L, PT of 11 s, and albumin of 3.3 mg/dL. Hepatitis serology results were negative. Symptoms resolved and laboratory tests normalized over the 4 mo following discontinuation of chaparral (Batchelor et al., 1995).

A case of chaparral-associated hepatotoxicity requiring liver transplant developed in a 60-yr-old woman who took one or two capsules of chaparral daily for 10 mo. Three weeks prior to hospital admission she developed a flulike syndrome and increased consumption to six capsules daily. Jaundice, right upper quadrant tenderness, and anorexia occurred 2 wk later. Past medical history was negative for liver disease, blood transfusions, and alcohol use. Medications included diltiazem, atenolol, aspirin, nitroglycerin, and occasional acetaminophen. Laboratory results were bilirubin, 12.4 mg/dL (normal is 0.1–1.2 mg/dL); AST, 1191 U/L (normal is 15–77 U/L); ALT, 341 U/L (normal is 15–37 U/L); ALP, 186 U/L (normal is 36–125 U/L); albumin, 2.4 mg/dL (normal is 3.2–5 mg/dL); and PT, 15.9 s (normal is 10.9–13.7 s). Hepatitis serology was negative, and autoantibody titers were normal. Ultrasound and CT scan showed a contracted gallbladder with a thickened multilaminated wall. Exploratory laparotomy, done 1 wk later because of persistent abdominal pain, showed ascites and a nodular liver. Liver biopsy revealed severe acute hepatitis with areas of lobular collapse and nodular regeneration, mixed portal inflammation, and marked bile duct proliferation. She became encephalopathic and more deeply jaundiced. After suffering aspiration pneumonia, sepsis, and renal failure necessitating dialysis, her bilirubin increased to 35.5 mg/dL, and PT increased to 28 s. Despite aggressive supportive therapy, an orthotopic liver transplantation was required 5 wk after initial admission. The hepatectomy specimen weighed 1.1 kg. Microscopy revealed large areas of lobular necrosis and collapse, nodular regeneration, marked portal inflammation, and bile duct proliferation. Eighteen months after transplantation liver function tests were normal and the patient was doing well (Gordon et al., 1995).

In addition to hepatotoxicity, chaparral-associated renal cell carcinoma and cystic renal disease have also been reported in humans. An asymptomatic 56-yr-old woman with a serum creatinine level of 1.5 mg/dL (normal is is 0.5–1.1 mg/dL) was found to have bilateral renal cystic disease on ultrasound. CT confirmed the presence of bilateral renal cystic disease with two complex cysts in the left kidney, and multiple bilateral simple cysts. Peripheral calcification with an irregular cyst wall was noted. Wedge excision of the midpole caliceal cyst and unroofing and biopsy of the superomedial cyst revealed low-grade cystic clear cell carcinoma. Left radical nephrectomy was performed. Examination of the excised kidney revealed numerous micro- and macroscopic cysts. A residual cyst wall at the biopsy sites contained collections of stratified epithelial cells with clear cystoplasm and mildly enlarged hyperchromatic irregular nuclei. There were 17 other grossly obvious cysts in the cortex, as well as many microscopic cysts measuring 100–300 μm in diameter. An 8-mm cyst had a fibrotic wall with one or two layers of atypical clear cells, similar to those in the two largest cysts. The microscopic cysts were ringed by flattened epithelial cells and appeared to originate as dilatations and outpouchings of the Bowman's capsule and the proximal and distal tubules. Most were glomerular and at the same stage of development. With questioning the patient admitted to consuming three to four cups daily of chaparral tea for a 3 mo period approx 18 mo prior to presentation. On postsurgical follow-up of almost 2 yr, serum creatinine stabilized at 1.7 mg/dL, and periodic renal ultrasound revealed no changes in the right kidney (Smith et al., 1994).

Sixteen cases of contact dermatitis have been attributed to chaparral or NDGA (Sheikh et al., 1997). In a case series of acute dermatitis caused by exposure to chaparral (Leonforte, 1986), six men developed dermatitis from exposure to chaparral as a bath additive; from using chaparral to make a fire for a barbecue; and through occupational exposure. Clinical presentation included scales, erythema, prutitus, edema, vesicles, and papules. An elevated white blood cell count and eosinophilia were noted in one patient. Biopsy, performed in one patient, revealed suprabasal, multiloculated blisters containing a net of fibrin, neutrophils, eosinophils, and mononuclear cells. An inflammatory infiltrate and congested capillaries were seen at the base of the dermis. Patch test to chaparral leaves was positive in the four patients in whom it was performed. Although the clinical presentation suggested a photodermatitis in four patients, a photopatch test was negative in another patient in whom it was performed.

In one of the cases reviewed by Sheikh and colleagues, a patient developed a generalized urticarial rash, nausea, and abdominal pain after ingestion of chaparral, but had been taking chaparral for 1 yr, had a history of allergies, and was also taking naproxen and ketorolac. Miscellaneous adverse effects associated with chaparral use include sudden unilateral loss of vision, tachycardia, electrolyte abnormalities with cardiac arrest, and syncopal episodes (Sheikh et al., 1997).

## 16.6 Drug Interactions

Although drug interactions with chaparral have not been reported, NDGA is an inhibitor of CYP450 microsomal enzymes in vitro (Capdevila et al., 1988; Agarwal et al., 1991). Its ability to inhibit drug metabolizing isoforms of CYP450 in vivo remains to be seen.

## 16.7 Pharmacokinetics

In rats, NDGA is metabolized in the lower third of the ileum and cecum to its *o*-quinone metabolite. It is absorbed into the bloodstream, is filtered by the glomeruli, then reabsorbed and retained by the proximal tubule epithelial cells

(Grice et al., 1968), where it accumulates with repeated exposure (Goodman et al., 1970). NDGA also has an *o*-methylated metabolite that has been detected in rat kidney. Free NDGA is not found in the rat kidney, but is found in the feces (Goodman et al., 1970).

## 16.8 Chemical Analysis/Analysis of Biofluids

Extraction of NDGA and its metabolites from kidney tissue and fecal material is described in the cited reference. The *o*-quinone metabolite gives a strong oxidation product with Schiff reagent. The product has an absorption peak at 505 μm. This metabolite reacts with Alcian blue, and a strong dark blue color develops with Schmorl's ferri-ferricyanide method. NDGA does not react with Schiff reagent or Alcian blue, but gives a deep blue precipitate with Schmorl's reagent and reacts with ammoniacal silver nitrate to produce a black precipitate (Goodman et al., 1970). Thin-layer chromatography (TLC) analysis of both NDGA and its *o*-quinone metabolite has been described (Grice et al., 1968). TLC has been used to quantitate NDGA and its *o*-quinone and *o*-methoxylated metabolites in the rat kidney. NDGA is not detected in the kidney using TLC. The *o*-methoxylated metabolite has been detected in the rat kidney but not quantified. NDGA cannot be detected in the feces using TLC owing to interference with bile salts (Goodman et al., 1970).

## 16.8 Regulatory Status

Chaparral is considered a dietary supplement in the United States. The FDA has warned the public about the dangers of consuming chaparral (Stone, 1992). Chaparral is not listed in the German Commission E monographs (Blumenthal, 1998).

## References

Agarwal R, Wang ZY, Bik DP, Mukhtar H. Nordihydroguaiaretic acid, an inhibitor of lipoxygenase, also inhibits cytochrome P-450 mediated monooxygenase activity in rat epidermal and hepatic microsomes. Drug Metab Dispos 1991;19:620–4.

Alderman S, Kailas S, Goldfarb S, Singaram C, Malone DG. Cholestatic hepatitis after ingestion of chaparral leaf: confirmation by endoscopic retrograde cholangiopancreatography and liver biopsy. J Clin Gastroenterol 1994;19:242–7.

Anonymous. Chaparral-induced toxic hepatitis—California and Texas, 1992. Morbid Mortal Wkly Rep 1992;41:812–4.

Anonymous. The Lawrence review of natural products. St. Louis, MO: Facts and Comparisons, 1993.

Batchelor WB, Heathcote J, Wanless IR. Chaparral-induced hepatic injury. Am J Gastroenterol 1995;90:831–3.

Blumenthal M. The complete German Commission E monographs. Austin, TX: American Botanical Council, 1998.

Burk D, Woods M. Hydrogen peroxide, catalase, glutathione peroxidase, quinones, nordihydroguaiaretic acid, and phosphopyridine nucleotides in relation to x-ray action on cancer cells. Radiat Res 1963;3(Suppl):212–46.

Capdevila J, Gil L, Orellana M, Marnett LJ, Mason JI, Yadagiri P, Falck JR. Inhibitors of cytochrome P-450-dependent arachidonic acid metabolism. Arch Biochem Biophys 1988;261:257–63.

Evan AP, Gardner KD. Nephron obstruction in nordihydroguaiaretic acid-induced renal cystic disease. Kidney Int 1979;15:7–19.

Goodman T, Grice HC, Becking GC, Salem FA. A cystic nephropathy induced by nordihydroguaiaretic acid in the rat. Light and electron microscopic investigations. Lab Invest 1979;23:93–107.

Gordon, D, Rosenthal G, Hart J, Sirota R, Baker A. Chaparral ingestion. The broadening spectrum of liver injury caused by herbal medications. JAMA 1995;273:489–90.

Grice HC, Becking G, Goodman T. Toxic properties of nordihydroguaiaretic acid. Food Cosmet Toxicol 1968;6:155–61.

Kemal C, Louis-Flamberg P, Krupinski-Olsen R, Shorter AL. Reductive inactivation of soybean lipoxygenase 1 by catechols: a possible mechanism for regulation of lipoxygenase activity. Biochemistry 1987;26:7064–72.

Leonforte J. Contact dermatitis from *Larrea* (creosote bush). J Am Acad Dermatol 1986;14:202–7.

Luo J, Chuang T, Cheung J, Quan J, Tsai J, Sullivan C, et al. Masoprocol (nordihydroguaiaretic acid): a new antihyperglycemic agent isolated from the creosote bush (*Larrea tridentata*). Eur J Pharmacol 1998;346:77–9.

Obermeyer WR, Musser SM, Betz JM, Casey RE, Pohland AE, Page SW. Chemical studies of phytoestrogens and related compounds in dietary supplements: flax and chaparral. Proc Soc Exp Biol Med 1995;208:6–12.

Pavani M, Fones E, Oksenberg D, Garcia M, Hernandez C, Cordano G, et al. Inhibition of tumoral cell respiration and growth by nordihydroguaiaretic acid. Biochem Pharmacol 1994;48:1935–42.

Robison T, Sevanian A, Forman H. Inhibition of arachidonic acid release by nordihydroguaiaretic acid and its antioxidant action in rat alveolar macrophages and Chinese hamster lung fibroblasts. Toxicol Appl Pharmacol 1990;105:113–22.

Salari H, Braquet P, Borgeat P. Comparative effects of indomethacin, acetylenic acids, 15–HETE, nordihydroguaiaretic acid and BW755C on the metabolism of arachidonic acid in human leukocytes and platelets. Prostagland Leukatr Med 1984;13:53–60.

Sheikh NM, Philen RM, Love LA. Chaparral associated hepatotoxicity. Arch Intern Med 1997;157:913–9.

Smart CR, Hogle HH, Robins RK, Broom AD, Bartholomew D. An interesting observation on nordihydroguaiaretic acid (NSC-4291; NDGA) and a patient with malignant melanoma—a preliminary report. Cancer Chem Rep 1969;53:147–51.

Smith AY, Feddersen RM, Gardner KD, Davis CJ. Cystic renal cell carcinoma and acquired renal cystic disease associated with consumption of chaparral tea: a case report. J Urol 1994;152:2089–91.

Stone B. Chaparral consumption warning. HHS News P92-38. Rockville, MD: Food and Drug Administration, December 10, 1992.

Tyler V. The honest herbal, 3rd edit., Binghamton, NY: Pharmaceutical Products Press, 1993.

Waller C, Gisvold O. A phytochemical investigation of *Larrea divaricata* Cav. J Am Pharm Assoc 1945;34:78–81.

Chapter 17

# Coltsfoot

*Amanda Dailey and Melanie Johns Cupp*

*Tussilago farfara* (L.), coughwort, feuilles de tussilage, horse-hoof, huflattichblatter, kuandong hua (Anonymous, 1996), *Petasites japonicus* Maxim ("fuki-no-toh") (Hirono et al., 1973)

## 17.1 History and Traditional Uses

Coltsfoot is a perennial yellow flower that reaches heights of 30 cm. The hoof-shaped, toothed leaves, which are green on top with white hairs on the underside, do not appear until the flower and stem begin to die in the spring. Coltsfoot is native to Europe, but can also be found in the northeastern and north central United States, southern Canada, and China (Anonymous, 1996; Berry, 1996).

The flowers and leaves of coltsfoot have long been used to treat all kinds of respiratory disorders, but its use to prevent coughs and soothe the throat is well documented (Anonymous, 1996; Berry, 1996). In addition to treatment of respiratory ailments, coltsfoot has also been used to treat diarrhea, to purify the blood, to stimulate metabolism, to cause diuresis and sweating, and topically as a wound treatment (Blumenthal, 1998).

Coltsfoot has been served cooked; raw in salads; fried in batter; and used to make beer, wine (Salvador, 1996), and candy (Anonymous, 1996).

## 17.2 Current Promoted Uses

Products containing coltsfoot are promoted as antihistamines, decongestants, and as expectorants. Respiratory ailments such as cough and hoarseness,

From Forensic Science: *Toxicology and Clinical Pharmacology of Herbal Products*
Edited by: M. J. Cupp © Humana Press Inc., Totowa, New Jersey

sore throat, allergies and colds, and acute mild inflammation of the oral mucosa are said to benefit. Coltsfoot is also touted as nourishment for the endocrine system, providing rejuvenation of hormones, the adrenal system, pancreas, pituitary, thyroid, and reproductive system. It is also purported to rejuvenate and rebuild the respiratory system, cleansing drugs, mucus, and toxins from lungs and bronchioles in patients with emphysema, silicosis, and chronic bronchitis.

## 17.3 Products Available

Despite the fact none of coltsfoot's constituents are volatile and any active ingredient would be destroyed by burning, herbal tobaccos with blends of coltsfoot, lavender, rosemary, thyme, chamomile, and other herbs are smoked to treat asthma and bronchial congestion, particularly in Britain (Salvador, 1996). Coltsfoot leaves can be mail-ordered via the World Wide Web as a chelated extract, capsules, powder, or cut and sifted. Intact plants are also available through on-line purchasing from nurseries. Bronchostad® is an instant tea made from coltsfoot leaves, which can also be used to prepare liquid and solid extracts. Dried flower heads and tablets are other available dosage forms. Syrups may be prepared by adding boiling sugar water to a coltsfoot tincture, and an external ointment can also be prepared.

Several combination products contain coltsfoot. Hormone Rejuvenator® is a capsule containing bilberry bark, cascara sagrada, chamomile, chickweed, coltsfoot, comfrey root, dandelion root, golden seal root, hyssop, juniper berries, licorice root, and wild cherry bark. Respiratory Rejuvenator® contains pleurisy root, horehound, lobelia, fenugreek, eucalyptus, coltsfoot, comfrey, mullein, lady slipper, marshmallow, white pine bark, myrrh, and hyssop. Alvita Teas, Herb Pharm, and Nature's Answer are all manufacturers that provide coltsfoot products.

## 17.4 Pharmacologic/Toxicologic Effects

### 17.4.1 Respiratory Effects

Mucilage is the sole ingredient responsible for coltsfoot's pharmacologic action as a demulcent (Salvador, 1996). It is a hydrophilic colloid that forms a viscous solution when mixed with water. As a viscous solution, often in the form of tea, mucilage creates a protective barrier over the pharynx, larynx, and trachea. Therefore, it soothes the throat and suppresses coughs by preventing irritation (Tyler, 1994).

Components of coltsfoot have also been noted to increase the activity of epithelial cilia in the frog esophagus, possibly giving credence to use of coltsfoot as an expectorant (Anonymous, 1996).

Tussilagone, a sesquiterpene compound found in coltsfoot, has been identified as a potent respiratory stimulant. Doses ranging from 0.02 to 0.03 mg/kg were administered via the femoral vein to anesthetized dogs. Low to moderate doses of tussilagone increased respiratory rate and tidal volume, while large doses elevated respiratory rate to the point that tidal volume decreased. The effects of tussilagone were short in duration (approx 5 min) and appeared to be centrally mediated (Li and Wang, 1988).

L-652,469, an analog of tussilagone isolated from the methylene chloride extract of the bud of coltsfoot, has been shown to weakly inhibit receptors for platelet-activating factor (PAF) and to weakly block $Ca^{2+}$ channels, thus inhibiting platelet aggregation and inflammation. Unlike tussilagone, L-652,469 is orally active, as demonstrated by its ability to inhibit PAF-induced rat foot edema and carrageenan-induced rat paw edema (Hwang et al., 1997). By virtue of these effects, coltsfoot may elicit efficacy against certain inflammatory respiratory diseases such as asthma.

### *17.4.2 Cardiovascular Effects*

Tussilagone has cardiovascular stimulant effects. Tussilagone was injected into the femoral vein of anesthetized cats (0.02–0.5 mg/kg), dogs (0.02–0.3 mg/kg), and rats (0.4–4 mg/kg). The pressor response was immediate, and blood pressure returned to normal within 6 min. Dose-related changes in blood pressure were similar to the effect elicited by 0.01–0.03 mg/kg of dopamine, but tachyphylaxis was not observed. There was also a dose-related decrease in the heart rate of the anesthetized dogs. Other studies suggest that the effects of tussilagone on the cardiovascular system are peripheral and more similar to that of dopamine than norepinephrine (Li and Wang, 1988).

### *17.4.3 Antimicrobial Effects*

In vitro antibacterial activity limited to Gram-negative bacteria has been demonstrated using aqueous leaf extracts and phenolic components of coltsfoot (Anonymous, 1996).

### *17.4.4 Hepatotoxicity*

The hepatotoxic pyrrolizidine alkaloids (PAs) present in coltsfoot pose the greatest concern regarding use of coltsfoot. (*see also* Chapter 18 for additional discussion of the pyrrolizidine alkaloids). Hepatic venoocclusive disease is characteristic of PA intoxication. The specific histologic findings are described in Section 17.5, but generally include endothelial edema, sclerosis and occlusion of the small vessels, necrosis, progressive fibrosis, and eventually cirrhosis (Roulet et al., 1988). PAs are not hepatotoxic themselves, but are converted by the liver by dehydrogenation to highly reactive, electrophilic pyrrole-like compounds capable of binding to tissues (Mattocks, 1968). Molecular characteristics of those PAs that are metabolized to reactive metabolites include lipid solubility, allowing access to the hepatic microsomal enzymes; ester groups, which act as highly reactive alkylating groups; branching chains, which interfere with ester hydrolysis to nontoxic metabolites (Mattocks, 1981); and the presence of a double bond in the five-membered ring structure of the molecule (Frei et al., 1992). PAs present in coltsfoot that are metabolized to reactive metabolites that covalently bind to hepatic, renal, and pulmonary macromolecules such as DNA and RNA include senecionine and seneciphylline (Eastman et al., 1982). Senkirkine, another PA present in coltsfoot, has been shown to be hepatotoxic in rats (Schoental, 1970). Tussiglione, discussed in Sections 17.4.1 and 17.4.2, does not have the molecular features that would predict hepatotoxicity (Li and Wang, 1988).

The risk of hepatotoxicity from PA consumption is likely dependent upon dose and individual characteristics (Kumana et al., 1985). For example, female rats appear to be more susceptible to PA toxicity than male rats (Candrian et al., 1985).

### *17.4.5 Carcinogenicity/Genotoxicity*

Dried coltsfoot flowers fed to rats induced hemangioendothelial carcinoma (Hirono et al., 1976). These observations prompted further carcinogenicity studies of the PAs. The PA senkirkine has proved to be carcinogenic, causing nonmalignant liver cell adenomas in rats (Hirono et al., 1979). Proliferation of intrahepatic bile ducts and oval cells, blood lagoons, and cirrhosis was found, even in rats that did not develop tumors. Senkirkine and senecionine were shown to be genotoxic carcinogens based on studies showing damage to DNA in rodent hepatocytes (Mori et al., 1985). Dried flower stalks of *Petasites japonicus*, a kind of coltsfoot found in Japan, fed to rats induced liver cell adenoma, hepatocellular carcinoma, and hemangioendothelial sarcoma of the liver, which appeared as soft, hemorrhagic nodules (Hirono et al., 1973). Petasitenine, a PA found in *Petasites japonicus* Maxim, was later isolated and given to rats (Hirono et al., 1977). Liver cell necrosis, hemorrhage, bile duct proliferation, liver cell adenomas, and hemangioendothelial sarcomas appearing as multicentric hemorrhagic nodules were documented. One rat had metastasis of hemangioendothelial sarcoma to the lung.

In a study (Candrian et al., 1985) using radiolabeled senecionine and seneciphylline, the ability of senecionine to bind to liver DNA in female rats was four times higher than that in males, suggesting that females are more susceptible to the carcinogenic effects of these compounds.

The molecular features that predict hepatotoxicity, discussed previously, also predict carcinogenicity (Frei et al., 1992); thus, the two effects are closely related, as evidenced by the hepatotoxic changes noted in the carcinogenicity studies, and the carcinogenicity noted in the hepatotoxicity studies.

## 17.5 Case Reports of Toxicity Due to Commercially Available Products

Death attributed to hepatic venoocclusive disease was reported in the newborn infant of a woman who drank herbal tea throughout her pregnancy (Roulet et al., 1988). The 5-d-old infant was admitted to the hospital because of jaundice, massive hepatomegaly, and ascites. During pregnancy, her mother had experienced a pruitic eruption of unknown etiology beginning in the fourth month of pregnancy, and vaginal bleeding during the last 3 d of pregnancy, which prompted cesarean section at 36 wk because of suspicion of abruption. Physical exam upon admission revealed an icteric, apathetic infant with a distended abdomen, hard liver palpated 5 cm below the right costal margin, and moderate ascites. Ultrasound revealed homogeneous normoechogenic hepatosplenomegaly, moderate ascites, and large kidneys. Abnormal laboratory values included aspartate aminotransferase (AST) 3725 U/L, alanine aminotransferase (ALT) 760 U/L, fibrinogen 0.4 g/L (normal is 1.8–4 g/L), prothrombin time 13% (normal is 70–140 %), plasma ammonia 133 µmol/L (normal is <100 mmol/L), serum albumin 27.9 g/L (normal is 30–42 g/L), and total bilirubin 164 µmol/L (normal is < 21 mmol/L). Sodium, potassium, urea, glucose, and blood pH values were normal. The hemoglobin value was 168 g/L, white blood cell (WBC) count was 10,600/µL, and platelet count was 270,000/µL. An open liver biopsy done at age 27 d showed marked centrilobular fibrosis, neovascularization, and iron deposition, associated with widespread circumferential connective tissue occlusion of small and medium size hepatic veins, strongly suggested a diagnosis of hepatic venoocclusive disease. The infant expired 11 d later. Postmortem examination revealed an icteric female infant with 500 mL of yellow ascitic fluid and a firm, green 120-g liver. Microscopic examination of the liver showed centrilobular congestion and necrosis, neovascularization, atrophy of liver cords, fibrosis with bridging between adjacent central veins, and extensive deposition of hemosiderin. Calcium deposits were found in areas of centrilobular fibrosis. Most of the central and sublobular veins were partially occluded by subintimal circumferential proliferation of connective tissue. Budd–Chiari syndrome was ruled out based on the absence of thrombosis in the large hepatic veins. Because hepatic venoocclusive disease is a rare disorder seen mainly in children who have consumed toxic pyrrolizidine alkaloids, the composition of the expectorant tea consumed by the mother was investigated. Chemical analysis by thin-layer chromatography (TLC) revealed a concentration of 0.6 mg of senecionine (measured as the *N*-oxide) per kilogram dry weight. According to the manufacturer, the tea contained 9% *Tussilago farfara* plus nine other plants.

Hepatic venoocclusive disease was also reported in an 18-mo-old boy after daily ingestion of up to 500 mL of a homemade herbal tea since the age of 3 mo (Sperl et al., 1995). After experiencing vomiting, diarrhea, subfebrile temperature, and abdominal pain for 3 d, the patient was admitted to the hospital. The liver was palpated 3 cm below the costal margin. Abnormal laboratory values included sodium 128 mEq/L; platelet count 15,000/mm$^3$; WBC 17,700/mm$^3$; AST 269 U/L (normal is < 23 U/L), and ALT 124 U/L (normal is i.e. less than 28 U/L), which increased over 5 d to 1079 U/L and 923 U/L, respectively; serum protein 4.14 mg/dL (normal is 5.8–8.6 mg/dL), prothrombin time 55% (normal is 80–100%), fibrinogen 55 mg/dL (normal is 150–500 mg/dL), and total bilirubin 2.78 mg/dL (normal is 0.3–1.0 mg/dL) . Ultrasonography revealed severe ascites and hepatomegaly with slit-like hepatic veins and compression of the vena cava. Magnetic resonance imaging (MRI) showed that the vena cava and portal vein were patent, although the intrahepatic veins were markedly narrowed, and parenchymal edema was suggested by the low signal intensity in the periportal area. Liver biopsy revealed severe distortion of the liver cell plates by massive hemorrhagic congestion affecting zones II and III of the acinus, extending almost into zone I in some areas. Although the lobular architecture of the liver was preserved, the central veins were not discernible. The diagnosis of venoocclusive disease was made, which led to investigation of the homemade herbal tea. The mother had been preparing the tea from plants she believed to be coltsfoot and peppermint. Chemical analysis of a methonolic extract of the plant leaves revealed the presence of 0.16% seneciphylline, isolated using column chromatography and identified by TLC, mass spectroscopy, and nuclear magnetic resonance (NMR) spectroscopy. The plant was determined to be *Adenostyles alliariae* (Aldendost), which, like coltsfoot, contains the PA seneciphylline. The patient was treated with sodium and fluid restriction, spironolactone, furosemide, and paracentesis, and the signs and symptoms resolved over 6 wk. Assuming a fixed concentration the herbal tea, the exposure dose was calculated to be at least 60 μg/kg/d.

In an additional case series (Kumana, 1985), three young adult women were admitted to the hospital with features of venoocclusive disease 61–68 d after beginning a daily herbal tea regimen prescribed by their dermatologist for the treatment of psoriasis. Symptoms of hepatomegaly and ascites began 19–45 d after start of tea consumption. With onset of symptoms, two patients discontinued taking the tea. The third patient continued to take the tea for an additional 16 d, against medical advice, and ultimately died of hepatic failure, gastrointestinal hemorrhage, and portal hypertension despite treatment with diuretics and paracentesis. The fourth patient discontinued the tea after 21 d because she developed a rash. When evaluated 77 d later, she was found to have mild hepatomegaly only. Pertinent initial laboratory values for the four patients included normal serum albumin in all four. The patient who later died presented with an elevated bilirubin of 55 μmol/L (normal is < 26 μmol/L), which increased to 402 mmol/L after 12 d. Bilirubin was within normal limits in the other three patients. AST and ALT were initially elevated (52–232 U/L) in all but the fourth patient, and decreased over time in all but the patient who died, in which they increased slightly. An elevated prothrombin time (PT) ratio of 1.2, which increased to 1.7 after 12 d, was documented in the patient who later died. Ultrasonography revealed hepatomegaly with patent hepatic and portal veins, even in the two patients who had portal hypertension, reflecting the short duration of the disease. Liver biopsy was performed on all four patients, and in all four cases the histologic features of venoocclusive disease were evident. The biopsy from the patient who eventually died showed areas of intense centrilobular sinusoidal dilatation with hemorrhage, cell atrophy, and necrosis. Intimal edema and loose fibrosis significantly narrowed many central and sublobular hepatic veins. Liver biopsies from two of the three patients who survived were similar, but congestion and liver cell changes in the centrilobular zone were not as severe. The liver biopsy from the patient who discontinued the tea after only 3 wk revealed only slight residual sclerosis of some of the sublobular veins with dilatation of the feeding venules. Postmortem examination of the patient who died revealed a slightly enlarged liver with "nutmeg" appearance and reverse lobulation, extensive centrilobular hemorrhagic necrosis, and scarring around severely narrowed, sclerotic sublobular and central veins. Other findings included 3 L of ascitic fluid, esophageal varices, and bloody mucus in the stomach.

The tea consumed by these four women was analyzed using spectrophotometry after reaction with Ehrlich's reagent revealed unsaturated PAs that were determined to be senecionine and the corresponding *N*-oxide in concentrations of 0.42 mg/g and 1.4 mg/g, respectively. The leaves were determined to be from the family Compositae, to which coltsfoot belongs, although their exact identity could not be determined because of their chopped condition. Cumulative doses of these alkaloids were calculated to be 1350 mg over 45 d for one patient, 1380 mg over 46 d for the patient who died, 570 mg over 19 d for another patient, and 630 mg over 21 d for the patient with the mildest symptoms. The cumulative dose was 15 mg/kg in the patient who exhibited mild symptoms, while the mean cumulative dose was 18 mg/kg in the other three patients.

## 17.6 $LD_{50}$

The $LD_{50}$ of the cardiovascular–respiratory stimulant tussilagone in mice was determined to be 28.9 mg/kg (Li and Wang, 1988). The $LD_{50}$ of senkirkine in rats is 220 mg/kg (Hirono et al., 1979).

## 17.7 Pharmacokinetics/Toxicokinetics

### 17.7.1 Absorption

Mucilage, the component of coltsfoot responsible for its soothing effect on the throat and oral mucosa, is not absorbed; it produces a local effect only (Tyler, 1994).

### 17.7.2 Distribution

Radiolabeled senecionine and seneciphylline were administered to rats via stomach tube, and radioactivity was measured in tissues and biofluids (Candrian et al., 1985). Senecionine and seneciphylline were noted to concentrate in the liver, but also distributed to the lungs and kidneys in small amounts. At 6 h post-dose, on average 60.3% of the administered radioactivity administered as radio-labeled senecione was detected in the liver of male rats, 0.4% in the lung, and 3% in the kidney. For females, these same data were 43.9%, 1%, and 4.2%, respectively. Data on the same order of magnitude were obtained for seneciphylline.

Radiolabeled senecionine and seneciphylline were detected throughout the body after intraperitoneal administration to mice (Eastman et al., 1982). Sixteen hours after administration an average of 75% of the radioactivity administered as radiolabeled senecionine was detected in the urine, 14% in feces, 3.6% in the intestines with contents, 1.92% in the liver, and <1% each in the blood, kidney, lung, heart, brain, expired $CO_2$, and remaining carcass. Average values for radioactivity measured 16 h after radiolabeled seneciphylline administration were similar. Only 0.04% of each PA was found in the milk of lactating mice, suggesting this would be a minor route of exposure for neonates of women drinking herbal teas.

Senecionine subcutaneously administered to pregnant rats has been shown to cross the placenta and cause severe liver damage and death in fetuses. Likewise, senecionine intravenously administered to fetal rats crossed the placenta and caused liver damage in the mother (Sundareson 1942).

### 17.7.3 Metabolism/Elimination

As discussed in Sections 17.4.4 and 17.4.5, senkirkine (Schoental, 1970), senecionine, seneciphylline (Eastman et al., 1982) and petasitenina (Hirono et al., 1977) are pyrrolizidine alkaloids (PAs) present in coltsfoot that are activated through dehydrogenation in the liver to form pyrrole metabolites (Mattocks, 1981). Pyrrole metabolites possess chemically reactive alkylating groups that can form covalent bonds with nucleophilic groups on tissue. Hepatotoxicity and genotoxicity of a PA is directly related to the extent of pyrrole metabolite formation by the liver and the degree to which the pyrrole can bind to tissue. Physical and chemical properties of PAs that promote hepatotoxicity include lipophilicity, which makes hepatic enzymes more accessible, a structural shape that promotes *C*-hydroxylation rather than *N*-oxidation, and resistance to ester hydrolysis (Mattocks, 1981). The presence of a double bond between the no. 1 and 2 carbons in the necine ring structure of the molecule is also necessary for metabolism to the toxic metabolite (Frei et al., 1992). The *N*-oxide metabolites are less hepatotoxic and genotoxic than their parent compounds when administered intraperitoneally, but *N*-oxides formed in vivo are excreted into the bile and transformed back into the parent compound by intestinal microorganisms (Frei et al., 1992). Another metabolite is excreted in the urine as an *N*-acetylcysteine conjugate (Estep et al., 1990a).

Radioactivity was measured in the bile, urine, and blood after intravenous administration of radiolabeled senecionine to rats (Estep et al., 1990b). Bile, urine, and blood samples were collected over 7 h. Collection of bile and urine was shown to decrease the plasma concentration compared to when only blood and urine were collected, suggesting enterohepatic recirculation. Total excretion over 7 h resulted in 43% of the administered radioactivity appearing in urine and 44% in bile. Absence of bile collection led to a significant increase in urine excretion (59% of dose). Senecionine *N*-oxide represented 52% of the radioactivity in the bile and 30% of the radioactivity in the urine, accounting for >35% of the total administered radioactivity.

In the study by Candrian and colleagues, an average of 3.3% (males) and 11.2% (females) of the radioactivity administered as radiolabeled senecionine was detectable in the livers of rats 4 d after the dose was administered. An average of 3.6% and of the dose of the radioactivity administered as radiolabeled seneciphylline was detectable in the livers of female rats 5 d after administration. These data suggest slow elimination of the compounds from the liver, reflecting the ability of the compounds to covalently bind to liver DNA, especially in female rats.

## *17.8 Analysis of Biofluids/Chemical Analysis*

A simple check for the presence of PAs metabolites in urine and tissues using Ehrlich reagent has been described (Mattocks, 1968). Tissue samples are sliced into small pieces, rinsed in distilled water and in ethanol, homogenized in absolute ethanol, centrifuged, and shaken with a modified Ehrlich reagent (3 g of 4-dimethylaminobenzaldehyde in 60 mL of absolute ethanol and 40 mL of 14% methanolic boron trifluoride). Modification of the reagent with acid is required to overcome tissue buffering activity. The mixture is heated for 1–2 min at 80–95°C and then the reagent is decanted and exchanged with new ethanol. Ehrlich reagent gives a mauve color in the presence of tissue samples containing PA metabolites. Demonstration of PA metabolites in the liver by color change can be accomplished by making thin liver slices, fixing them with alcohol, heating for a few minutes in Ehrlich reagent, then replacing the reagent with clean ethanol. Because PA metabolites are highly bound to tissues, Ehrlich reagent works for fresh tissues that have been frozen, ethanol-fixed slices, ethanolic homogenates that are 2 wk old, and perhaps even on older tissues. Ehrlich reagent will also give a mauve color when added to urine containing pyrrolizidine metabolites. Quantification of PAs and metabolites can be done using spectrophotometry (Mattocks, 1968; Kumana et al., 1985). PAs in herbal products can also be quantified using this method (Kumana et al., 1985).

TLC analysis of PAs (Sharma et al., 1965; Mattocks, 1967; Mattocks, 1986) and their N-oxides (Mattocks, 1967) has been described. Seneciphylline and its N-oxide metabolite have been detected in herbs using TLC, fast atom bombardment mass spectrometry, NMR spectrometry, gas chromatography–mass spectroscopy (GC–MS), and co-chromatography (thin-layer and gas chromatography) (Sperl et al., 1995). Senkirkine was detected in dried, milled flowers using GC–MS (Hirono et al., 1976). Alternatively, senkirkine can be extracted from the milled buds (Koekemoer and Warren, 1951), then its melting point, TLC, and infrared (IR) spectrum can be compared to an authentic sample (Hirono et al., 1979). Boiling point, melting point, retention time ($R_T$) for gas chromatography, and retention factor ($R_F$) for TLC have been published for senecionine, seneciphylline, and senkirkine, along with procedural details of these analyses (Chalmers et al., 1965).

High-performance liquid chromatography (HPLC) was used to measure seneciphylline and senecionine in rat lung, liver, and kidney (Candrian et al., 1985). Details of HPLC detection of these compounds using a reversed-phase styrene–divinylbenzene resin column and Schoeffel SF-770 detector set at 220 nm have been described (Ramsdell and Buhler, 1981). Metabolites of senecionine in rat urine have been detected using HPLC and mass spectrometry (Estep et al., 1990a).

## 17.9 Regulatory Status

The German Commission E recommends limiting the use of coltsfoot leaf to 4–6 wk per year. Furthermore, the daily dosage of PAs with the 1,2-unsaturated necine structure plus their corresponding *N*-oxides in teas, extracts, pressed juices, and ointments should not exceed 10 μg, 1 μg, and 100 μg, respectively. The fact that the concentrations of PAs are not standardized in available coltsfoot's products presents a safety problem with its use. Coltsfoot leaf is approved for use in acute catarrh of the respiratory tract with cough and hoarseness, and acute, mild inflammation of the oral and pharyngeal mucosa. The efficacy of coltsfoot flower, herb, and root for any indication is undocumented, and in consideration of the toxicity of the PA component, are unapproved for use (Blumenthal, 1998).

Coltsfoot is classified as a dietary supplement, and as an "herb of undefined safety" by the FDA (Anonymous, 1996).

## References


Anonymous. Coltsfoot. The Lawrence review of natural products. St. Louis, MO: Facts and Comparisons, 1996.

Berry M. Herbal products. Coltsfoot. Pharmaceut J 1996;256:234–5.

Blumenthal M. The complete German Commission E monographs. Austin, TX: American Botanical Council, 1998.

Candrian URS, Luthy J, Schlatter C. In vivo covalent binding of retronecine-labelled [$^3$H] senecionine to DNA of rat liver, lung and kidney. Chem Biol Interact 1985;54:57–69.

Chalmers AH, Culvenor CCJ, Smith LW. Characterization of pyrrolizidine alkaloids by gas, thin-layer and paper chromatography. J Chromatogr 1965;20:270–7.

Eastman DF, Dimenna GP, Segall HJ. Covalent binding of two pyrrolizidine alkaloids, senecionine and seneciphylline, to hepatic macromolecules and their distribution, excretion, and transfer into milk of lactating mice. Drug Metab Dis 1982;10:236–40.

Estep JE, Lame MW, Jones AD, Segall HJ. *N*-Acetylcysteine-conjugated pyrrole identified in rat urine following administration of two pyrrolizidine alkaloids, monocrotaline and senecionine. Toxicol Lett 1990a;54:61–9.

Estep JE, Lame MW, Segall HJ. Excretion and blood radioactivity levels following [$^{14}$C]senecionine administration in the rat. Toxicology 1990b;64:179–89.

Frei H, Luthy J, Brauchili J, Zweifel U, Wurgler FE, Schlatter C. Structure/activity relationships of the genotoxic potencies of sixteen pyrrolizidine alkaloids assayed for the induction of somatic mutations and recombination in wing cells of *Drosophila mealnogaster*. Chem Biol Interact 1992;83:1–22.

Hirono I, Shimizu M, Fushimi K, Mori H, Kato K. Carcinogenic activity of *Petasites japonicus* Maxim., a kind of coltsfoot. Gann 1973;64:527–8.

Hirono I, Mori H, Culvenor CCJ. Carcinogenic activity of coltsfoot, *Tussilago farfara* (L.). Gann 1976;67:125–9.

Hirono I, Mori H, Yamada K, Hirata Y, Haga M, Takematsu H, Kanie S. Carcinogenic activity of petasitenine, a new pyrrolizidine alkaloid isolated from *Petasites japonicus* Maxim. J Natl Cancer Inst 1977;58:1155–6.

Hirono I, Haga M, Fujii M, Matsuura S, Matsubara N, Nakayama M et al. Induction of hepatic tumors in rats by senkirkine and symphytine. J Natl Cancer Inst 1979;63:469–71.

Hwang S, Chang MN, Garcia ML, Han QQ, Huang L, King VF, et al. L-652,469—a dual receptor antagonist of platelet activating factor and dihydropyridines from *Tussilago farfara* L. Eur J Pharmacol 1987;141:269–81.

Koekemoer MJ, Warren FL. The senecio alkaloids. VIII. The occurrence and preparation of the N-oxides. An improved method of extraction of the senecio alkaloids. J Chem Soc 1951;47:66–8.

Kumana CR, NG M, Lin HJ, Ko W, Wu P, Todd D. Herbal tea induced hepatic veno-occlusive disease: quantification of toxic alkaloid exposure in adults. Gut 1985;26:101–4.

Li Y, Wang Y. Evaluation of tussilagone: a cardiovascular-respiratory stimulant isolated from Chinese herbal medicine. Gen Pharmacol 1988;19:261–3.

Mattocks AR. Detection of pyrrolizidine alkloids on thin layer chromatography. J Chromatogr 1967;27:505–8.

Mattocks AR. Toxicity of pyrrolizidine alkaloids. Nature 1968;217:723–8.

Mattocks AR. Relation of structural features to pyrrolic metabolites in livers of rats given pyrrolizidine alkaloids and derivatives. Chem Biol Interact 1981;35:301–10.

Mattocks AR. Chemistry and toxicology of the pyrrolizidine alkaloids. London: Academic Press, 1986.

Mori H, Sugie S, Yoshimi N, Asada Y, Furuya T, Williams GM. Genotoxicity of a variety of pyrrolizidine alkaloids in the hepatocye primary culture-DNA repair test using rat, mouse, and hampster hepatocytes. Cancer Res 1985;45:3125–9.

Ramsdell HS, Buhler DR. High-performance liquid chromatrographic analysis of pyrrolizidine (senecio) alkaloids using a reveresed-phase styrene-divinylbenzene resin column. J Chromatrogr 1981;210:154–8.

Roulet M, Laurini R, Rivier L, Calame A. Hepatic veno-occlusive disease in newborn infant of a woman drinking herbal tea. J Pediatr 1988;112:433–6.

Salvador RL. Coltsfoot. Can Pharmaceut J 1996;(July–Aug):48–50.

Schoental R. Hepatotoxic activity of retrorsine, senkirkine and hydroxysenkirkine in newborn rats, and the role of epoxides in carcinogenesis by pyrrolizidine alkaloids and aflatoxins. Nature 1970;227:401–2.

Sharma RK, Khajuria GS, Atal CK. Thin-layer chromatography of pyrrolizidine alkaloids. J Chromatogr 1965;19:433–4.

Sperl W, Stuppner H, Gassner I, Judmaier W, Dietze O, Vogel W. Reversible hepatic veno-occlusive disease in an infant after consumption of pyrrolizidine-containing herbal tea. Eur J Pediatr 1995;154:112–6.

Sundareson AE. An experimental study on placental permeability to cirrhogenic poisons. J Pathol Bacteriol 1942;54:289–98.

Tyler, V. Herbs of choice: the therapeutic use of phytomedicinals. New York: Haworth Press, 1994.

# Chapter 18

# Comfrey

*David Burch and Melanie Johns Cupp*

*Symphytum officinale* (L.), *S. tuberosum*, *Sympytum* × *uplandicum* Nyman (Russian comfrey, a hybrid of *S. officinale* and *S. asperum*) (Anonymous, 1995), *Symphytum asperum* Lepech (prickly comfrey) (USP, 1998), boneset, knitback, knitbone (Awang, 1987), consound, common comfrey, blackwort, bruisewort, slippery root, yalluc, gum plant, consolida, ass ear (Grieve, 1971)

## *18.1 History and Traditional Uses*

Comfrey is a perennial herb that has a thick root and white, hairy, branching stems (Leung, 1980). The plant is native to Europe and Asia and grows to about 1 m high (Leung, 1980). Over the past 2000 yr, people from all over the world have been using comfrey to heal their ailments. Comfrey use was first documented by the ancient Romans and Greeks (Wiesner, 1984). Around 200 AD, the Greek physician Dioscorides praised the therapeutic uses of comfrey in his book *Materia Medica* and coined the genus name *Symphytum* from the Greek word *syuphuo*, which means "to make to grow together." During the Middle Ages, comfrey in the form of an external poultice became popular for healing broken bones (Awang, 1987). It was during this time that comfrey received nicknames such as boneset, knitbone, and knitback. As the popularity of comfrey grew over the centuries so did its indications for use. Comfrey has been used to treat respiratory problems (bronchitis, catarrh, hemoptysis, pleurisy, whooping cough), gastrointestinal diseases (cholecystitis, colitis, dysentery, diarrhea, ulcers, hematemesis), metorrhagia, phlebitis, and tonsillitis (USP, 1998). Comfrey has also been touted for its nutritional value; it has been considered a good source of protein and vitamin $B_{12}$, which is unusual for a plant.

From Forensic Science: *Toxicology and Clinical Pharmacology of Herbal Products*
Edited by: M. J. Cupp © Humana Press Inc., Totowa, New Jersey

However, recent studies have concluded that >4 lbs of comfrey would have to be ingested to meet daily requirements for $B_{12}$ (Teynor et al., 1998). Furthermore, comfrey has lower amounts of eight essential amino acids when compared to turnip greens or spinach.

## 18.2 Current Promoted Uses

Comfrey is currently promoted for prevention of kidney stones, for treatment of rheumatic and pulmonary disorders, and for treatment of injuries such as burns and bruises. Combination products containing comfrey for internal use are promoted for nourishing and repairing bone and muscle. Several cosmetic products contain comfrey and claim to remove excess oil from the skin, as well as to moisturize and exfoliate dry skin.

## 18.3 Products Available

Many different commercial forms of comfrey are marketed including oral and external products. Comfrey can be bought in bulk as dried leaf or whole root to be used in preparing teas or poultices (Awang, 1987). Powdered comfrey root is packaged in gelatin capsules, in tablets, or in tablets that may also contain acacia gum, silica, and calcium stearate. Combination products containing pepsin in tablets or capsules are promoted to aid digestion, and can contain as much as 2.9 mg/g of toxic alkaloids (Bach, 1989). In Europe, a company called Kytta makes preparations of comfrey including poultice paste (Kytta-Plasma®) and ointment (Kytta-Salbe®) (Bisset, 1994). In Great Britain, Potter's Comfrey ointment contains comfrey root extract.

Bone™ is a capsule that contains a 310 mg net wt combination of oatstraw, horsetail, comfrey, and pan pien lien. It is recommended that two capsules of Bone™ be taken with a large glass of water three times a day. BM&C™ is a capsule that contains a 380 mg net wt combination of white oak bark, marshmallow root, mullein herb, wormwood herb, lobelia herb, scullcap herb, comfrey root, black walnut bark, and gravel root. The recommended daily use of BM&C™ is two capsules with a large glass of water three times daily. Simply Clean® Combination/Oily Skin is a cosmetic cream that contains five hydroxy acids, chamomile, comfrey, and aloe. Delicate Cleanser® Dry Skin is a cosmetic cream that contains five hydroxy acids, chamomile, comfrey, yarrow, aloe, and ginseng.

## 18.4 Pharmacological/Toxicologic Effects

An excellent resource for toxicology information pertaining to comfrey is Mattocks (1986).

### 18.4.1 Gastrointestinal Effects

In an in vitro study using rat gastric tissue, researchers showed that an extract of 10 mg of dried comfrey leaves (*S. officinale*) homogenized in 1 mL of Kreb's solution increased the release of prostaglandin $F_{2\alpha}$ and 6-keto-prostaglandin $F_{1\alpha}$ (Stamford and Tavares, 1983). As numerous prostaglandins have been found to protect the gastric mucosa, there may be a biologic basis for use of comfrey as a treatment for peptic ulcers.

### 18.4.2 Hepatotoxicity

Commercial comfrey is usually derived from the leaves or roots of *Symphytum officinale* (common comfrey) (USP, 1998). However, some products are derived from *Symphytum* × *uplandicum* Nyman (Russian comfrey) or *Symphytum asperum* Lepech (prickly comfrey), which appear to be more toxic than common comfrey (Anonymous, 1998). Russian comfrey and prickly comfrey contain a very toxic pyrrolizidine alkaloid (PA) called echimidine that common comfrey does not contain (Tyler, 1994). Although common comfrey does not contain echimidine, it does contain other hepatotoxic PAs. These alkaloids include 7-acetylintermedine, 7-acetyllycopsamine, their unacetylated precursors, and symphytine (Tyler, 1993).

These PAs can cause hepatic venoocclusive disease with zonal or focal hemorrhagic hepatic necrosis, damage to the endothelium of the central and sublobular veins, hepatocyte swelling, biliary hyperplasia, and marked fibrosis (Abbott, 1988). These alkaloids can also cause pulmonary fibrosis (Svoboda and Reddy, 1972).

Several studies in rats have shown liver damage caused by comfrey. In one study (Yeong et al., 1991), three groups of mice received different doses of PAs derived from the fresh roots and leaves of *Symphytum* × *uplandicum* Nyman (Russian comfrey). A single dose of 200 mg/kg was given to group I rats, a dose of 100 mg/kg three times a week was given to group II rats, and dose of 50 mg/kg three times a week for 3 wk was given to group III rats. All of the rats developed dose-dependent liver damage evident by light and electron microscopy. Group I rats showed swelling of hepatocytes and hemorrhagic necrosis of perivenular cells with preservation of sinusoidal walls and endothelial cells. Group I rats also developed noticeable extravasation of red blood cells. Group II and III rats had similar changes but with more severe necrosis. Loss of sinusoidal lining cells and disruption of hepatocyte cellular margins was found in both group II and group III rats. All of these histologic changes are indicative of hepatic venoocclusive disease caused by PAs.

Another study examined the activity of various hepatic drug-metabolizing enzymes in liver homogenates of three groups of six male Long-Evans rats fed a 5%, 10%, or 30% comfrey diet ad libitum for 3 wk (Garrett et al., 1982). The activity of aminopyrine N-demethylase was found to be increased, but the activity of glutathione S-transferase and epoxide hydrolase was not affected by comfrey. Epoxide hydrolase activity has previously been reported to be increased by carcinogens, and is thought to play a role in the neoplastic process.

Another study involved injecting eight adult rats (four male, four female) with 50 mg/kg of comfrey (*Symphytum* × *uplandicum* Nymann leaves, roots, and stems) derived alkaloids per week for 6 wk (Yeong et al., 1993). One week after the last dose was given, the rats were killed and their livers were examined with light and electron microscopy. Light microscopy showed excessive sinusoidal congestion, loss of definition of hepatocyte cellular membranes, and mild zone 3 necrosis. Ultrastructural damage such as endothelial sloughing and loss of hepatocyte microvilli was evident. The most significant finding in this study was florid bleb formation. Formation of blebs is an indicator of impending irreversible liver damage. Blebs were observed in the sinsoidal borders of hepatocytes. Some of these blebs occluded the sinusoidal lumina. The space of Disse was damaged by deposition of collagen and was extensively dilated. These findings were not found in the two control groups. All eight experimental rats showed the same liver damage described previously.

Some have also questioned the safety of comfrey externally. According to one toxicologic researcher (Mattocks, 1980), external use of comfrey should not be hazardous because the PAs must be converted to the toxic free PAs by the liver (Mattocks, 1968).

An animal study supports Mattock's hypothesis. The absorption of comfrey through unbroken skin is very low and should not cause toxicity. A Swiss experiment with rats showed that 0.1–0.4% of a dermal dose of 194 mg of alkaloid *N*-oxides/kg (extracted from the roots of Polish *S. officinale*) was recovered in the urine 48 h later (Brauchli et al., 1982). The researchers noted that the orally ingested alkaloids showed up in the urine at 20–50 times the concentration of the alkaloids found in the urine after dermal administration. Of the dermally absorbed alkaloids, only a small amount was converted to the toxic free alkaloids. These researchers concluded that short-term dermal use of comfrey should not be dangerous.

### *18.4.3 Carcinogenicity/Mutagenicity*

Long-term studies in animals have shown that comfrey is carcinogenic (USP, 1998). This carcinogenicity has been associated with the PAs found in comfrey. Several studies involving rats have made this correlation.

In 1978, the results of a study involving *Symphytum officinale* were published in the Journal of the National Cancer Institute (Hirono et al., 1978b).

Over a 480- to 600-d period, seven groups of inbred strain ACI rats were fed dried comfrey leaves (*S. officinale*) or dried comfrey roots (*S. officinale*). Three groups of rats consisting of 19–22 rats were fed comfrey leaves as 0.5–33% of their diet, and four groups consisting of 15–24 rats were fed comfrey roots as 1–4% of their diets. A control group was fed a normal diet. All groups of rats fed comfrey roots or leaves developed hepatocellular adenomas, while the rats in the control groups did not develop liver tumors. The results also showed that the highest incidence of liver tumors occurred in those rats being fed comfrey roots.

A study published almost 1 yr later showed very similar results. Twenty rats were injected with 13 mg/kg of symphytine (a PA common in comfrey) (10% of the $LD_{50}$) extracted from dried comfrey roots, while a control group received intraperitoneal injections of 0.9% sodium chloride (Hirono et al., 1978a). Of the rats injected with symphytine, four developed liver tumors; three developed hemangioendothelial sarcomas, and one developed liver cell adenoma. The rats in the control group developed no liver tumors. This pattern of carcinogenicity was similar to that seen in the previous study using comfrey leaves.

Lasiocarpine is another carcinogenic PA. Lasiocarpine has been detected in *S. officinale* roots by thin-layer chrommatography (TLC) at a concentration of 0.0058% (Winship, 1991). An experiment conducted by Northwestern University Medical School involved feeding 20 male inbred strain F-344 rats lasiocarpine at a concentration of 50 ppm over 55 wk (Rao and Reddy, 1978). Ten control rats were fed a diet without lasiocarpine. At the end of 59 wk, necropsies were performed on all animals (survivors were killed along with the control animals). None of the control rats had any abnormalities based on light and electron microscopy. Of the 20 experimental rats, 17 developed malignancies. Forty-five percent (nine) developed angiosarcomas while 35% (seven) developed hepatocellular carcinomas. One rat developed malignant adnexal tumor of the skin and one developed lymphoma. Four rats with angiosarcoma developed lung mestases while one rat with hepatocellular carcinoma developed lung metastases.

Mutagenicity has been demonstrated by many PAs using several standard tests (Mattocks, 1986).

### *18.4.4 $LD_{50}$*

It has been stated that humans appear more sensitive to the toxic affects of the alkaloids than are rats, meaning that human deaths have occurred at much lower $LD_{50}$s when compared to rats (Huxtable, 1989). However, it is important to note that the $LD_{50}$ varies among the alkaloids, and because the plant contains multiple alkaloids, calculations based on administration of a single alkaloid might not apply clinically (Mattocks, 1986). In addition, the extent to which the alkaloids are toxic in a given species depends on the extent to which the hepatic enzymes can convert the alkaloids to their toxic metabolites. As an example, the $LD_{50}$ of one alkaloid, retrosine, is 34 mg/kg in male rats, but 800 mg/kg in guinea pigs.

## 18.5 Case Reports of Toxicity Due to Commercially Available Products

In 1994, Joseph Betz, an FDA pharmacognosist, analyzed the PA content of 11 products containing comfrey that were bought throughout the Washington, DC area. Of the 11 products purchased, 9 had measurable levels of alkaloids (Betz et al., 1994). The levels of alkaloids present in these products could provide an explanation of the hepatotoxicities attributable to comfrey seen over the last 30 yr. It is estimated that comfrey root tea can contain up to 26 mg of alkaloid per cup (Bach, 1989). Although the comfrey root contains a much higher amount of alkaloids than the comfrey leaves, teas made with comfrey leaves contain measurable amounts of alkaloids because PAs are water soluble (Betz et al., 1994). Case reports of hepatotoxicity associated with comfrey tea contradict proponents who claim that the tea is safe because the alkaloid content of the leaf is low, and the alkaloids are not water soluble.

A 10-yr-old British boy was diagnosed with Crohn's disease and was treated with an herbal tea containing comfrey leaf. Other medications included sporadic use of prednisolone and sulfasalazine. Three years later, he presented with weight loss, diarrhea, fever, abdominal pain, ascites, tender hepatomegaly, and fatigue. Laboratory tests revealed mild iron deficiency anemia (Hgb 117 g/L), elevated bilirubin (26 mmol/L) and aspartate aminotransferase level (87 IU/L), and low serum albumin. Ascitic fluid protein concentration was 27 g/L. Liver biopsy showed the thrombotic variant of venoocclusive disease. He was treated with salt restriction and spironolactone, with good response. After excluding other etiologies, his liver disease was attributed to chronic use of comfrey tea (Weston et al., 1987).

A 47-yr-old woman suffering from abdominal pain, fatigue, and allergies began consuming 10 cups of comfrey tea and handfuls of comfrey pills each day (Bach, 1989). Four years later, her aminotransferase levels were documented to be twice normal. After 4 more years, she presented to the hospital with confusion, hyponatremia, and ascites. Liver biopsy 1 mo after admission revealed a normal lobular structure with thickening of the terminal hepatic venules and narrowing of their lumens confirmed by trichrome stain. Perivenular fibrosis surrounded atrophic hepatocytes, and had replaced necrotic hepatocytes. Portal tracts were mildly fibrotic, and a few scattered glycogenated nuclei were seen. She was diagnosed with hepatic venoocclusive disease attributed to comfrey consumption. A repeat liver biopsy 20 mo later showed dense fibrosis of portal tracts with proliferating bile ductules and minimal inflammatory cells. Areas of collapse also contained proliferating bile ductules and isolated hepatocytes. Thin, fibrous septa compressed by regenerating nodules radiated from small, occluded terminal hepatic venules. Most of the terminal hepatic venules were patent, although some had thickened walls. The bile ducts were unremarkable.

In another case report (Yeong et al., 1990), a 23-yr-old man was diagnosed with venoocclusive disease. Symptoms began 1–2 wk after ingestion of four to five comfrey leaves each day for 1–2 wk. He presented with a 3-mo history of flulike symptoms followed by malaise and night sweats, and a 3-wk history of abdominal distension and peripheral edema. He was hypoalbuminemic (22 g/L) with a bilirubin of 28 μmol/L, markedly elevated alkaline phosphatase (475 U/L,) glutamyl transferase of 99 U/L, and aspartate transferase markedly elevated (365 U/L). The prothrombin time (PT) ratio was 1.4, partial thromboplastin time (PTT) was 38 s, and platelet count was mildly decreased ($148 \times 10^9$/L). Two tricut liver biopsies on two separate occasions showed centrilobular hemorrhagic necrosis and platelet plugging of the central and sublobular veins. Sinusoidal dilatation and congestion was also evident. Cellular infiltrate in the necrotic areas consisted of fibroblasts, lymphocytes, and macrophages. Liver angiography revealed luminal narrowing in the small hepatic vein radicles associated with nonhomogeneous filling of the hepatic sinusoids. Hepatic venous wedge pressure was elevated at 30 mm Hg. The main hepatic veins and portal vein were patent, but the lumen of the inferior vena cava was narrowed by the enlarged liver. He later died of liver failure attributed to comfrey-induced hepatic venoocclusive disease. Contributing factors included ingestion of young comfrey leaves, which have a relatively high alkaloid content, and the protein-deficient diet that the young man had followed for the 4 yr preceding his death.

In the first published case of venoocclusive disease associated with consumption of a comfrey-containing preparation, a 49-yr-old woman presented with swelling of the abdomen and extremities that had begun 4 mo prior. Liver biopsy showed centrilobular necrosis and congestion. During hepatic venography, a wedge pressure of 23 mm Hg and a corrected sinusoidal pressure of 17 mm Hg were recorded, suggesting moderate portal hypertension. No outflow obstruction in the vena cava or hepatic veins was appreciated. The smaller hepatic venules were seen to be nearly obliterated on films taken during balloon distention of one of the intrahepatic venous tributaries. The patient's condition required placement of a side-to-side portacaval shunt. During surgery, portal pressures and postshunt preportal pressure confirmed postsinusoidal block.There was no evidence of a hypercoagulable state or outlet obstruction, and the patient had not been taking any medications; however, the patient had, for the 6 mo prior to presentation, consumed approx 1 quart per day of a tea known as MU-16, and had taken two comfrey-pepsin pills with meach meal for the past 4 mo. Other food supplements taken by the patient included vitamins C, K, E, A, and B complex; calcium, magnesium, zinc, iron, lecithin, sterotrophic adrenal bovine extract, and approx 3 cups of chamomile tea per week. After analyzing the MU-16 tea and comfrey-pepsin pills for PAs and pyrrolizidine *N*-oxides, the investigators calculated that the patient had consumed 14.1 µg/kg/d pyrrolizidines from the capsules, and 0.49–1.45 µg/kg/d from the tea (Ridker et al., 1985).

Comfrey tea from a particular distributor in Britain was found to be contaminated with the anticholinergic *Atropa belladonna* (deadly nightshade) (Anonymous, 1983). Three patients experienced anticholinergic symptoms including hallucinations, erythema, thirst (Galizia, 1983), light-headedness, agitation, confusion, difficulty in urination, dry mouth, sinus tachycardia, dilated pupils, and warm dry skin (Routledge and Spriggs, 1989) after drinking comfrey tea. In these case reports, belladonna was not definitively identified as the contaminant, but the tea consumed by one patient was found to contain atropine at a concentration of 0.014% (Routledge and Spriggs, 1989).

## 18.6 Drug Interactions

A study involving rats showed that phenobarbital induces the metabolism of PAs to their lethal metabolites (Lafranconi and Huxtable, 1984). The USP recognizes this as a possible drug interaction and also suggests that patients on any medications avoid taking comfrey (USP, 1998).

## 18.7 Pharmacokinetics/Toxicokinetics

### 18.7.1 Absorption

Comfrey is absorbed through the skin as well as the gastrointestinal tract (Abbott, 1988). A experiment conducted by Swiss researchers on rats showed that 0.1–0.4% of the dermal dose of 194 mg of alkaloid *N*-oxides/kg (extracted from the roots of Polish *S. officinale*) was absorbed and was recovered in urine within 48 h (Brauchli et al., 1982).

## *18.7.2 Distribution*

The pyrrole metabolites are distributed throughout the body (Abbott, 1988). No data is available on the distribution of PAs into human breast milk. Rats suckled by mothers fed lasiocarpine, a PA found in comfrey, developed liver damage (Schoental, 1959). Cows that ate PA-containing plants (*Sencio* sp. [tansy ragwort] — not comfrey) secreted milk that contained 9.4–16.7 μg of a PA called jacoline (which is not found in comfrey) per 100 mL of milk (Dickinson et al., 1976). The investigators measured blood leukocyte counts, serum protein levels, serum albumin levels, and globulin content in both the calves and the cows. Liver biopsy and sorbitol dehydrogenase levels were used to determine liver damage in both the calves and the cows. The four cows were shown to have marked sorbitol dehydrogenase (an indicator of liver function) levels, leukocytosis, and decreased albumin levels. Biopsy of cow livers revealed megalocytosis, portal fibroplasia, and centrolobular necrosis indicative of PA-induced toxicity. No abnormalities were found in the calves. Although no harmful effects were found in calves or rats to which cow milk was fed, the author of a similar study did not feel that his results exclude the possibility of toxicity to humans who drink milk from cows who graze on PA-containing plants (Johnson, 1976).

## *18.7.3 Metabolism/Elimination*

The PAs are not toxic until they are metabolized in the liver. Dehydrogenation by P-450 enzymes forms toxic pyrrolic metabolites. These pyrrolic metabolites either undergo hydrolysis to pyrrolic alcohols or destroy surrounding tissues. Both the pyrrolic esters (primary metabolites) and the pyrrolic alcohols (secondary metabolites) have antimitotic effects and are responsible for the damage to cells in the liver (Abbott, 1988).

In animals, the PAs are rapidly metabolized and eliminated such that they are not detectable in biofluids more than 24 h post-ingestion (Winship, 1991).

# *18.8 Analysis of Biofluids*

In a study (Brauchli et al., 1982) in which urine from rats exposed to PAs via dermal application was analyzed for PA content, TLC and gas chromatographyy–mass spectroscopy (GC–MS) were used. Details are available in the cited reference.

PA content of cow milk was determined using a spectrophotometric technique (Dickinson et al., 1976) as described by a previous investigator (Mattocks, 1967).

## 18.9 Chemical Analysis

HPLC (Ramsdell and Buhler, 1981), GC–MS (Betz, 1994), and TLC analyses of the PAs has been described (Sharma et al., 1965).

## 18.10 Regulatory Status

The German E Commission approves only the use of comfrey root, herb, and leaf for external use (Blumenthal, 1998). It is recommended that external poultices be applied only to intact skin, and pregnant women should not apply or take comfrey internally without consulting a physician. Product labels must include a warning that the daily dosage should not exceed 100 μg. Also, it is recommended that the duration of administration not to exceed 4–6 wk per year.

The USP discourages the internal use of comfrey because of studies showing hepatotoxicity and carcinogenicity, and no studies have shown the benefit of taking comfrey orally (USP, 1998). The Delaney Clause of the Food, Drug and Cosmetic Act establishes no tolerance for carcinogens in foods. Even so, comfrey is considered a dietary supplement, and can be sold if labeled as such.

In Australia, comfrey is classified as a poison, and its sale has been restricted in several states (USP, 1998). In Austria, medicinal preparations of comfrey must be registered with the Federal Ministry of Health and Environmental Protection, and can be sold only in pharmacies. A similar situation exists in Sweden, where comfrey products must be registered. Sale for medicinal use is prohibited in Belgium, the United Kingdom, and Indonesia. In Canada, the Health Protection Branch of Health does not accept comfrey root as an ingredient in medicinal products, and it is listed as unacceptable as a food. In France, as in Germany, the root is permitted for external use only.

## References


Anonymous. Coe's comfrey. Available from: www.geocitoes.com/RainForest/Canopy/4809/whatiscomfrey.html. Accessed 1998 Oct 22.

Anonymous. Comfrey. The Lawrence review of natural products. St. Louis, MO: Facts and Comparisons, 1995.

Anonymous. Poisoned comfrey tea warning. Pharm J 1983;230:173.

Abbott P. Comfrey: assessing the low-dose health risk. Med J Austr 1988;149:678–81.

Awang DVC. Herbal medicine: comfrey. Can Pharmaceut J 1987;120:101–4.

Bach N, Thung S, Schaffner F. Comfrey herb tea-induced hepatic veno-occlusive disease. Am J Med 1989;87:97–9.

Betz J, Eppley R, Taylor W, Andrzejewski D. Determination of pyrrolizidine alkaloids in commercial comfrey products. J Pharmaceut Sci 1994;83:649–52.

Bisset N. Herbal drugs and phytopharmaceuticals. Stuggart: Medpharm, 1994.

Blumenthal M. The complete German Commission E Monographs: therapeutic guide to herbal medicines. Austin, TX: American Botanical Council, 1998.

Brauchli J, Luthy J, Zweifel U, Schlatter C. Pyrrolizidine alkaloids from *Symphytum officinale* L. and their percutaneous absorption in rats. Experientia 1982;38:1085–7.

Dickinson JO, Cooke MP, King RR, Mohamed PA. Milk transfer of pyrrolizidine alkaloids in cattle. J Am Vet Med Assoc 1976;169:1192–6.

Galizia EJ. Clinical curio: hallucinations in elderly tea drinkers. Br Med J 1983;287:979.

Garrett B, Cheeke P, Miranda C, Goeger D, Buhler D. Consumption of poisonous plants (*Senecio jacobaea, Symphytum officinale, Pteridium aquilinum, Hypericum perforatum*) by rats: chronic toxicity, mineral metabolism, and hepatic drug-metabolizing enzymes. Toxicol Lett 1982;10:183–188.

Grieve, M. A modern herbal. New York, NY: Dover, 1971.

Hirono I, Masanobu H, Fujii M, Shin M, Matsubara N, Nakayama M, Furuya T, Hikichi M, Takanashi H, Uchida E, Hosaka S, Ueno I. Induction of hepatic tumors in rats by senkirkine and symphytine. J Natl Cancer Inst 1978a;63:469–71.

Hirono I, Mori H, Haga M. Carcinogenic activity of *Symphytum officinale*. J Natl Cancer Inst 1978b;61:85–9.

Huxtable RJ. Human embryotoxicity of pyrrolizidine-containing drugs. Hepatology 1989;9:510–1.

Johnson AE. Changes in calves and rats consuming milk from cows fed chronic lethal doses of *Senecio jacobaea* (tansy ragwort). Am J Vet Res 1976;37:107–10.

Lafranconi WM, Huxtable RJ. Hepatic metabolism and pulmonary toxicity of monocrotaline using isolated perfused liver and lung. Biochem Pharmacol 1984;33:2479–84.

Leung A. Encyclopedia of common natural ingredients. New York: John Wiley & Sons, 1980.

Mattocks AR. Spectrophotometric determination of unsaturated pyrrolizidine alkaloids. Analyt Chem 1967;39:443–7.

Mattocks A. Toxicity of pyrrolizidine alkaloids. Nature 1968;217:723–8.

Mattocks A. Toxic pyrrolizidine alkaloids in comfrey. Lancet 1980;2:1136–7.

Mattocks, AR. Chemistry and toxicology of pyrrolizidine alkaloids. Orlando, FL: Academic Press, 1986.

Ramsdell HS, Buhler DR. High-performance liquid chromatographic analysis of pyrrolizidine (*Senecio*) alkaloids using a reversed-phase styrene-divinylbenzene resin column. J Chromatogr 1981;210:154–8.

Rao MS, Reddy JK. Malignant neoplasms in rats fed lasiocarpine. Br J Cancer 1978;37:289–92.

Ridker PM, Ohkuma S, McDermott W, Trey C, Huxtable R. Hepatic venocclusive disease associated with the consumption of pyrrolizidine-containing dietary supplements. Gastroenterology 1985;88:1050.

Routledge PA, Spriggs TLB. Atropine as a possible contaminant of comfrey tea. Lancet 1989;I:963–4.

Schoental R. Liver lesions in young rats suckled by mothers treated with the pyrrolizidine (Senecio) alkaloids, lasiocarpine and retrosine. J Pathol Bacteriol 1959;77:485–95.

Sharma RK, Khajuria GS, Atal CK. Thin-layer chromatography of pyrrolizidine alkaloids. J Chromatogr 1965;19:433–34.

Stamford IF, Tavares IA. The effect of an aqueous extract on prostaglandin synthesis by rat isolated stomach. J Pharmaceut Pharmacol 1983;35:816–7.

Svoboda D, Reddy J. Malignant tumors in rats given lasiocarpine. Cancer Res 1972;32:908–12.

Teynor TM, Putnam DH, Doll JD, Kelling KA, Oelke EA, Undersander DJ, Oplinger ES. Alternative Field Crops Manual: Comfrey. Available from: www.hort.purdue.edu/newcrop/articles/comfrey.html. Accessed 1998 Oct 22.

Tyler, V. The honest herbal, 3rd edit., Binghamton, NY: Pharmaceutical Products Press, 1993.

Tyler, V. Herbs of choice. The therapeutic use of phytomedicinals. Binghamton, NY: Pharmaceutical Products Press, 1994.

United States Pharmacopeial Convention (USP). Comfrey. Botanical monograph series. Rockville, MD: United States Pharmacopeial Convention, 1998.

Weston CF, Cooper BT, Davies JD, Levine JD. Veno-occlusive disease of the liver secondary to ingestion of comfrey. Br Med J 1987;295:183.

Wiesner D. Pharmacists and Comfrey. Austr J Pharm 1984;65:959–63.

Winship KA. Toxicity of comfrey. Adverse Drug React Toxicol Rev 1991;10:47–59.

Yeong ML, Clark SP, Waring JM. The effects of comfrey derived pyrrolizidine alkaloids on rat liver. Pathology 1991;23:35–8.

Yeong ML, Swinburn B, Kennedy M, Nicholson G. Hepatic veno-occlusive disease with comfrey ingestion. J Gastroenterol Hepatol 1990;5:211–4.

Yeong ML, Wakefield SJ, Ford H. Hepatocyte membrane injury and bleb formation following low dose comfrey toxicity in rats. Int J Exp Pathol 1993;74:211–7.

*Chapter 19*

# Scullcap

*Jennifer Schumacher and Melanie Johns Cupp*

Virginian scullcap, mad-dog scullcap, madweed (*Scutellaria laterifolia)*; common scullcap, greater scullcap, helmet flower, toque, hoodwort (*Scutellaria galericulata*); lesser scullcap (*Scutellaria minor*) (Grieve, 1971), mad-dog weed (Anonymous, 1993), monkey-flower (Crellin and Philpott, 1990), *Scutellaria baicalensis* Georgi (Tyler, 1993).

## *19.1 History and Traditional Uses*

Scullcap is a perennial that grows mainly in temperate regions and tropical mountains near rivers, lakes (Grieve, 1971), and moist woods (Anonymous, 1993). It is found in the United States (*Scutellaria laterifolia*), Mexico (*Scutellaria coccinea*), Europe (*Scutellaria galericulata, Scutellaria minor*) (Grieve, 1971), and Asia (*Scutellaria baicalensis*) (Tyler, 1993). Reaching about 3 ft in height, the plant blooms from July to September and has blue, pink, purple or red flowers (Grieve, 1971; Anonymous, 1993). Scullcap was introduced into American medicine in 1773 by Dr. Lawrence Van Derveer who used it to treat rabies (Tyler, 1993); hence the common name mad-dog weed (Anonymous, 1998b). It was believed that *Scutellaria lateriflora* relieved muscle spasm associated with rabies, but was not found to cure it. Scullcap later came to be recognized as a tonic, tranquilizer, and antispasmodic, and was therefore used as an ingredient in many "patent medicines" for "female weakness" (Tyler, 1993). Scullcap was also combined with other reputedly calming herbs such as hop and valerian and promoted as a sedative or anxiolytic (Anonymous, 1993, 1998b). Other traditional uses include epilepsy, headache, insomnia, various other neurologic and psychiatric disorders, hypertension, fever, rheumatism, and stress (Anonymous, 1998a).

From Forensic Science: *Toxicology and Clinical Pharmacology of Herbal Products*
Edited by: M. J. Cupp © Humana Press Inc., Totowa, New Jersey

## 19.2 Current Promoted Uses

Scullcap is promoted commercially in the United States as a sedative, anxiolytic, and spasmolytic and is promoted for the treatment of premenstrual syndrome (PMS), menstrual cramps, depression, exhaustion, and muscle pain caused by stress (Israel and Youngkin, 1997). Other purported uses include headache (Grieve, 1971) and epilepsy (Anonymous, 1998b).

## 19.3 Products Available

Scullcap is currently commercially available in the United States as capsules, tea, liquid extract, tincture, and bulk root. Capsules are commonly available in bottles of 100; the strengths sold include 425 mg and 429 mg and the usual instructions are to take one capsule one to three times a day as needed. The liquid extract is available in a small brown bottle containing either 1 or 2 oz; instructions are to put 10–12 drops in a glass of water per day and drink. If the dried herb is used, 1–2 teaspoons of dried leaf are placed in hot water to make a tea. The products are not sold under a specific brand name and are labeled as "scullcap" or "skullcap." Scullcap can be found either alone or in combination with other psychoactive herbs such as valerian or St. John's wort.

## 19.4 Pharmacologic/Toxicologic Effects

### 19.4.1 Antispasmodic Effects

A study by Pilcher in 1916 found scullcap extract to have very weak ability to inhibit the contractility of excised guinea pig uterus, and no effect on the uterus in living animals that received what was considered to be a normal dose (Tyler, 1993). Two species of scullcap (*S. galericulata* and *S. scordiifolia*) studied in 1957 by Kurnakov were also found to show no antispasmodic activity in various small animals (Tyler, 1993).

### 19.4.2 Hepatotoxicity

*See* Section 19.5.

### 19.4.3 Cardiovascular Effects

Neither *S. galericulata* nor *S. scordiifolia* was found by Kurnakov to affect blood pressure in cats or rabbits (Tyler, 1993). A tincture of *S. baicalensis* was reported by Ursow in 1958 to cause a decline in blood pressure in dogs. However, this report requires verification (Tyler, 1993).

## *19.4.4 Antimicrobial Activity*

Scullcap has in vitro antimicrobial activity. *Scutellaria baicalensis* root was boiled, filtered, lyophylized, and diluted with sterile water to a concentration of 16 mg/mL. Sufficient quantities of this solution were added to Mueller Hinton Medium to yield final concentrations of 100 μg/mL, 200 μg/ mL, 400 μg/mL, 800 μg/mL, and 1600 μg/mL. Activity against *Klebsiella pneumoniae*, *Proteus vulgaris*, *Alcaligenes calcoaceticus*, *Staphylococcus aureus*, and *Mycobacterium smegmatis* was noted. The minimum inhibitory concentration (MIC), defined as the lowest concentration resulting in complete absence of growth at 36 h post-incubation, was 200 μg/mL, 200 μg/mL, 800 μg/mL, 400 μg/mL, and 1600 μg/mL for each organism, respectively (Franzblau and Cross, 1986). Whether the antimicrobial principles of scullcap prepared as a tea, tincture, or dried herb could achieve concentrations necessary for antimicrobial activity in vivo is unknown.

## *19.4.5 Anti-Inflammatory Activity*

Sialic acids, which are present in cell membranes and mucous secretions, are thought to allow viruses and other substances to enter cells. Serum sialic acid levels have been shown to increase in certain disease states such as cancers, rheumatic diseases, other inflammatory diseases, and infections (Anonymous, 1993). Elevated serum sialic acid levels have also been found in men with coronary artery disease and type II diabetes mellitus (Pickup et al., 1995). It has been hypothesized that inhibition of the enzyme sialidase, which is involved in the formation of sialic acid, could be of therapeutic importance (Anonymous, 1993).

The anti-inflammatory activity of the Asian species *S. baicalensis* has been studied by Japanese researchers (Anonymous, 1993). An in vitro study with the *Scutellaria* components wogonin and isoscutellarein glucuronide demonstrated significant inhibition of the enzyme sialidase whereas baicalein, baicalin, and wogonin glucuronide showed no inhibition (Nagai et al., 1989a). Another study (Nagai et al., 1989b) demonstrated that a hot water extract of the root of *Scutellaria baicalensis* had potent mouse liver sialidase inhibition. Flavonoid content for the study was measured by high-performance liquid chromatography (HPLC). The flavonoids wogonin, wogonin glucuronide, baicalein, and baicalin all demonstrated similar inhibition at higher concentrations (50–125 μg/mL); inhibitory activity of wogonin and baicalein was more potent than that of wogonin glucuronide or baicalin at lower concentrations (10 μg/mL). The differences between the two studies may be explained by differences in the sialidase substrates used (Nagai et al., 1989a). However, baicalin and wogonin glucuronide are metabolized to baicalein and wogonin in mammals, so in vivo the differences in activity among these compounds may be insignificant (Nagai et al., 1989a).

### 19.4.6 Chemotherapeutic Activity

Preliminary animal studies have demonstrated the possibility that scullcap may improve the tolerability and efficacy of some chemotherapeutic agents. *Scutellaria baicalensis* Georgi was found to decrease tumor cell viability and ameliorate myelosuppression when used with cyclophosphamide and 5–fluorouracil in both mice and rats (Razina et al., 1987).

## 19.5 Case Reports of Toxicity Due to Commercially Available Products

Although an herbal reference (Grieve, 1971) states that high doses of scullcap tincture have been reported to cause giddiness, stupor, confusion, twitching, arrhythmias, and epilepsy, case reports in the medical literature involve only hepatotoxicity.

One report from Scotland (MacGregor et al., 1989) documents hepatotoxic effects in four women ranging in age from 41 to 57 who had been taking herbal remedies containing scullcap to relieve stress. Three were taking Kalms® tablets and one woman took Neurelax® tablets. Each woman presented with jaundice, and three with dark urine and pale stools. None of the women had a history of drug or alcohol abuse, but one woman drank approximately the equivalent of 120 g of alcohol per week. One patient had taken one tablet of indapamide daily for many years, and another had taken a low-dose oral contraceptive for the previous 5 yr. All had been in good health previously, and none had traveled abroad, received blood or blood products, or been in contact with persons with jaundice or hepatitis. None of the women presented with fever or abdominal pain. Save for one woman who had mild hepatomegaly on exam, none had signs of chronic liver disease on physical exam. In one case a liver scan was performed with normal results, and in three women ultrasonography was performed with normal results. Liver biopsy revealed severe acute hepatitis with centrilobar and bridging necrosis in one case, moderately active acute hepatitis in another, and chronic aggressive hepatitis with advanced fibrosis in a third case (this biopsy was performed 3 mo after presentation); biopsy was unsuccessful in the fourth case. Plasma bilirubin ranged from 232 mmol/L to 484 mmol/L (normal is 2–17 mmol/L), alanine aminotransferase (ALT) from 293 IU/L to 1165 IU/L (normal is 10–40 IU/L), aspartate aminotransferase (AST) from 581–617 mg/L (normal is 10–35 IU/L), alkaline phosphatase from

97 to 730 IU/L (normal is 40–100 IU/L), and prothrombin ratio from 1.3 to 1.9. In one patient, antinuclear antibody and rheumatoid factor were tested and found to be positive. Upon discontinuation of the herbal medication, liver function tests (LFTs) returned to normal values within 2–19 mo. The rapid onset of liver damage after beginning the herbal therapy in three of the women (ranging from 3 d in one case to 3 wk in two cases) may suggest a hypersensitivity type reaction. The herbal remedies these women took contained the common ingredients of valerian and scullcap prior to October, 1984; after this time, Kalms® was reformulated to contain valerian, asafetida, hops, and gentian. The authors of this case study were uncertain if the Kalms® tablets taken by their patients were the reformulated products or the older scullcap-containing formulation. Personnel from the Welsh Drug Information Center communicated that they had received several reports of jaundice associated with ingestion of Kalms®, Neurolax®, Box's Nerve Tablets® (which also contained scullcap), scullcap tablets, scullcap in combination with valerian, and scullcap in combination with mistletoe. Because of the presence of coingestants and questions about the ingredients in the Kalms® tablets ingested, it is not possible to definitively implicate scullcap as the cause of hepatotoxicity in these four cases.

Another report (Harvey and Colin-Jones, 1981) describes a case of acute hepatitis associated with use of a preparation containing both mistletoe and scullcap. A 49-yr-old woman presented with nausea, malaise, and a dull ache in the lower right quadrant. Liver function tests revealed serum albumin levels of 34 g/L, bilirubin of 42 mmol/L, alkaline phosphatase of 123 U/L, lactate dehydrogenase (LDH) of 395 U/L, and AST of >250 U/L. Liver biopsy revealed light inflammatory infiltration of the portal tracts with preservation of liver architecture. Hepatitis B and cholelithiasis were ruled out. Liver function tests returned to normal over 6 mo. Twenty-eight months later she again presented with the same symptoms. It was then that it was discovered that she had been taking tablets containing motherwort, kelp, wild lettuce, scullcap, and mistletoe for several weeks before this presentation as well as prior to the previous admission. LFTs on this admission included an albumin level of 37 g/L, bilirubin of 14 mmol/L, alkaline phosphatase of 55 U/L, LDH of 235 U/L, and AST of 23 U/L. Liver biopsy revealed light inflammatory infiltrate with occasional focal necrosis, but with preservation of architecture. LFTs returned to normal over 6 wk. Upon rechallenge with the same herbal medicine, nausea and malaise appeared after 10 d, and after 14 d liver biopsy showed heavy infiltration of lymphocytes and plasma cells, considerable focal necrosis, and distortion of liver architecture. LFTs were albumin 41 g/L, bilirubin 38 mmol/L, alkaline phosphatase 144 U/L, LDH 381 U/L, and AST > 250 U/L. An increase in serum IgG with no increase in complement concentrations was also noted. With discontinuation of the product, the patient's LFTs and liver histology normalized over the next 9 mo. The hepatotoxicity experienced by this woman was attributed to the mistletoe component of the product because no record of toxic reactions to kelp, motherwort, or scullcap were found. Although the same was true of mistletoe, the authors believed mistletoe to contain several potential hepatotoxins.

There is currently no experimental data that document liver toxicity of scullcap (Larrey, 1997). Studies of scullcap products available in the United Kingdom in the early 1980s revealed that some products contained a species of *Teucrium* in place of scullcap (Phillipson and Anderson 1984, Anonymous, 1985). The genus *Teucrium* is of the same family (Lamiaceae) as scullcap but is associated with hepatotoxicity. Several cases of liver toxicity and injury have been associated with *Teucrium chamaedrys* (Germander) in France, where it has been used as an herbal weight loss product (Larrey et al., 1992).

In light of these facts, it is important be aware of the toxicities of other herbs that may be included in scullcap products. It is difficult to attribute hepatotoxicity to scullcap because it has not been reported with products containing only scullcap. Be aware that many herbal products contain multiple ingredients, and some ingredients may not even be listed on the label. For example, scullcap is often formulated with valerian (Foster, 1998). Perhaps an interaction between scullcap and other herbs is responsible for some of the cases of hepatotoxicity.

## 19.6 Chemical Analysis

Flavonoid content of scullcap hot water extract has been determined using HPLC with a UV detector (Nagai et al., 1989b).

Interestingly, melatonin, the human pineal gland hormone, has been detected in scullcap at a concentration of 0.09 μg/g (Murch et al., 1997).

## 19.7 Regulatory Status

Scullcap is approved as a nonprescription medication in Canada and is on the General Sales List in the United Kingdom. *Scutellaria baicalensis* can be found in the Japanese Pharmacopoeia (Anonymous, 1998b). The drug is not regulated in France. In the United States, scullcap is regulated as a dietary supplement, and has been classified as an "Herb of Undefined Safety" by the FDA (Duke, 1985). A scullcap monograph was listed in the United States Pharmacopoeia from 1863 to 1916 but is currently not included (Tyler, 1993). Scullcap is not listed in the German Commission E monographs.

## *REFERENCES*

Anonymous. Herbal review: an educational service of sequential healing health services. Available from: URL: http://www.sequentialhealing.com/herbs/skullcap.html. Accessed on 1998a Oct 23.

Anonymous. Scullcap. The Lawrence review of natural products. St. Louis, MO: Facts and Comparisons, 1993.

Anonymous. Scullcap substitution. Herbal Gram 1985;2:3.

Anonymous. The Wampole family guide to nutritional supplements. Compiled from Reader's Digest "Family guide to natural medicine." Available from: URL: http://www.wampole.ca/english/scullcap.htm. Accessed on 1998b Oct 23.

Crellin JK, Philpott J. Herbal medicine past and present. Vol. II. Durham, NC: Duke University Press, 1990.

Duke JA. Handbook of medicinal herbs. Boca Raton, FL: CRC Press, 1985.

Foster, S. Germander toxicity and scullcap adulteration [letter]. Med Herbal 1994;6(1). Available from: URL: http//www.medherb.com/sample.htm. Accessed on 1998 Oct 23.

Franzblau SG, Cross C. J Ethnopharmacol 1986;15:279.

Grieve M. A modern herbal. New York, NY: Dover, 1971.

Harvey J, Colin-Jones DG. Mistletoe hepatitis. Br Med J 1981;282:186–7.

Israel D, Youngkin EQ. Herbal therapies for perimenopausal and menopausal complaints. Pharmacotherapy 1997;17:970–84.

Larrey D. Hepatotoxicity of herbal remedies. J Hepatol 1997;26(Suppl. 1):47–51.

Larrey D, Vial T, Pauwels A, Castot A, Biour M, David M, Michel H. Hepatitis after germander (*Teucrium chamaedrys*) administration: another instance of herbal medicine hepatotoxicity. Ann Intern Med 1992;117:129–32.

MacGregor FB, Abernethy VE, Dahabra S, Cobden I, Hayes PC. Hepatotoxicity of herbal remedies. Br Med J 1989;299:1156–7.

Murch SJ, Simmons CB, Saxena PK. Melatonin in feverfew and other medicinal plants. Lancet 1997;350:1598–9.

Nagai T, Miyaichi Y, Tomimori T, Yamada H. Inhibition of mouse liver sialidase by plant flavonoids. Biochem Biophys Res Commun 1989a;163:25–31.

Nagai T, Yamada H, Otsuka Y. Inhibition of mouse liver sialidase by the root of *Scutellaria baicalensis*. Planta Med 1989b;55:27–9.

Phillipson JD, Anderson LA. Herbal remedies used in sedative and antirheumatic preparations: Part 1. Pharmaceut J 1984;233:80–2.

Pickup JC, Mattock MB, Crook MA, Chusney GD, Burt D, Fitzgerald AP. Serum siliac acid concentration and coronary heart disease in NIDDM. Diabetes Care 1995;18:1100–3.

Razina TG, Udintsev SN, Prishchep TP, Iaremenko KV. Enhancement of the selectivity of the action of the cytostatics cyclophosphane and 5–fluorouracil by using an extract of the Baikal skullcap in an experiment. Vopr Onkol 1987;33:80–4.

Tyler VE. The honest herbal, 3rd edit., Binghamton, NY: Pharmaceutical Products Press, 1993.

# Chapter 20

# Licorice


## Michael Newton and Melanie Johns Cupp


*Glycyrrhiza glabara* (L.), *G. uralensis, G. palidiflora,* licorice, Spanish licorice, Russian licorice (Anonymous, 1998)

## 20.1 History and Traditional Uses

Licorice is harvested from the roots of *Glycyrrhiza glabara*, a 4–5 ft shrub found in subtropical climates with rich soil (Anonymous, 1998). The plant is native to Greece, Turkey, Spain, Iraq, Caucasian and Transcaspian Russia, and northern China (Davis and Morris, 1991). Its use dates back thousands of years to ancient Egyptian rituals that enabled the spirits of pharaohs to prepare a sweet drink known as mai sus in the afterlife. A beverage called mai sus is still consumed today as an iced beverage in Egypt. Theophrastus, an ancient Greek botanist, referred in his writings to the ability of licorice to treat asthma and heal wounds. In writings from the first century BC, licorice was purported to abate hunger and thirst, clear the voice, heal sores of the mouth and genitals, and treat kidney and bladder ailments. Western herbalists recognized licorice as a remedy for "dropsy," as did Pliny, and asserted that the root had emollient, demulcent, expectorant, and diuretic effects. Licorice was probably introduced to Native Americans by the early English settlers, and was subsequently used by medicine men to treat diabetes. In traditional Chinese medicine licorice was considered to benefit all organs of the body.

## 20.2 Current Promoted Uses

Today, licorice is employed in many capacities around the world. In China, licorice is used to treat a variety of symptoms and diseases, including Addison's


From Forensic Science: *Toxicology and Clinical Pharmacology of Herbal Products*
Edited by: M. J. Cupp © Humana Press Inc., Totowa, New Jersey

disease (Davis and Morris, 1997), sore throats, carbuncles, diarrhea due to "spleen deficiency," thirst due to "stomach deficiency," cough due to "dry lungs," and palpitations (Blumenthal, 1997). Other modern uses include bronchitis and other "catarrhal conditions," gastritis, colic, arthritis, and hepatitis (Blumenthal, 1997). Licorice contains the natural sweetener glycyrrhizic acid (Gunnarsdottir and Johannesson, 1997), and is used to flavor soy sauce in China and Japan (Davis and Morris, 1991).

In the United States, licorice is used to cure and flavor tobacco products. Most licorice-flavored candies and other products in the United States today actually contain anethole from the aniseed plant as a substitute for licorice (Davis and Morris, 1991); however, licorice may still be found in some imported confections, gums, cough mixtures and lozenges, and Belgian beers (De Klerk et al., 1997).

## 20.3 Products Available

Aside from its use as a flavoring, licorice root can be found in some herbal supplements, usually those touted for their antiinflammatory effects. One product, for example, contains licorice root and several other "natural" substances such as shark cartilage, and is promoted to meet the complex nutritional needs of the musculoskeletal system. Another product utilizing licorice in combination with other herbal components claims to increase production of digestive juices, thereby reducing gas, cramping, bloating, upset stomach, heartburn, and nausea.

Licorice may also be found in herbal teas. For example, one tea product is touted as a "women's tonic," and in addition to licorice contains dong quai, astragalus, and ginseng to "combat stress, nourish the adrenals, pancreas, liver, and endocrine system." The tea manufacturer also claims that their product helps with hormonal balance and relief of premenstrual syndrome.

## 20.4 Pharmacologic/Toxicologic Effects

### 20.4.1 Respiratory Effects

Licorice has often been touted as an expectorant and cough suppressant. Extracts of licorice are found in herbal cough mixtures and cough drops in Europe (De Klerk et al., 1997). However, literature supporting these claims is lacking.

### 20.4.2 Anti-Inflammatory Effects

Some components of licorice may have anti-inflammatory effects. One such component is glycyrrhetinic acid, a metabolite of glycyrrhizin (glycyrrhizic acid), the major saponin of licorice root (Inoue et al., 1989). This study assessed the antiinflammatory activity of glycyrrhetinic acid and its synthetic derivatives on mouse ear edema induced by application of 12-*O*-tetradecanoylphorbol-13-acetate (TPA), the irritant principle of croton oil. This inflammatory model has been used to assess the antiinflammatory activity of other substances by other investigators as well. Inoue and colleagues concluded that the dihemiphthalate derivatives of glycyrrhetinic acid are useful antiinflammatory agents both topically and orally. Glycyrrhetinic acid itself was a less potent antiinflammatory than its derivatives topically, and produced no antiinflammatory effect when administered orally. These findings were substantiated by a later study that compared glycyrrhetinic acid to its derivative dihemiphthalate compounds in the inhibition of carrageenan-induced rat paw edema, and inhibition of mouse paw edema induced by the vasoactive substances histamine, bradykinin, platelet activating factor (PAF), and serotonin (Inoue et al., 1993). In addition, the effects of these compounds on the contraction of isolated guinea pig ileum in response to histamine, serotonin, and bradykinin were examined. The dihemiphthalate compounds attenuated vascular permeability caused by histamine, PAF, and bradykinin, while glycyrrhetinic acid had little effect on paw swelling induced by these vasoactive substances. Both glycyrrhizin and its derivatives were effective in reducing carrageenan-induced edema. These findings suggest that glycyr rhetinic acid has a different mechanism of antiinflammatory action than its derivatives, which apparently modulate vascular permeability. Glycyrrhizin is thought to inhibit the generation of reactive oxygen species by neutrophils (Akamatsu et al., 1991). Glycyrrhetinic acid may also possess an inhibitory effect upon the human complement cascade at the level of complement component C2 (Kroes et al., 1997).

The results of these studies cannot be extrapolated to oral ingestion of licorice, such as is found in dietary supplements.

### *20.4.3 Adrenocorticotropic Effects*

Licorice has a well-documented mineralocorticoid-like effect. This effect occurs not because licorice mimics mineralocorticoid action, but rather is due to the inhibition of 11-β-hydroxysteroid dehydrogenase (11β-OHSD), the enzyme that catalyzes the conversion of cortisol to cortisone (Stewart et al., 1987). Deficiency or inhibition of this enzyme leads to an increase in renal cortisol, which can bind to mineralocorticoid receptors (Stewart et al., 1987). The inhibiting substance in licorice appears to be 3-monoglucuronylglycyrrhetinic acid, a metabolite of glycyrrhetinic acid (Kato et al., 1995). This resultant mineralocorticoid effect may cause sodium retention, hypertension, hypokalemia, and suppression of plasma renin activity (Epstein et al. 977).

The inhibition of 11β-OHSD by licorice can mimic the syndrome of apparent mineralocorticoid excess produced by congenital deficiency of this enzyme. For example, there is a rise in free urinary cortisol, and a decreased urinary ratio of cortisone to cortisol metabolites in both situations (Stewart et al., 1987). However, the elevated urinary ratio of 5β-tetrahydrocortisol to 5α-tetrahydrocortisol that occurs with licorice ingestion is the opposite of the finding expected in children with the syndrome of apparent mineralocorticoid excess (Stewart et al., 1987).

Plasma atrial natriuretic peptide levels increased in healthy volunteers who ingested 100 g of licorice daily for 8 wk (Forslund et al., 1989). This effect is thought to be a physiologic response to prevent licorice-induced fluid retention and hypertension.

### 20.4.4 Gastrointestinal Effects

Carbenoxolone, the semisynthetic succinic acid ester of 18-β-glycyrrhetic acid, has been used in many countries other than the United States for the treatment of peptic ulcer disease, gastroesophageal reflux disease, and oral ulcers (Lewis, 1974). The exact mechanism of action is unknown, but it is thought to enhance mucus secretion, increase the life span of gastric epithelial cells, inhibit back-diffusion of hydrogen ions induced by bile, and to inhibit peptic activity (Lewis, 1974). It can cause edema, hypertension, hypokalemia, myopathy, and myoglobinuria (Lewis, 1974). Although these adverse effects can be ameliorated with spironolactone, the therapeutic effects are also negated (Lewis, 1974). Newer drugs have largely supplanted the use of carbenoxolone. Deglycyrrhizinated licorice (DGL; licorice from which glycyrrhizin has been removed) has also been investigated as an antiulcer agent, but results have been inconclusive (Anonymous, 1998).

### 20.4.5 Antimicrobial Activity

Glycyrrhizin may exhibit antiviral effects. It has been shown to protect mice exposed to a lethal dose of influenza virus (Utsunomiya et al., 1997). This effect may be produced through the stimulation of interferon-γ production by T cells (Abe et al., 1982; Utsinomiya et al., 1997). Glycyrrhizin also demonstrated an ability to inhibit the replication of varicella-zoster virus in human embryonic fibroblasts in vitro (Baba and Shigeta, 1987).

In vivo and in vitro studies have shown glycyrrhizin to have an antiviral effect on the human immunodeficiency virus (HIV). A Japanese study found that glycyrrhizin sulfate, a slightly modified form of glycyrrhizin, inhibited HIV reverse transcriptase in vitro (Nakashima and Matsui, 1987). Another study (Hattori et al., 1989) evaluated glycyrrhizin's utility in three hemophiliacs with AIDS. Researchers administered 400–1600 mg/d of glycyrrhizin intravenously for periods of at least 1 mo, for a total of six treatment courses. Viral p24 antigen was not detected at the end of or during three of the five treatment courses in which the antigen was measured, and decreased in the other two courses. The effect of glycyrrhizin treatment on CD4 count was equivocal. Note that this study was performed prior to the availability of antiretroviral drugs.

Preliminary studies suggest that glycyrrhizin may also be effective for the treatment of other viruses. Intravenous glycyrrhizin decreased liver function tests in three infants with cytomegalovirus-associated liver dysfunction (Numazaki et al., 1994). In addition, a retrospective chart review (Arase et al., 1997) of hepatitis C patients revealed that long-term treatment with an intravenous Japanese medicine called Stronger Neo-Minophagen (0.2% glycyrrhizin, 0.1% cysteine, and 2% glycine) was associated with a decreased incidence of hepatocellular carcinoma and stabilization of alanine aminotransferase (ALT) levels. Because patients were not randomized to treatment vs nontreatment, it is possible that some other factor was responsible for the study outcome. Glycyrrhizin may also be effective in altering the course of hepatitis B (Eisenburg, 1992). Whether glycyrrhizin's effects in these hepatic diseases can be attributed to its antiviral activity, antiinflammatory effect, or some other effect remains to be seen.

The antimicrobial effects of licorice may extend beyond antiviral activity. Licochalcone A, a flavonoid component of licorice found in alcoholic root extracts, has been found to inhibit the growth of *Leishmania major* and *Leishmania donovani* promastigotes and amastigotes in vitro (Chen et al., 1993). Licochalcone A appears to elicit its toxic effects upon the protozoal mitochondria in concentrations that do not harm human leukocytes.

Licochalcone A and C have been shown to possess activity in vitro against Gram-positive bacteria (Haraguchi et al., 1998). The mechanism of this effect is hypothesized to be inhibition of oxygen consumption and NADH oxidation in susceptible bacterial cells through inhibition of mitochondrial NADH-cytochrome *c* reductase.

## 20.5 Case Reports of Toxicity Due to Commercially Available Products

Several reports of toxicity due to licorice ingestion exist in the medical literature. In most of the cases, there is a common finding of hypokalemia. Rhabdomyolysis, acute renal failure, pseudoaldosteronism, pulmonary edema, hypertension, and any combination thereof have also been reported.

In one case (De Klerk et al., 1997), a 21-yr-old woman presented to her primary care physician with a headache. She was in the habit of eating approx

100 g of licorice daily and was taking oral contraceptives. Examination was normal except for an elevated blood pressure of 190/120 mm Hg. She was advised to stop eating licorice and to discontinue oral contraceptives. Her blood pressure remained elevated and did not return to normal even after treatment with a combination of atenolol, lisinopril, hydrochlorothiazide, and amlodipine. Drug treatment was discontinued. Two weeks later her blood pressure was 180/110 mm Hg, and plasma concentrations of sodium, potassium, and bicarbonate were 143 mmol/L (normal is 136–146 mmol/L), 2.6 mmol/L (normal is 3.8–5 mmol/L), and 35.9 mmol/L (23–29 mmol/L), respectively. Plasma renin activity was 0.096 ng/(L × s) (normal is is 0.96–3.61 ng/L), and plasma aldosterone concentration was 160 pmol/L. After a more thorough history, she was found to have been using two packets of Stimorol Sugar Free® (Warner Lambert Confectionery) chewing gum per day. This gum contained 585 mg of licorice (8–12% glycyrrhizinic acid) per 15-g packet. Based on this information, her daily intake of glycyrrhizinic acid was approx 120 mg. Three weeks after discontinuation of the gum, her blood pressure was 110/80 mm Hg and her potassium concentration was 5.3 mmol/L.

In a second case reported by these same authors, a 35-yr-old woman was found to have a serum potassium concentration of 2.2 mmol/L. Her medications included oral contraceptives, and 500 mg of chlorothiazide twice daily for treatment of pretibial edema. Other clinical findings included blood pressure of 140/80 mm Hg, pitting edema, and plasma bicarbonate concentration of 30.8 mmol/L. One week after stopping chlorothiazide and starting 600 mg of oral potassium chloride three times daily, her sodium, potassium, and bicarbonate levels were still abnormal at 146 mmol/L, 2.0 mmol/L, and 37 mmol/L, respectively. One week later, the electrolyte abnormalities persisted, with a plasma potassium level of 1.5 mmol/L, sodium of 144 mmol/L, and bicarbonate of 39 mmol/L. She was admitted to the hospital for evaluation and intravenous potassium chloride replacement. In the hospital, she was found to have plasma renin activity of 0.036 ng/(L × s) (normal is 1.08–4.32 ng/[L × s]), plasma aldosterone level of 80 pmol/L, and daily sodium excretion of 57 mmol. These findings suggested exogenous mineralocorticoid administration. It was found that she had been using three packets of BenBits Cool Mint® chewing gum daily, which contained 160 mg of licorice (10% glycyrrhizinic acid) in each 16-g packet. The gum was discontinued, intravenous potassium was discontinued after 2 d, and oral potassium was stopped after 15 d. Three weeks later, her blood pressure had fallen to 110/80 mm Hg, her potassium concentration had risen to 4.2 mmol/L, and all other electrolytes had normalized (De Klerk et al., 1997).

A life-threatening arrhythmia was reported secondary to licorice-induced hypokalemia (Bryer-Ash et al., 1987). A 69-yr-old Cambodian woman presented to the Stanford Hospital Emergency Room with a history of four syncopal episodes lasting up to 15 min over the preceding 24 h. A family member witnessed each episode. These episodes consisted of abrupt collapse of the patient without warning or complaint. They were independent of posture, and did not resemble seizures. For the past few days, the patient had been taking several tablets daily of a traditional Chinese herbal medicine called chui-feng-su-ho-wan for relief of upper respiratory symptoms. On admission, her serum potassium level was 3.0 mmol/L and her serum sodium was 148 mmol/L. Serum chloride, bicarbonate, creatinine, and calcium were normal, and blood pressure was 140/90 mm Hg. Her tongue, however, was stained black. Soon after electrocardiographic monitoring leads were attached, she developed a characteristic torsades de pointes rhythm. She was asymptomatic, and her blood pressure was 150/90 mm Hg. She was treated with 75 mg of lidocaine, and she converted to normal sinus rhythm. Lidocaine infusion was continued for the next 24 h, and potassium was corrected to 4.7 mmol/L with intravenous and oral supplementation. She had no further episodes of torsades, and was discharged 3 d after admission. Because the Chinese remedy she had been taking contained glycyrrhizic acid, it was implicated as the cause of her tongue discoloration, hypokalemia, and subsequent torsades. She was advised to discontinue the herbal remedy, and had no further difficulties.

Another case report (Brayley and Jones, 1994) cites life-threatening hypokalemia due to excessive licorice ingestion. A 29-yr-old woman with a history of anorexia nervosa with bulimia presented to the hospital with a complaint of weakness and muscle pain over the preceding 2 wk. This patient had increased her licorice candy consumption over the past month from 300 g to 600 g/d in the month before admission. Concurrently, she had also been decreasing the intake of other foods and water, and was taking 40 mg of furosemide in the morning for premenstrual edema. She was dehydrated, had a serum potassium level of 0.9 mmol/L (normal is 3.8–4.9 mmol/L), and serum sodium of 134 mmol/L (normal is 135–145 mmol/L). Vital signs included a pulse of 92 beats/min, blood pressure of 125/80 mm Hg, temperature 36°C, and respiratory rate 24 breaths/min. She was experiencing severe proximal muscle weakness in her arms and legs. Her ECG showed marked S–T segment depression and a prolonged Q–T interval consistent with hypokalemia. The woman was admitted to the intensive care unit and recovered completely after receiving intravenous normal saline and potassium. Muscle weakness resolved, and she was discharged from the hospital. Her serum potassium level rose to 3.1 mmol/L after she stopped taking both licorice and furosemide.

Ingestion of glycyrrhizin-containing products can also lead to myopathy, rhabdomyolysis, acute renal failure and death. In one atypical case (Saito et al.,

1994), a 78-yr-old man was hospitalized because of muscle weakness and acute renal failure. The man had been taking 280 mg of glycyrrhizin per day for the last 7 yr, and had a history of hypertension. Serum potassium level was 1.9 mEq/L with metabolic alkalosis, and hyporeninemic hypoaldosteronism. Serum myoglobin peaked at 46 μg/mL and there was massive myoglobinuria. During the hospital course, blood urea nitrogen (BUN) rose from 20.9 mg/dL to 87 mg/dL and serum creatinine rose from 1.3 mg/dL to 6.7 mg/dL. Lactic dehydrogenase (LDH) and creatine phosphokinase (CPK) were also markedly elevated. Autopsy revealed marked calcium deposition in the quadriceps femoris, axillar, neck, and cardiac muscles.

In another case (Farese et al., 1991) in which rhabdomyolysis was reported, a 70-yr-old man was admitted to the hospital for evaluation for hypertension and hypokalemia. He had had hypertension for 4 yr, and blood pressure had been difficult to control over the past year. He also complained of weakness, mental slowness, and a 15-kg weight loss during this time. Nine months prior to evaluation, treatment of a thiazide diuretic had resulted in hypokalemia (plasma potassium, 1.9 mmol/L) and rhabdomyolysis. He required 20 mmol of potassium chloride three times daily, 240 mg of verapamil daily, and 25 mg of spironolactone four times daily for blood pressure control and normalization of plasma potassium. Before referral, plasma aldosterone, renin activity, and 18-hydroxycortisone were normal. History revealed that for the past 4–5 yr, he had been eating 60–100 g daily of a licorice candy (Panda, Vaajakoski, Finland; 0.3% glycyrrhizin), but that he had stopped eating it 1 wk prior to admission. Upon admission, physical exam revealed a thin gentleman with a blood pressure of 124/63 mm Hg. His plasma sodium was 137 mmol/L, and plasma potassium was 5.7 mmol/L. In the hospital, the patient was rechallenged with 100 g/d of the candy for 2 wk. During this time, his dietary sodium and potassium were held constant, and verapamil was continued. Sodium balance became positive, potassium balance became negative, body weight increased, blood pressure increased to 154/72 mm Hg, and plasma cortisol and deoxycorticosterone remained normal. Plama renin activity, plasma aldosterone, and urinary aldosterone were elevated upon admission, but fell while he was taking licorice. At the end of the first week of licorice treatment, urinary cortisol was elevated and the ratio of urinary tetrahydrocortisone to 5α-tetrahydrocortisol plus 5β-tetrahydrocortisol was low, indicating 11β-hydroxysteroid dehydrogenase inhibition. Urinary glycyrrhetinic acid was detected for the first 3 d after licorice discontinuation, but was undetectable 15 d later. Urinary cortisol excretion normalized in parallel to decline in urinary glycyrrhetinic acid excretion. These findings are in agreement with those of Stewart and colleagues, described in Section 20.4.3.

## 20.6 Pharmacokinetics/Toxicokinetics

### 20.6.1 Absorption

Glycyrrhizin (glycyrrhizic acid) is biotransformed in the large intestine to the active glycyrrhetinic acid (glycyrrhetic acid) by the glucuronidase activity of anaerobic bacteria in the large intestine (Hattori et al., 1983; Gunnarsdottir and Johannesson, 1997). Absorption is independent of dose (Krahenbuhl et al., 1994b), but the bioavailability of glycyrrhetic acid in plasma has been found to be greater after ingestion of pure glycyrrhizic acid than after ingestion of licorice (Cantelli-Forti, 1994). In one human study, the mean $C_{max}$ of glycyrrhetic acid after ingestion of 200 mg of glycyrrhizic acid in licorice was 794 ng/mL (range 466–1636 mg/mL), occurring at a mean $T_{max}$ of 13 h (range 8–30 h) (Gunnarsdottir and Johannesson, 1997).

### 20.6.2 Distribution

Glycyrrhizic acid, when administered intravenously, has been found to have a volume of distribution of approx 80 mL/kg, and is undetectable in plasma after oral administration (Yamamura et al., 1992). The likely reason for this latter finding is biotransformation by intestinal bacteria, as mentioned in the previous section. After oral administration of 500 mg, 1000 mg, and 1500 mg of glycyrrhetinic acid, volume of distribution was calculated to be 2300 mL/kg, 3100 mL/kg, and 3800 mL/kg, respectively (Krahenbuhl et al., 1994a).

### 20.6.3 Metabolism/Elimination

The elimination half-life of glycyrrhizic acid after intravenous administration is 3.5 h, and is independent of the dose in human studies (Yamamura et al., 1992).

As mentioned in the preceding discussion of absorption, glycyrrhetinic acid is the active principle after oral administration owing to cleavage of two glucuronic acid moieties from glycyrrhizic acid by intestinal flora (Hattori et al., 1983; Hattori et al., 1989; Krahenbuhl et al., 1994b). The elimination half-life of glycyrrhetinic acid in humans was found to be 11.5 h after a dose of 100 mg, and 38.7 h after a dose of 1500 mg. The terminal half-life could not be calculated after a dose of 500 mg. This dose-dependent elimination likely reflects extensive tissue binding and has been hypothesized be the reason toxicity may take weeks to resolve after cessation of chronic licorice ingestion (Krahenbuhl et al., 1994b). Urinary elimination of glycyrrhetinic acid is negligible; rat studies suggest the majority of its elimination is achieved through elimination of glucuronide or sulfate conjugates in the bile. Human studies suggest that enterohepatic recirculation occurs (Krahenbuhl et al., 1994a).

### 20.6.4 Analysis of Biofluids

The presence of glycyrrhizin (glycyrrhizic acid) and glycyrrhetinic acid in biological fluids and tissue can be determined through high-performance liquid chromatography (HPLC), thin-layer chromatography (TLC) (Parke et al., 1963), enzyme immunoassay (Kanaoka et al., 1988a), radioimmunoassay (Kanaoka et al., 1988b), and gas chromatography-selected ion monitoring (Itoh et al., 1985). Most pharmacokinetic studies have been performed using HPLC; thus, Krahenbuhl and colleagues have written a review of HPLC methods of bioanalysis of glycyrrhizin and glycyrrhetinic acid. These compounds are readily extracted using methanol, acetonitrile, chloroform, or acetoacetate–*n*-heptane with or without prior addition of inorganic salts. These extracts can be used directly for HPLC. Determination of urine and bile concentrations can be difficult owing to the presence of interfering endogenous compounds. Extraction using a combination of ion-pairing with organic solvent extraction or with solid-phase extraction using C18 columns is more time consuming than direct solvent extraction, but recovery is in excess of 90% (Krahenbuhl et al., 1994b). The latter technique has been described for detection in plasma using commercially available 18-β-glycyrrhetinic acid as the internal standard and the use of a Bond Elut C2 (ethyl) extraction column to minimize the amount of organic solvent required (Russel et al., 1998).

A micellar electrokinetic chromatographic technique for determining glycyrrhizin and glycyrrhetinic acid in human plasma and urine has limits of detection of glycyrrhizin in urine and plasma of 1.6 μg/mL and 0.8 μg/mL, respectively, and limits of 2 μg/mL and 1 μg/mL for glycyrrhetinic acid in urine and plasma (Wang et al., 1998). In contrast, an HPLC technique has been described with a limit of detection of both compounds in plasma of 0.1 μg/mL (de Groot and Koops, 1988).

## 20.7 Regulatory Status

Licorice is approved by the German Commission E to treat peptic ulcer, in doses of 200–600 mg glycyrrhizin daily (Blumenthal, 1998). They also recommend that treatment not exceed 6 wk because of the known side effects of licorice. It is recommended that patients with cardiovascular or renal disease use licorice only under the care of a physician. Patients prone to potassium deficiency are also advised not use licorice.

In the United States licorice is regulated as a dietary supplement (Blumenthal, 1997). It is Generally Recognized as Safe (GRAS) (Blumenthal, 1997), a designation that refers only to its use as a food additive.

## *References*

Abe N, Ebina T, Ishida N. Interferon induction by glycyrrhizin and glycyrrhetinic acid in mice. Microbiol Immunol 1982;26:535–9.

Akamatsu H, Komura J, Asada Y, Niwa Y. Mechanism of antiinflammatory action of glycyrrhizin: effect on neutrophil functions incuding reactive oxygen species generation. Planta Med 1991;57:119–21.

Anonymous. Licorice. The review of natural products. St. Louis, MO: Facts and Comparisons, 1998.

Arase Y, Ikeda K, Murashima N, Chayama K, Tsubota A, Koida I, et al. The long term efficacy of glycyrrhizin in chronic hepatitis C patients. Cancer 1987;79:1494–500.

Baba M, Shigeta S. Antiviral activity of glycyrrhizin against varicella-zoster virus in vitro. Antiviral Res 1987;7:99–107.

Blumenthal, M. Popular herbs in the U.S. market. Licorice root. Austin, TX: American Botanical Council, 1997.

Blumenthal M. Licorice root. The complete German Commission E monographs. Austin, TX: American Botanical Council, 1998.

Brayley J, Jones J. Life-threatening hypokalemia associated with excessive licorice ingestion. Am J Psychiatry 1994;151:617–8.

Bryer-Ash M, Zehnder J, Angelchik P, Maisel A. Torsades de pointes precipitated by a Chinese herbal remedy. Am J Cardiol 1987;60:1186–7.

Cantelli-Forti G, Maffei F, Hrelia F, Bugamelli F, Bernandi P, D'Intino P, et al. Interaction of licorice on glycyrrhizin pharmacokinetics. Environ Health Perspect 1994;102(Suppl 9):65–8.

Chen M, Christensen SB, Blom J, Lemmich E, Nadelmann L, Fich K, et al. Licochalcone A, a novel antiparasitic agent with potent activity against human pathogenic protozoan species of *Leishmania*. Antimicrob Agent Chemother 1993;37:2550–6.

Davis EA, Morris DJ. Medicinal uses of licorice through the milennia: the good and plenty of it. Mol Cell Endocrinol 1991;78:1–6.

De Groot G, Koops R. Improvement of selectivity and sensitivity by column switching in the determination of glycyrrhizin and glycyrrhetic acid in human plasma by high-performance liquid chromatography. J Chromatogr 1988;456:71–81.

De Klerk GJ, Nieuwenhuis MG, Beutler JJ. Hypokalaemia and hypertension associated with use of liquorice flavoured chewing gum. Br Med J 1997;314:731–2.

Eisenburg J. Treatment of chronic hepatitis B. Part 2: Effect of glycyrrhizic acid on the course of illness. Fortschr Med 1992;110:395–8.

Epstein MT, Espiner EA, Donald RA, Hughes H. Effect of eating liquorice on the renin–angiotensin aldosterone axis in normal subjects. Br Med J 1977;1:488–90.

Farese RV, Biglieri EG, Shackleton CHL, Irony I, Gomez-Fontes R. Licorice-induced hypermineralcorticoidism. New Engl J Med 1991;325:1223–7.

Forslund T, Fyhrquist F, Froseth B, Tikkanen I. Effects of licorice on plasma atrial natriuretic peptide in healthy volunteers. J Intern Med 1989;225:95–9.

Gunnarsdottir S, Johannesson T. Glycyrrhetic acid in human blood after ingestion of glycyrrhizic acid in licorice. Pharmacol Toxicol 1997;81:300–2.

Haraguchi H, Tanimoto K, Yamura Y, Mizutani K, Kinoshita T. Mode of antibacterial action of tertrochalcones from *Glycyrrhiza inflata*. Phytochemistry 1998;48:125–9.

Hattori M, Sakamoto T, Kobas K, Namba T. Metabolism of glycyrrhizin by human intestinal flora. Planta Med 1983;48:38–42.

Hattori T, Ikematsu S, Koito A, Matsushita S, Maeda Y, Hada M, et al. Preliminary evidence for inhibitory effect of glycyrrhizin on HIV replication in patients with AIDS. Antiviral Res 1989;11:255–62.

Inoue H, Moir T, Shibata S, Koshihara Y. Modulation by glycyrrhetinic acid derivatives of TPA-induced mouse ear oedema. Br J Pharmacol 1989;96:204–10.

Inoue H, Inoue K, Takeuchi T, Nagata N, Shibata S. Inhibition of rat acute inflammatory paw oedema by dihemiphthalate of glycyrrhetinic acid derivatives: comparison with glycyrrhetinic acid. J Pharm Pharmacol 1993;45:1067–71.

Itoh M, Asakawa N, Hashimoto Y, Ishibashi M, Miyazaki H. Quantitative analysis of glycyrrhizin and glycyrrhetinic acid in plasma after administration of FM-100 by using gas chromatography-selected ion monitoring. Yakugaku Zasshi 1985;105:1150–4.

Kanaoka M, Yano S, Kato H, Nakada T, Kawamura K. Studies on the enzyme immunoassay of bio-acitve constituents contained in oriental medicinal drugs. IV. Enzyme immunoassay of glycyrretic acid. Chem Pharmaceut Bull 1985a;36:8–14.

Kanaoka M, Yano S, Kato H. Preparation of [$^3$H]-3β-hydroxy-18β- and 3α-hydroxy-18β and α-glycyrrhetic acid and radioimmunoassay of glycyrrhetic acid. Chem Pharmaceut Bull 1985b;36:3264–70.

Kato H, Kanaoka M, Yano S, Kobayashi M. 3-Monoglucuronyl-glycyrrhetinic acid is a major metabolite that causes licorice-induced pseudoaldosteronism. J Clin Endocrinol Metab 1995;80:1929–33.

Krahenbuhl S, Hasler F, Frey BM, Frey FJ, Brenneisen R, Krapf R. Kinetics and dynamics of orally administered 18 beta-glycyrrhetinic acid in humans. J Clin Endocrinol Metab 1994a;78:581–5.

Krahenbuhl S, Hasler F, Krapf R. Analysis and pharmacokinetics of glycyrrhizic acid and glycyrrhetinic acid in humans and experimental animals. Steroids 1994b;59:121–6.

Kroes BH, Beukelman CJ, Van den Berg AJJ, Wolbink GJ, Van Dijk H, Labadie RP. Inhibition of human complement by β-glycyrrhetinic acid. Immunology 1997;90:115–20.

Lewis J. Carbenoxolone sodium in the treatment of peptic ulcer. JAMA 1974;229:460–2.

Nakashima H, Matsui T. A new anti-human immunodeficiency virus substance, glycyrrhizin sulfate: endowment of glycyrrhizin with reverse transcriptase-inhibitory activity by chemical modification. Jpn J Cancer Res 1987;11:225–61.

Numazaki K, Umetsu M, Chiba S. Effect of glycyrrhizin in children with liver dysfunction associated with cytomegalovirus infection. Tohoku J Exp Med 1994;172:147–53.

Parke DV, Poilock S, Williams RT. The fate of tritium-labelled β-glycyrrhetic acid in the rat. J Pharm Pharmacol 1963;15:500–6.

Russel FG, van Uum S, Tan Y, Smits P. Solid-phase extraction of I 8beta-glycyrretinic acid from plasma and subsequent analysis by high-performance liquid chromatography. J Chromatogr B Biomed Sci Appl 1998;710:223–6.

Saito T, Tsuboi Y, Fujisawa G, Sakuma N, Honda K, Okada K, et al. An autopsy case of licorice-induced hypokalemic rhabdomyolysis associated with acute renal failure:

special reference to profound calcium deposition in skeletal and cardiac muscle. Nippon Jinzo Gakkai Shi 1994;36:1308–14.

Stewart PM, Wallace AM, Valentino R, Burt D, Shackleton CHL, Edwards CRW. Mineralocorticoid acitivity of liquorice:11–beta-hydroxysteroid dehydrogenase deficiency comes of age. Lancet 1987;ii:821–3.

Utsunomiya T, Kobayashi M, Pollard RB, Suzuki F. Glycyrrhizin, an active component of licorice roots, reduces morbidity and mortality of mice infected with lethal doses of influenza virus. Antimicrob Agent Chemother 1997;41:551–5.

Wang P, Li SF, Lee KII. Determination of glycyrrhizic acid and 18–beta-glycyrrhetinic acid in biological fluids by micellar electrokinetic chromatography. J Chromatogr A 1998;811:219–24.

Yamamura Y, Kawakami J, Santa T, Kotaki H, Uchino K, Sawada Y, et al. Pharmacokinetic profile of glycyrrhizin in healthy volunteers by a new high-performance liquid chromatographic method. J Pharmaceut Sci 1982;81:1042–1046.

# Chapter 21

# Pokeweed

## A. Heather Knight-Trent and Melanie Johns Cupp

*Phytolacca americana, P. decandra, P. rigida,* American night shade, coakum, crowberry, pokeberry, inkberry, pigeonberry, garget, poke, red ink plant, cancer jalap, cancer root, chongras, and scoke (Anonymous, 1991)

## 21.1 History and Traditional Uses

Pokeweed grows in several parts of the world, including the eastern United States, Canada, California, and Hawaii along roadsides and fences, in fields and woods, and along coastal dunes and marshes (Hardin and Arena, 1974; Anonymous, 1991). It is a large perennial herb reaching heights of up to 12 ft (Macht, 1937). The leaves are green and approx 1 ft long (Hardin and Arena, 1974). Stems vary in color from green to red or purple (Hardin and Arena, 1974) and can resemble that of horseradish, resulting in accidental poisoning (Macht, 1937). The flowers are white and sag toward the ground. The purple berries are round and about ½ in. in diameter. Pokeweed has various traditional uses from medicinal to industrial. It has been used as a cathartic, emetic, narcotic, and gargle (Macht, 1937). Additional medicinal uses included treatment of various skin diseases, conjunctivitis, syphilis, cancer, parasitic infestations of the scalp, chronic rheumatism, ringworm (Macht, 1937), dyspepsia, swollen glands, scabies, ulcers (Tyler, 1993), edema, dysmenorrhea, mumps, and tonsillitis (Anonymous, 1991). The immature leaves and stems were boiled twice and eaten as greens (Hardin and Arena, 1974). The berries have been cooked in pies without harm, and the Europeans used their juice as a dye for wine (Macht, 1937). In the 19th century poisonings were common in the eastern United States because pokeroot tinctures were used to treat rheumatism (Lewis and Smith,

From Forensic Science: *Toxicology and Clinical Pharmacology of Herbal Products*
Edited by: M. J. Cupp © Humana Press Inc., Totowa, New Jersey

1979). Eating uncooked berries or mistaking the root for that of an edible plant were other causes of poisoning.

## 21.2 Products Available

The immature leaves, or poke greens, have been commercially canned and sold under the name "poke salet" (Lewis and Smith, 1979; Anonymous, 1991), which resembles spinach. Pokeroot and pokeberries are commercially available as powder, capsules, and cut pieces. The whole berries are also available.

## 21.3 Pharmacologic/Toxicologic Effects

### 21.3.1 Antimicrobial Activity and Antineoplastic Activity

Purified pokeweed antiviral protein has been investigated as an inhibitor of cellular and viral protein synthesis. Three lectins (PL-A, PL-B, and PL-C) were purified from the pokeweed root. All three lectins exhibited mitogenic actions. PL-B's hemagglutinating and mitogenic performance are greater than those of PL-A and PL-C (Kino et al., 1995). Investigators have also linked pokeweed antiviral protein to murine monoclonal antibodies for the treatment of B-lineage acute lymphoblastic leukemia (ALL) (Myers et al., 1995). The mechanism of action involves inactivation of ribosomes by enzymatic cleavage of a single adenine from the 3' terminus of all large ribosomal RNAs. Pharmacodynamic and pharmacokinetic studies of this preparation have been done in mice and rabbits.

### 21.3.2 Anti-Inflammatory Activity (see also Section 21.4)

Triterpenoid saponins named phytolaccosides exhibit anti-inflammatory activity (Woo et al., 1978).

### 21.3.3 Cardiovascular Effects

Mobitz type I heart block was reported after ingestion of uncooked pokeweed leaves (Hamilton et al., 1995). Hypotension, bradycardia, tachycardia, and ventricular fibrillation have also been reported after pokeweed consumption (French, 1900; Lewis and Smith, 1979; Jaeckle and Freeman, 1981; Roberge et al., 1986). These cardiovascular effects of pokeweed have been attributed to nonspecific vagal or sympathetic stimulation secondary to gastrointenstinal irritation (Roberge et al., 1986; Hamilton et al., 1995). Of note, however, is the observation that pokeroot evaporated fluid extract administered intravenously to cats produced circulatory depression at a dose of 1 mL, and at 4 mL "paralyzed … the heart " (Macht, 1937).

### 21.3.4 Musculoskeletal Effects (see also Section 21.4)

Musculoskeletal effects of pokeweed include muscle weakness and spasms (French, 1900; Hardin and Arena, 1974; Jaeckle and Freeman, 1981).

### 21.3.5 Gastrointestinal Effects (see also Section 21.4)

Nausea, vomiting, watery and bloody diarrhea, abdominal pain with cramping, and hematemesis were associated with ingestion of pokeroot tea (Lewis and Smith, 1979).

Emesis was also induced in cats given 5–10 mL of fluid pokeroot extract diluted in water via stomach tube (Macht, 1937). These effects were attributed to a nonspecific irritant effect, rather than to a central effect on the vomiting center.

### 21.3.6 Respiratory Effects

Bradypnea and dyspnea were described as effects of pokeweed ingestion (French, 1900; Jaeckle and Freeman, 1981; Tyler, 1993). Intravenous administration of 4 mL of an evaporated fluid extract of the root caused respiratory arrest in cats (Macht, 1937).

### 21.3.7 Neurologic Effects

Diaphoresis, tremor, confusion, incontinence, and convulsions have been reported after pokeroot ingestion (Jaeckle and Freeman, 1981).

### 21.3.8 Hematologic Effects

Extracts of whole ripe and unripe berries, seed, pulp, root, leaf, and stem produce erythrocyte agglutination and leukocyte mitosis (Farnes et al., 1964). A glycoprotein known as pokeweed mitogen is responsible for leukocyte mitosis, and in pokeweed poisonings, plasmacytosis variable in onset and lasting 2 mo or longer is seen (Barker et al., 1966; Roberge et al., 1986).

## 21.4 Case Reports of Toxicity

Clinical clues that a patient has ingested pokeweed include purple stains from pokeberry juice on the hands and face, lymphocytosis caused by pokeweed mitogens (lectins), and foamy diarrhea caused by glycoside (triterpenoid) saponins, or phytolaccosides, that cause a sudsing effect on the colon contents (Roberge et al., 1986). The phytolaccosides are also the components responsible for emesis and diarrhea associated with pokeweed ingestion (Anonymous, 1981; Roberge et al., 1986). Although all parts of the pokeweed plant should be considered toxic, the root is generally thought to be the most toxic part. Toxicity increases with plant maturity, with the exception of the berries; green berries are more toxic than red berries. Ripe pokeberries are the least toxic part of the plant, but as few as 10 ripe berries can lead to toxicity in children. Although immature leaves, collected before turning red and boiled for 5 min, rinsed, and reboiled, are considered edible (Anonymous, 1991), symptoms of toxicity have been associated with properly cooked shoots (Anonymous, 1981). The following case reports illustrate the clinical course of pokeweed poisoning.

A 43-yr-old woman drank one cup of tea made with ½ teaspoon of powdered pokeweed root (Lewis and Smith, 1979). Thirty minutes later she experienced nausea, vomiting, abdominal cramping and pain, and watery diarrhea. When hematemesis and bloody diarrhea began, she went to the emergency department. She was hypotensive and tachycardiac. Treatment included crystalloids, nasogastric lavage and suction, and fluid replacement. The condition stabilized within a day of presentation.

One of two family members who ate uncooked "pork salad" leaves developed Mobitz type 1 heart block associated with vomiting and watery diarrhea (Hamilton et al., 1995). A complete blood count (CBC) revealed a white blood cell (WBC) count of 14,600/mm$^3$ with 80% polymorphonulear leukocytes (PMNS), 10% lymphocytes, and 10% monocytes. Hematocrit and platelets were normal. Promethazine in a dose of 25 mg IV was given to facilitate administration of charcoal. Within 15 min of promethazine administration vomiting stopped, and 1 h later, the Mobitz type I block had disappeared, and a first-degree AV block remained. The patient was discharged 36 h later; EKG and WBC had normalized.

Twenty (43%) of 46 campers who ate a salad prepared from young pokeweed leaves that had been boiled, drained, and reboiled experienced nausea, stomach cramps, vomiting, headache, dizziness, burning in the stomach or mouth, and diarrhea (Anonymous, 1981). Illness was associated with consumption of more than 1 teaspoonful of the salad. Symptoms began 30 min to 5 h (mean 3 h) after ingestion of the salad, and lasted from 1 to 48 h (mean 24 h). Four campers required hospitalization for 1 or 2 d for treatment protracted vomiting and dehydration.

A 68-yr-old man drank pokeweed tea as a treatment for constipation. He experienced a loose bowel movement, diaphoresis, confusion, tremor, muscle weakness, salivation, vomiting, urinary incontinence and syncope (Jaeckle and Freemon, 1981). He became unconscious for 10 or 15 min. Breathing was deep and rapid at 22 breaths per minute. After arrival at the hospital his blood pressure increased from 74/54 mm Hg to 120/80 mm Hg over the course of an hour.

Normal findings included electrolytes, liver and renal function tests, WBC count, ECG, computed tomography (CT) scan, EEG, and 24-h Holter monitoring. Physical exam revealed generalized weakness and a broad-based gait. He recovered fully the following day.

A 65-yr-old Laotian woman arrived at the hospital with complaints of crampy abdominal pain, vomiting, profuse watery diarrhea, and generalized weakness after chewing on pokeroot that she found in her backyard (Roberge et al., 1986). Although she had used this remedy in the past for relief of sore throat and cough, in this instance she failed to boil the root before consumption. She exhibited hypotension (SBP 80 mm Hg), hypoactive bowel sounds, pink foamy diarrhea that tested guiac-positive, ST–T segment depressions in all precordial leads, Q waves in leads II and III, and ventricular fibrillation. Hematocrit was 54%, and WBC count was 15,400/mm$^3$ with 37 PMNs, 51 band forms, and 8 metamyelocytes. Lymphocyte count increased fourfold within 1 wk of ingestion. The patient was admitted to the ICU with supplemental oxygen by nasal cannula and IV fluid challenge of 500 mL of normal saline solution over 1 h. Cardiac isoenzyme tests did not show evidence of myocardial infarction. She was discharged in good condition after 7 d.

Dr. Cecil French D.V.S. reported in 1900 his own poisoning with pokeroot, which he had mistaken for horseradish. He consumed the pokeroot at 1:00 PM, at dinner, and promptly spit it out when he experienced a burning sensation and bitter taste. He estimated that he had swallowed only "as much as would fill a thimble." At 2:30 PM he experienced a dry, burning sensation in his throat, and inspection of his pharynx with the aid of a mirror revealed erythema. He was overcome by a general lassitude, started yawning repeatedly, and had vision problems, a dry hacking cough, and profuse salivation. He then experienced a "warm" sensation in his stomach, followed by severe abdominal cramps and retching, with six or seven occurrences of vomiting. The burning sensation then extended from his mouth to his stomach, and he had difficulty breathing. By 3:15 PM vomiting and gastralgia had become very severe, especially with movement, and he experienced vertigo and almost complete loss of vision. Other symptoms included tremors; prickly sensations, especially on the palms, soles, and flexor surface of the arms; coldness; clammy perspiration; profuse salivation; a feeling of suffocation; and an aching in the lumbar region. At 3:30 PM a doctor examined Dr. French and found a weak pulse, slow and labored respirations, cold perspiration, vomiting of mucus and blood, and small pupils. The physician administered one half a grain of morphine sulfate and one-fiftieth of a grain of atropine subcutaneously. In a few minutes the pulse and respirations quickened and breathing was not as labored. The physician took Dr. French to the hospital, where he was given coffee and half an ounce of whiskey with water. He was sent home 2 h later where he experienced vomiting every hour. The vomiting ceased at 2:00 AM when he drank an ounce of diluted brandy. He experienced diarrhea and a bitter taste for 48 h.

## 21.5 Pharmacokinetics/Toxicokinetics

Pokeweed is absorbed in the gastrointestinal tract and through abrasions on the skin (Lewis and Smith, 1979).

## 21.6 Chemical Analysis

Pharmacologically/toxicologically important components of the plant include triterpenoid saponins (phytolaccosides) (Woo et al., 1978), mitogenic lectins (Kino et al., 1995), and pokeweed antiviral protein (PAP) (Myers et al., 1995). Isolation of lectins A, B, and C from pokeroot using Q-Sepharose column chromatography followed by gel filtration on a Sephadex G-75 column, hydrophobic chromatography using a Butyl-Toyopearl column, FPLC on a Mono-Q column, and sodium dodecyl sulfate-polyacrylamide gel electrophoresis (SDS-PAGE) have been described (Kino et al., 1995). Phytolaccosides A, B, D, E, and G have also been isolated from pokeweed root using chromatographic techniques (Woo et al., 1978)

## 21.7 Regulatory Status

In 1979, the Herb Trade Association recommended that members should stop selling pokeroot as an herbal food or beverage, and that except for the immature leaves, all pokeweed products should be withdrawn from sale in the United States (Lewis and Smith, 1979).

## References

Anonymous. Pokeweed. Lawrence review of natural products, April 1991.

Anonymous. Plant poisonings—New Jersey. Mortal Morbid Wkly Rep 1981;30:65–7.

Barker BE, Farnes P, LaMarche PH. Peripheral blood plasmacytosis following systemic exposure to *Phytolacca americana* (pokeweed). Pediatrics 1966;38:490–3.

Farnes P, Barker BE, Brownhill LE, Fanger H. Mitogenic activity in *Phytolacca americana* (pokeweed). Lancet 1964;ii:1100–1.

French C. Pokeroot poisoning. NY Med J 1900;72:653–4.

Hamilton RJ, Shih RD, Hoffman RS. Mobitz type I heart block after poke weed ingestion. Vet Hum Toxicol 1995;37:66–7.

Hardin JW, Arena JM. Human poisoning from native and cultivated plants. Durham, NC: Duke University Press, 1974.

Jaeckle KA, Freemon FR. Pokeweed poisoning. South Med J 1981;74:639–40.

Kino M, Yamaguchi K, Umekawa H, Funatsu G. Purification and characterization of three mitogenic lectins from the roots of pokeweed (*Phytolacca americana*). Biosci Biotechnol Biochem 1995;59:683–8.

Lewis WH, Smith PR. Pokeroot herbal tea poisoning. JAMA 1979;242:2759–60.

Macht D. A pharmacological study of *Phytolacca*. JAMA 1937;26:594–9.

Myers DE, Yanishevski Y, Masson E, Irvin JD, Evans WE, Uckun FM. Favorable pharmacodynamic features and superior anti-leukemic activity of B43 (anti-CD 19) immunotoxins containing two pokeweed antiviral protein molecules covalently linked to each monoclonal antibody molecule. Leukem Lymphoma 1995;18:93–102.

Roberge R, Brader E, Martin ML, Jehle D, Evans T, Harchelroad F, Magreni G, et al. The root of evil—pokeweed intoxication. Ann Emerg Med 1986;15:470–3.

Tyler VE. The honest herbal, 3rd edit., Binghamton, NY: Pharmaceutical Products Press, 1993.

Woo WS, Kang SS, Wagner H, Seligmann, Chari M. Triterpenoid saponins from the roots of *Phytolacca americana*. Planta Medica 1978;34:87–92.

# *Chapter 22*

# Sassafras

*David Hutson and Melanie Johns Cupp*

*Sassafras albidum* (Nuttal) Nees (a.k.a. *S. officinale* Nees et Erbem and *S. varifolium* Kuntze), saxifras, ague tree, cinnamon wood, saloop (Anonymous, 1997)

## 22.1 History and Traditional Uses

*Sassafras* is a small tree native to eastern North America and eastern Asia. Native Americans used sassafras for centuries and encouraged settlers to employ it for a variety of ailments (Anonymous, 1997). According to the Spanish physician Monardes, sassafras could "comfort" the liver and stomach, and dissolve obstructions in the body to "engender good humors" because it was capable of moving the stools and urine. In 1617, John Woodall claimed sassafras was the "great opener of all obstructions or stoppings in the body." Sassafras was used for stomach ache, vomiting, urinary retention, lameness, gout, dropsy, syphilis, scurvy, and jaundice. The claim was made that sassafras could even promote pregnancy because it aided menstrual flow. Demand for sassafras was high and expeditions were sent to New England in the early 1600s to scout for English entrepreneurs who envisioned selling the root bark for £50 per ton (Estes, 1995). Sassafras was also listed in medical texts in the 18th and 19th centuries as a cure for various types of cancer (Hartwell, 1969).

Over the years, people have experimented with each part of the sassafras plant. Oil from the wood and roots has been used in perfumes and soaps as a scenting agent. After being dried and powdered, the leaves and pith have been used as soup thickeners. Extracts were used as flavoring in root beer until the latter part of this century (Anonymous, 1997).

From Forensic Science: *Toxicology and Clinical Pharmacology of Herbal Products*
Edited by: M. J. Cupp © Humana Press Inc., Totowa, New Jersey

## 22.2 Current Uses

Sassafras oil, sassafras bark, and safrole (80% of the oil) are prohibited by the FDA as food additives and flavorings because of their carcinogenic properties. A safrole-free extract is available on the market, but studies have shown that the product still produces tumors in rats (Tyler, 1993). Nevertheless, sassafras is touted in herbal home remedy books and continues to be available in health food stores. Sassafras still enjoys a reputation as a spring tonic, stimulant, antispasmodic, blood purifier, and sudorific (sweat producer), and as a cure for rheumatism, skin diseases, syphilis, typhus, and dropsy (congestive heart failure) (Tyler, 1993). Unfortunately, sassafras seems to be nothing more than a folk medicine; for more than 200 yr it has been known to be without therapeutic utility (Tyler, 1994).

## 22.3 Pharmacologic/Toxicologic Effects

### 22.3.1 Anti-Inflammatory Activity

As part of a research program to develop therapeutically active compounds from raw materials in nature, researchers have synthesized a potentially useful nonsteroidal anti-inflammatory drug (NSAID) structurally similar to sulindac from safrole (Pereira et al., 1989; Barreiro and Lima, 1992). In addition, sassafras itself has been used for relieving eye inflammation (Duke, 1989).

### 22.3.2 Antineoplastic Activity

*Sassafras albidum* has been reported to have antineoplastic activity. Over the years many different preparations, including teas, salves, and fluid extracts have been utilized for breast, cervical, and other types of cancer. In the 1787 edition of *Materia Medica Americana* sassafras root was listed as a remedy for cancerous ulcers. In 1833 *The American Practice of Medicine* listed sassafras oil as a cure for osteosarcomatous tumors (Hartwell, 1969). It is now known that sassafras has no antineoplastic activity and has itself been identified as carcinogenic.

### 22.3.3 Carcinogenicity

Based on studies conducted by the Food and Drug Administration (FDA) showing that safrole is a hepatocarcinogen in rats, the sale of sassafras has been prohibited since 1960 (Segelman et al., 1976). Since this ruling by the FDA, more investigations have supported these earlier findings. One study (Epstein et al., 1970) found a high incidence of hepatomas in infant Swiss mice administered various subcutaneous doses of safrole weekly for the first 4 wk of life. Of 12 mice that received a total dose of 0.66 mg of safrole, 50% had developed hepatomas by the time they were killed at 1 yr of age. Of 31 male mice that received a total safrole dose of 6.6 mg, 58% developed hepatomas and 6% developed multiple pulmonary adenomas. Ten percent of the safrole-treated male mice developed large (>5 mm) pulmonary adenocarcinomas, but only one in 38 females developed pulmonary adenocarcinoma. Histologically, the pulmonary adenomas and hepatomas were well differentiated, while the pulmonary adenocarcinomas were less well differentiated with atypical cells, frequent mitotic figures, and local invasion. These animal data demonstrating carcinogenicity with exposure to very small sassafras doses (approx 66 mg/kg) is significant because a single sassafras tea bag may easily contain 3.0 mg/kg of safrole (Segelman et al., 1976).

Another study (Vesselinovitch et al., 1979) examined the cancer-causing effects of safrole in offspring after administration of the agent to pregnant and lactating female mice. Seven percent of female offspring, but none of the male offspring or controls, developed renal epithelial tumors due to exposure *in utero*. Thirty-four percent of nursed male offspring but none of the nursed female offspring or controls developed hepatocellular tumors. One group of mice was administered safrole orally twice weekly for 90 wk after weaning. Forty-eight percent of the females and 8% of the males in this group developed hepatocellular tumors. This is in contrast to the sex difference favoring males in the study by Epstein and colleagues. The data suggest that safrole crosses the placenta and is excreted in breast milk.

Despite these animal data, it is not entirely clear if safrole is carcinogenic in humans; documentation that humans can metabolize safrole to its carcinogenic metabolite is lacking (Benedetti et al., 1977). *See* Section 22.5 for further discussion of how pharmacokinetic differences between humans and rats might influence the interpretation of safrole carcinogenicity studies.

### *22.3.4 Antimicrobial Activity*

Two antimicrobial neolignans, magnolol and isomagnolol, have been isolated from the roots of *Sassafras randaiense*. These compounds were found in alcoholic extracts of the roots and displayed activity against *Staphylococcus aureus, Mycobacterium smegmatis, Saccharomycetales cerevisiae,* and *Trichophyton mentagrophytes* (El-Feraly et al., 1983). Another study (Clark et al., 1981) using magnolol isolated from *Magnolia grandiflora* L. suggests this chemical has activity comparable to streptomycin sulfate and amphotericin B against Gram-positive bacteria, acid-fast bacilli, and fungi. These compounds have not been found to have activity against Gram-negative bacteria.

## 22.4 Case Reports of Toxicity

A case of sassafras poisoning that occurred in 1888 was described in the U.S Dispensatory. The details are scanty, but apparently a young adult male took 1 teaspoonful of sassafras oil, vomited, collapsed with dilated pupils, lapsed into a stupor, and eventually died. By 1953 five cases of toxicity had been reported in children. Generally, symptoms were present within 10–90 min of ingesting the oil. Clinical presentation included vomiting in all five patients; four were described as being in shock; three experienced vertigo; two were described as being in a stupor; and one was aphasic. One subject responded dramatically to emesis, followed by an injection of nikethamide (a cardiovascular and respiratory stimulant) at the hospital. All ingestions were unwitnessed, so the amount taken may be overestimated; however, because 1 teaspoon killed an adult, it is assumed that a few drops would be toxic to a toddler (Craig, 1953).

A 47-yr-old woman called a regional poison center 1 h after accidentally ingesting 1 teaspoonful of sassafras oil. She described herself as "shaky" after having vomited spontaneously. She was instructed to go to the emergency department. Two hours post-ingestion, the subject was ambulatory, afebrile, anxious, and flushed but alert and oriented to person, place, and time. She was given activated charcoal with sorbitol, intramuscular prochlorperazine, and intravenous electrolyte replacement. Gradually her initial blood pressure (132/78 mm Hg) and pulse (100 beats/min) decreased to 118/78 mm Hg and 76 beats/min. After overnight observation the patient was released with normal kidney and liver function (Grande and Dannewitz, 1987).

An additional case report involved a 72-yr-old woman who presented to her physician complaining of perspiration and hot flashes, mostly during the day, which she likened to menopausal symptoms. She denied chest pain, dyspnea, dizziness, syncope, palpitations, fever, chills, or night sweats. Although the patient was obese (112.5 kg) and had hypertension, her blood pressure was controlled at 120/82 mm Hg. She was afebrile. She was taking furosemide, potassium chloride, and aspirin at the time, but denied smoking, drinking, or using over-the-counter medications. The patient admitted to drinking up to 10 cups of sassafras tea per day as a "tonic to purify the blood." The patient was instructed to stop drinking the herbal tea, and her symptoms promptly resolved (Haines, 1991).

Although details are unavailable, sassafras oil has been implicated in causing abortion and liver cancer. Additional alleged symptoms of sassafras oil overdose include hypothermia, exhaustion, spasms, hallucinations, and paralysis. Sassafras may also cause contact dermatitis (Anonymous, 1997).

## 22.5 Pharmacokinetics/Toxicokinetics

### 22.5.1 Absorption

The pharmacokinetics of different doses of [$^{14}$C] safrole were evaluated in humans and rats (Benedetti et al., 1977). Human volunteers received either a 0.163-mg or 1.655-mg dose of [$^{14}$C] safrole in 20 mL of a 9:1 sugar water–ethanol mixture. Doses in rats ranged from 0.63 to 750 mg/kg of [$^{14}$C] safrole. In both species, orally administered safrole was absorbed rapidly. In humans, maximum plasma levels were achieved at 30 min after the 1.655 mg dose.

### 22.5.2 Distribution

Accumulation of [$^{14}$C] safrole occurred in the kidneys and liver at a dose of 750 mg/kg in rats (Benedetti et al., 1977). The tissue/plasma radioactivity ratio was 2–3 times that produced by a 4.2 mg/kg dose, suggesting that accumulation in these tissues occurs. Further evidence of accumulation is reflected in the plasma concentrations of safrole vs total radioactivity at low vs high safrole doses. After a 4.2 mg/kg dose, plasma levels of total radioactivity were maximal within 1–3 h and decreased up to 8 h post-dose. Unchanged safrole accounted for only a minor part of total plasma radioactivity, and its levels decreased more rapidly than total radioactivity, suggesting the presence of metabolites with long half-lives. At the 750 mg/kg dose, plasma levels of radioactivity increased slightly up to 8 h post-dose, then remained constant up to 24 h post-dose. The safrole-to-total plasma radioactivity ratio was 50% between 1 and 24 h post-dose with the 750 mg/kg dose, but with the lower dose it was only 10% at 1 h and 2% at 24 h. Thus, in rats relatively larger amounts of unchanged [$^{14}$C] safrole were found in both tissues and plasma as the dosage was increased, suggesting that metabolism of safrole becomes saturated at higher doses in rats. Repeated high doses of safrole would be expected to accumulate in tissues, resulting in chronic toxicities such as cancer.

### 22.5.3 Metabolism/Elimination

The urinary and fecal elimination of safrole in rats and humans were also studied (Benedetti et al., 1977). In humans, detectable levels (2–3 ng/mL) of unchanged safrole were found only at 30 min post-dose, indicating rapid metabolism. Nearly complete recovery of the administered dose was obtained as metabolites in the urine. An average of 98% of the dose was recovered in the urine and feces within 5 d. No delay in elimination was detected with increasing dosage. The terminal half-life was 15 h.

In the rat, 20% of the radioactivity of a 0.8 mg/kg safrole dose, but only 3% of a 750 mg/kg dose, was excreted in the bile in the first 24 h post-dose

(Benedetti et al., 1977). Thirty percent of the radioactivity in the bile underwent enterohepatic recirculation in the rat, explaining the low recovery of metabolites in the feces. In rats, elimination was delayed as the dose was increased from 0.63 mg/kg to 60 mg/kg, and then to 745 mg/kg; 88%, 78%, and 25% of the radioactivity administered was recovered in the urine in 24 h, respectively. The total radioactivity recovered in the urine in 4 d did not differ among the three doses. The dose-dependent delay in elimination in rats suggests that a metabolic or excretory pathway becomes saturated at higher doses. In humans, either such saturation does not occur, or the administered dose was not high enough to saturate the pathway.

The major metabolite in both humans and rats is 1,2-dihydroxy-4-allylbenzene (Benedetti et al., 1977). This metabolite is excreted mainly as the glucuronide conjugate. The minor metabolite 1-methoxy-2-hydroxy-4-allylbenzene, is found in both rat and man. Eugenol was also detected in the urine in man. 1'-Hydroxysafrole, thought to be the carcinogenic metabolite of safrole, was found in the urine as the glucuronide conjugate in rats but not in humans. This finding has an important implication — if humans do not produce this carcinogenic metabolite, can the data from rat carcinogenicity studies be extrapolated to humans? The absence of 1'-hydroxysafrole in human urine in this study does not necessarily mean it is not produced in humans, only that it was not detected at the safrole doses used in this study. Another metabolite unique to the rat is 3'-hydroxysafrole, a product of 1'-hydroxysafrole hydrolysis and isomerization.

## 22.6 Drug and Food Interactions

Safrole is potent inhibitor of liver microsomal hydroxylating enzymes, and thus could increase plasma levels of certain drugs. In addition, eugenol, a safrole metabolite, is a moderate enzyme inhibitor (Jaffe et al., 1968). It appears that safrole acts as a substrate for cytochrome P-450 isoenzymes, and upon metabolism covalent bonds form between the reactive metabolites and the enzyme, resulting in enzyme inhibition (Ionnaides et al., 1985).

## 22.7 Analysis of Biofluids

Oil of sassafras has been reported to interfere with serum phenytoin concentration determination. A 4-mo-old boy was admitted to the hospital for failure to thrive and possible child abuse after an outpatient visit revealed that he was below the third percentile for height and weight, and had scattered bruises, including one above the left eye. The child's mother had a seizure disorder and was taking phenytoin and phenobarbital. It was suspected that she may have administered the medication to her infant son for its sedative effects. According to the method of Svensmark and Kristensen, the phenytoin level was 6.4 µg/mL, and by hospital d 4 it had declined to 2.8 mg/L. The mother denied giving the drug to her baby but mentioned using Dr. Hand's teething lotion and a multivitamin preparation. Adding increasing amounts of the teething lotion to a serum sample resulted in increasing phenytoin concentrations. These findings were confirmed by administering the teething lotion to a dog via gastric tube and measuring the resulting phenytoin concentration. Two ingredients of the lotion, clove and sassafras oil, were determined to have interfered with the phenytoin serum level. By using the more specific method of serum phenytoin determination described by Dill, phenytoin could not be detected in the patient's serum.

Thin-layer chromatography (TLC) was used to identify safrole, isosafrole, and dihydrosafrole in rat urine and bile (Fishbein et al., 1967). Gas chromatography–mass spectroscopy (GC–MS) and gas liquid chromatography–mass spectroscopy (GLC–MS) were utilized to identify the urinary metabolites of safrole in the rat (Klungsoyr and Scheline, 1983). Plasma and tissue safrole concentrations in rats and humans were measured by GC–MS. Urinary metabolites were identified using TLC and GC-MS (Benedetti et al., 1977).

## 22.8 Regulatory Status

As a result of data showing safrole caused hepatocarcinomas in rats, a regulation published in the Federal Register on December 3, 1960 prohibits the use of safrole in foods (Segelman et al., 1976).

## References

Anonymous. Sassafras. The review of natural products. St. Louis: Facts and Comparisons, 1997.

Barreiro EJ, Lima MEF. The synthesis and antiinflammatory properties of a new sulindac analogue synthesized from natural safrole. J Pharmaceut Sci 1992;81:1219–22.

Benedetti MS, Malnoe A, Broillet AL. Absorption, metabolism, and excretion of safrole in the rat and man. Toxicology 1997;7:69–83.

Clark AM, El-Feraly FS, Wen-Shyong L. Antimicrobial activity of phenolic constituents of *Magnolia grandiflora* L. J Pharmaceut Sci 1981;70:951–2.

Craig JO. Poisoning by the volatile oils in childhood. Arch Dis Child 1953;28:475–83.

Duke J. CRC Handbook of medical herbs. Boca Raton, FL: CRC Press, 1989.

El-Feraly FS, Cheatham SF, Breedlove RL. Antimicrobial neoligans of *Sassafras randaiense* roots. J Nat Prod 1983;46:493–8.

Epstein SS, Fujii K, Andrea J, Mantel N. Carcinogenicity testing of selected food additives by parenteral administration to infant Swiss mice. Toxicol Appl Pharmacol 1970;16:321–34.

Estes JW. The European reception of the first drugs from the new world. Pharm Hist 1995;37(1):3–23.

Fishbein L, Fawkes J, Falk HL, Thompson S. Thin-layer chromatography of rat bile and urine following intravenous administration of safrole, isosafrole, and dihydrosafrole. J Chromatogr 1967;29:267–73.

Grande GA, Dannewitz SR. Symptomatic sassafras oil ingestion. Vet Hum Toxicol 1987;29:447.

Haines JD. Sassafras tea and diaphoresis. Postgrad Med 1991;90:75–76.

Hartwell JL. Plants used against cancer. Lloydia 1969;32:247–96.

Ioannides C, Delaforge M, Parke DV. Interactions of safrole and isosafrole and their metabolites with cytochrome P-450. Chem Biol Interact 1985;53:303–11.

Jaffe H, Fujii K, Sengupta M, Guerin H, Epstein SS. In vivo inhibition of mouse liver microsomal hydroxylating systems by methylenedioxyphenyl insecticidal synergists and related compounds. Life Sci 1968;7:1051–62.

Klungsoyr J, Scheline RR. Metabolism of safrole in the rat. Acta Pharmacol Toxicol 1983;52:211–6.

Pereira EFR, Pereira NA, Lima MEF, Coelho FAS, Barreiro EJ. Antiinflammatory properties of new bioisosteres of indomethacin synthesized from safrole which are sulindac analogues. Brazilian J Med Biol Res 1989;22:1415–9.

Segelman AB, Segelman FP, Karliner J, Sofia RD. Sassafras and herb tea. Potential health hazards. JAMA 1976;236:477.

Tyler VE. The honest herbal, 3rd edit., Binghamton, NY: Pharmaceutical Products Press, 1993.

Tyler VE. Herbs of choice, Binghamton, NY: Pharmaceutical Products Press, 1994.

Tyler VE, Brady LR, Robbers JE. Pharmacognosy, 8th edit., Philadelphia: Lea and Febiger, 1981.

Vesselinovitch SD, Rao KVN, Mihailovich N. Transplacental and lactational carcinogenesis by safrole. Cancer Res 1979;39:4378–80.

# Chapter 23

# Hawthorn

## *Jennifer Annon and Melanie Johns Cupp*

*Crataegus oxyacantha* (L.), *C. laevigata, C. monogyna* Jacquin, English hawthorn, haw, maybush, whitethorn (Anonymous, 1994), may, mayblossom, hazels, gazels, halves, hagthorn, ladies' meat, bread and cheese tree (Grieve, 1971)

## *23.1 History and Traditional Uses*

Hawthorn is a spiny, small tree or bush with white flowers and red berries (haws), each containing one to three nuts, depending on the species (Anonymous, 1994). Hybridization is common among individual species, making them difficult to identify (Hamon, 1988). Hawthorn is a member of the rose family and is found in Europe, North Africa, and western Asia (Grieve, 1971). It can reach heights of 25–30 ft and is used as a hedge (Anonymous, 1994; Bigus et al., 1998). The flowers grow in clusters and bloom from April to June, and the deciduous leaves are divided into three, four, or five lobes (Anonymous, 1994). The use of hawthorn can be dated back to Dioscorides in the first century AD (Tyler, 1993). Uses for the herb have included high and low blood pressure, tachycardia, arrhythmias, atherosclerosis, and angina pectoris (Anonymous, 1994). Hawthorn is also purported to have spasmolytic and sedative effects (Anonymous, 1994). Native Americans used it as a diuretic for kidney and bladder disorders and to treat stomach aches, stimulate appetite, and improve circulation (Bigus et al., 1998). The flowers and berries have astringent properties and have been used to treat sore throats in the form of haw jelly or haw marmalade (Tyler, 1993).

From Forensic Science: *Toxicology and Clinical Pharmacology of Herbal Products*
Edited by: M. J. Cupp © Humana Press Inc., Totowa, New Jersey

## 23.2 Current Promoted Uses

Hawthorn preparations are popular in Europe, and are gaining popularity in the United States (Tyler, 1993; Anonymous, 1994). Hawthorn is promoted for use in heart failure, hypertension, arteriosclerosis, angina pectoris, Buerger's disease, paroxysmal tachycardia (Blumenthal, 1997), heart valve murmurs, sore throat, skin sores, diarrhea, and abdominal distention (Williamson and Wyandt, 1997).

## 23.3 Products Available

Available products include tea, 1:5 tincture in 45% alcohol, 1:1 liquid extract in 25% alcohol (Blumenthal, 1997) and capsules of 250 mg, 455 mg, and 510 mg. The French Pharmacopoeia requires 45% ethanol for the fluid extract and 60% ethanol for the tincture (Bahorun et al., 1996). It is recommended that 0.5 –1 mL of liquid extract or 1–2 mL of tincture be taken three times a day (Blumenthal, 1997). The tea is made from 0.3–1 g of dried berries infused in hot water and taken three times a day (Blumenthal, 1997; Bigus et al., 1998). A typical therapeutic dose of extract, standardized to contain 1.8% vitexin-4 rhamnoside, is 100–250 mg three times daily. A standardized extract containing 18% procyanidolic oligomers (oligomeric procyanidns) is dosed at 250–500 mg daily (Anonymous, 1998).

## 23.4 Pharmacologic/Toxicologic Effects

### 23.4.1 Cardiovascular Effects

Hawthorn extracts purportedly dilate coronary blood vessels, decrease blood pressure, increase myocardial contractility, and lower serum cholesterol (Anonymous, 1999). Benefits have been demonstrated in heart failure patients (Iwamoto et al., 1981). In patients with Stage II New York Heart Association (NYHA) heart failure, doses of 160–900 mg/d of the aqueous-alcoholic extract for up to 56 d showed an increase in exercise tolerance, decrease in rate/pressure product, and increased ejection fraction (Blumenthal, 1998). The active principles are thought to be flavonoids, including hyperoside, vitexin, vitexin-rhamnose, rutin, and oligomeric procyanidins (dehydrocatechins; catechins and/or epicatechins) (Tyler, 1993; Blumenthal, 1997; Blumenthal, 1998; Bigus, 1998).

Investigators attempted to elucidate the mechanism of action of the flavonoids hyperoside, luteolin-7-glucoside, rutin, vitexin, vitexin-rhamnoside, and monoacetyl-vitexin-rhamnoside in spontaneous beating Langenhoff preparations of guinea pig hearts (Schussler et al., 1995). Dose-dependent effects on contractility, heart rate, and coronary blood flow similar to that of theophylline were exhibited by luteolin-7-glucoside, hyperoside, and rutin, while vitexin and its derivatives were less potent. These results were different from those of previous investigators, who found a decrease in coronary blood flow, contractility, and heart rate with hyperoside, while vitexin decreased contractility and increased heart rate and coronary blood flow. Vitexin-rhamnoside increased coronary blood flow, heart rate, and contractility in the previous study. These differences were attributed to differences in the experimental device. The investigators concluded that the mechanism behind the cardiac effects of these flavonoids involved phosphodiesterase inhibition, causing an increase in cAMP concentration, as well as inhibition of thromboxane synthesis and enhancement of prostacyclin ($PGI_2$) synthesis, as described by previous researchers. The authors also concluded that despite previous studies showing that vitexin-rhamnoside protected cultured heart cells from oxygen and glucose deprivation, the role of antioxidant activity as a mechanism behind the antiischemic effect of these flavonoids requires further study, given that vitexin-rhamnoside exhibited only minor effects in their study.

Because reactive oxygen species may play a role in the pathogenesis of atherosclerosis, angina, and cerebral ischemia, the antioxidant activity of dried hawthorn flowers and flowering tops, fluid extract, tincture, freeze-dried powder, and fresh plant extracts was investigated (Bahorun et al., 1996). Antioxidant activity, determined by the ability of the preparations to scavenge hydrogen peroxide, superoxide anion, and hypochlorous acid (HOCL), was provided by all preparations, but was highest with the fresh young leaf, fresh floral buds, and dried flowers. The antioxidant activity was correlated to total phenolic proanthocyanidin and flavonoid content.

The effects of hawthorn extract LI 132 standardized to 2.2% flavonoids (Faros® 300, Lichtwer Pharma GmbH, Berlin, Germany) on contractility, oxygen consumption, and effective refractory period of isolated rat cardiac myocytes were studied (Popping et al., 1995). In addition, the effect of partially purified oligomeric procyanidins on contractility was also studied. The concentrations used in their study were chosen for their physiologic plausibility based on the assumption that the volume of distribution of both hawthorn extract and procyanidins in humans is 5 L, and that the daily dose is 900 mg and 5 mg, respectively. At concentrations of 30–180 μg/mL, the hawthorn extract increased myocardial contractility with a more favorable effect on oxygen consumption than β-1 agonists or cardiac glycosides. Hawthorn also prolonged the effective refractory period, indicating that it might be an effective antiarrhythmic agent. Oligomeric procyanidins at concentrations of 0.1–30 μg/mL had no detectable effect on contractility, suggesting that they are not responsible for the positive inotropic effect of hawthorn.

Tincture of crataegus (TCR), made from hawthorn berries, was shown to have a hypocholesterolemic effect on rats fed 0.5 mL/100 g body wt for 6 wk. These findings prompted a study that examined the ability of TCR to increase low-density lipoprotein (LDL) binding to liver plasma membranes in rats fed an atherogenic diet (Rajendran et al., 1996). The hypocholesterolemic effect of TCR appears to be caused by a 25% increase in LDL receptor activity, resulting in greater LDL uptake by the liver. This was due to an increased number of receptors, not an increase in receptor binding affinity. In addition, TCR suppressed *de novo* cholesterol synthesis in the liver, and enhanced the use of liver cholesterol to make bile acids. Despite LDL receptor up-regulation, the atherogenic diet fed to the rats offset the beneficial effects; LDL levels increased 104% and liver cholesterol increased by 231%. The investigators did not attempt to determine which TCR constituent was responsible for the hypocholesterolemic effect, but hypothesized that all contribute in some manner.

### 23.4.2 Neurologic Effects

The flavonoids present in hawthorn purportedly have a sedative effect (Hamon, 1988; Tyler, 1993).

### 23.4.3 $LD_{50}$

The $LD_{50}$ of an alcoholic extract of hawthorn leaves and fruit called Crataegutt® administered orally was 33.8 mL/kg in rats and 18.5 mL/kg in mice. This particular extract was manufactured by Schwabe and contained 2% or 10% oligomeric procyanidins. Death occurred after approx 30 min and was caused by sedation and apnea. (Ammon and Handel, 1981).

### 23.4.4 Teratogenicity/Mutagenicity/Carcinogenicity

The German Commission E reports that hawthorn effects are unknown during pregnancy and lactation. No experimental data have been reported concerning toxicity in the embryo or fetus, or the effects on fertility or postnatal development. Commission E also reports the lack of experimental data concerning carcinogenicity. Despite experiential data that hawthorn may be mutagenic, Commission E feels that the amount of mutagenic substances ingested would not be sufficient to pose a risk to humans. Available information presents no indication of carcinogenic risk (Blumenthal, 1998).

## 23.5 Case Reports of Toxicity Due to Commercially Available Products

Although several references mention that hawthorn in high doses may cause hypotension, arrhythmias, and sedation in humans (Hamon, 1988; Tyler,

1993; Anonymous, 1994; Bigus et al., 1998), no substantiative case reports can be located.

## 23.6 Pharmacokinetics/Toxicokinetics

Although the investigators of one study (Popping et al., 1995) assumed a volume of distribution of 5 L (approximately plasma volume) for purposes of calculating a concentration to use in their in vitro study, there are no pharmacokinetic data to confirm this.

## 23.7 Chemical Analysis

Bahorun and colleagues describe the use of thin-layer chromatography (TLC) to determine total proanthocynidins, phenol, and flavonoid content of hawthorn extracts. High-performance liquid chromatography (HPLC) analysis using a UV detector at 280 nm for proanthocyanidins and phenolic acids, and 360 nm for flavonoids is also described (Bahorun et al., 1996).

## 23.8 Drug Interactions

Drug interactions with hawthorn are theoretically possible with cardioactive medications, but have not been documented (Harmon, 1988). In addition, the flavonoid constituents have been shown to have inhibitory and inducible effects on the cytochrome P-450 enzyme system, making other drug interactions possible (Canivenc-Lavier et al., 1996).

## 23.9 Regulatory Status

Originally, all preparations of hawthorn were approved under one German Commission E monograph based on historical experience. However, in 1993, the preparations were reevaluated and it was concluded that sufficient scientific evidence was lacking to justify use of the flowers, leaves, and berries as individual compounds. As a result, there are currently four hawthorn monographs: three Unapproved monographs for the berry, flower, and leaf individually and an Approved monograph for the flower with leaves. In addition, the Approved monograph has only one approved indication: treatment of "decreasing cardiac output according to functional stage II of the NYHA (Blumenthal, 1998)."

In Canada, hawthorn carries new drug status and is not approved, as self-treatment of cardiovascular conditions is deemed inappropriate. Hawthorn is not on the General Sales List in the United Kingdom. In France, the flower and flowering top are permitted for oral use, and in Switzerland, the leaf and flower are permitted as herbal teas. In Sweden, hawthorn is classified as a natural product, whereas in the United States, it is considered a dietary supplement (Blumenthal, 1997).

## REFERENCES

Ammon HO, Handel M. *Crataegus* toxicology and pharmacology. Part I: toxicity. Planta Med 1981;43:105–20.

Anonymous. Hawthorn (*Crataegus monogyna*). Nat Med J 1999;2:5.

Anonymous. The Lawrence review of natural products, St. Louis, MO: Facts and Comparisons, 1994.

Bahorun T, Gressier B, Trotin F, Brunet C, Dine T, Luyckx M, Vasseur J, Cazin M, Cazin JC, Pinkas M. Oxygen species scavenging activity of phenolic extracts from hawthorn fresh plant organs and pharmaceutical preparations. Arzneim Forsch 1996;46:1086–9.

Bigus A, Massengil D, Walker C. Hawthorn. Available from: URL:http://www.unc.edu/~cebradsh/main.html. Accessed 1998 Oct 15.

Blumenthal M. Popular herbs in the U.S. Market. Austin, TX: American Botanical Council, 1997.

Blumenthal M. The complete German Commission E monographs. Austin, TX: American Botanical Council, 1998.

Canivenc-Lavier M, Vernavaut M, Totis M, Siess M, Magdolou J, Suschetet M. Comparative effects of flavonoids and model inducers on drug-metabolizing enzymes in rat liver. Toxicology 1996;114:19–27.

Grieve M. A modern herbal. New York, NY: Dover, 1971.

Hamon NW. Hawthorns. CPJ/RPJ 1998;(Nov):708, 724.

Iwamoto M, Sato T, Ishizaki T. The clinical effect of *Crataegus* in heart disease of ischemic or hypertensive origin. A multicenter double-blind study. Planta Med 1981;42:1–16.

Popping S, Rose H, Ionescu I, Fisher Y, Hammermeier H. Effect of a hawthorn extract on contraction and energy turnover of isolated rat caridiomyocytes. Arzneim Forsch 1995;45:1157–60.

Rajendran S, Deepalakshmi PD, Parasakthy K, Devaraj H, Niranjali S. Effect of tincture of *Crataegus* on the LDL-receptor activity of hepatic plasma membrane of rats fed an atherogenic diet. Atherosclerosis 1996;123:235–41.

Schussler M, Holzl J, Fricke U. Myocardial effects of flavonoids from crataegus species. Arzneim Forsch 1995;45:842–5.

Tyler VE. The honest herbal, 3rd edit., Binghamton, NY: Pharmaceutical Products Press, 1993.

Williamson JS, Wyandt CM. Herbal therapies: the facts and the fiction. Drug Topics 1997; (Aug 4);141:78–85.

# Chapter 24

# Aloe

*Tara Dalton and Melanie Johns Cupp*

*Aloe barbadensis* Miller, Curacao aloe, *A. vera* Linne, aloe vera, *A. vera* Tournefort ex Linne, Barbados aloe, *A. vulgaris* Lamark, Cape aloe, Zanzibar aloe, Socotrine aloe, *A. ferox* Miller (Anonymous, 1992), *A. perryi* Baker, *A. africana* Miller, *A. capensis*, *A. spicata* Miller, natal aloes, mocha aloes (Wichtl, 1994), burn plant, aloe, aloe gel, aloe mucilage, aloe juice, aloe latex, dried aloes (Briggs, 1995), Mediterranean aloe, bitter aloe (Morton, 1961), Carrisyn® (acemannan) (Kahlon et al., 1991), *A. vera* (L.) N. L. Burm (Blumenthal, 1998)

## 24.1 History and Traditional Uses

Aloe is derived from the Arabic word *alloeh* or the Hebrew word *halal*, which is translated as "a shining, bitter substance" (Tyler, 1981). The word *vera* is derived from the Latin *versus*, which means true. There are approx 500 species of the genus *Aloe*, which belongs to the family Lilaceae (Swanson, 1995). The species most widely used is *Aloe baradensis* Miller, also known as *A. vera* Tournefort ex Linne, *A. vulgaris* Lamark, Curacao aloe, aloe vera (Swanson, 1995), *A. vera* (L.) N. L. Burm (Blumenthal, 1998), and *A. vera* (L.) Webb et Berth non Miller (Wichtl, 1994). The term "cape aloe" refers to the dried latex of the leaves of several species of the *Aloe* genus, especially *A. ferox* Miller, its hybrids, and preparations made from them (Blumenthal, 1998). Aloe is native to Africa, southern Arabia, Madagascar, and areas surrounding the Red Sea and Mediterranean Sea (Morton, 1961). It is grown in the Caribbean, especially the West Indies, in Japan, and in coastal areas of Venezuela (Anonymous, 1992; Wichtl, 1994). It is also grown in the United States in the Rio Grande Valley of Texas, California, Arizona, Florida, and in greenhouses in

From Forensic Science: *Toxicology and Clinical Pharmacology of Herbal Products*
Edited by: M. J. Cupp © Humana Press Inc., Totowa, New Jersey

Oklahoma (Wichtl, 1994; Hennessee, 1998). Each plant has about 15–30 green, rigid, thorny leaves in a rosette pattern (Anonymous, 1992). The flowers are yellow to orange-red in color (Swanson, 1995). Aloe was mentioned in the Egyptian Book of Remedies (circa 1500 BC) as a laxative and dermatologic preparation (Anonymous, 1992). Mesopotamians were also aware of its medicinal properties by that time (Swanson, 1995). An Egyptian papyrus written about 1500 BC gave formulas for preparing aloe to treat external and internal ailments (Hennessee, 1998). Aloe was first mentioned in Greek literature as a laxative before the first century (Hennessee, 1998). In the first century, the Greek physician Dioscorides wrote of its use in treating wounds, chapping, hair loss, genital ulcers, hemorrhoids, boils, mouth irritation and inflammation (Shelton, 1991; Anonymous, 1992; Hennessee, 1998). In the seventh century, aloe was used in the Orient for eczema and sinusitis (Shelton, 1991). The introduction into Western culture began with its use in the 1930s to treat radiation burns (Tyler, 1981).

## 24.2 Current Promoted Uses

Aloe is promoted to heal wounds, burns, skin ulcers, frostbite, and dry skin (Briggs, 1995; Swanson, 1995). It is an ingredient in dieters' teas used for their laxative effect (Kurtzweil, 1997). Aloe is found in other laxative and "body cleansing" products also. It is used in areas around the world for wounds, ringworm, hemorrhoids, joint inflammation, edema, burns, hair loss, and constipation (Morton, 1961). A study in urban and rural clinics in southwestern West Virginia found that aloe vera was the third most common folk or herbal remedy, with 42 out of 124 people admitting use within the 12 mo prior to the study (Cook and Baisden, 1986).

## 24.3 Products Available

Aloe is available in a wide variety of dosage forms including red and white powders, injectables, tablets, suppositories, capsules (brown and red), gels, creams, aloe dressings, and juices (light to dark brown tinge). The oral dosage forms range in strengths from 100 to 200 mg. It is found as either an active or inactive ingredient in natural food flavorings, cosmetics, soaps, shampoos, suntan lotions, after-sun lotions, shaving gels, dry skin lotions, hydrocortisone products, bubble baths, burn relief products, and on disposable razors to soothe the skin (Swanson, 1995). It is also available as a houseplant from which the fluid gel can be expressed and applied to minor burns and wounds (Briggs, 1995; Swanson, 1995).

Aloe, 100 mg, is commonly available in the United States in combination with 150 mg of cascara sagrada in a product called Nature's Remedy®. It is a brown, round tablet with the logo "NR."

Aloe vera is the source of two products that have different content. Aloe gel, also called aloe vera gel, mucilage, or (incorrectly) aloe juice, is the thin, clear jelly obtained by crushing the cells in the parenchymal tissue found inside the leaves (Tyler, 1993; Swanson, 1995). The gel is used in cosmetics and topical products (Swanson, 1995). Although this gel does not contain laxative anthraquinones, contamination can occur, so a cathartic effect might occur if the gel is used internally (Tyler, 1993). Contents of the gel include glucomannan, a polysaccharide thought to possess emollient properties (Anonymous, 1992); bradykinase and an antiprostaglandin agent, which are thought to be responsible for the gel's antiinflammatory activity; and magnesium lactate, which is purported to block histamine release (Natow, 1986). Whether these substances are stable during storage is controversial (Tyler, 1993).

The aloe latex or aloe juice is obtained from the yellow latex of pericyclic cells found beneath the epidermis (Swanson, 1995). It is dried to yield a solid material called "aloe" that contains anthraquinones (Leung, 1980). The specific constituents of the latex include barbaloin, which is metabolized to the laxative aloe-emodin (Leung, 1980; Blumenthal, 1998), iso-barbaloin, chrysophanic acid (Leung, 1980), and aloin (Blumenthal, 1998). The term "aloin" also refers to a crystalline, concentrated form of the dried latex (aloe).

The term "aloe vera gel extract" sometimes is used to refer to the pulverized leaves, rather than to an actual extract (Leung, 1980). Two preparations that may contain only minimal amounts of aloe include "aloe extract," which may be highly diluted, and "reconstituted aloe vera," which is prepared from a powder or liquid concentrate (Tyler, 1993). Preparations that list "aloe" as an ingredient, but not near the top of the ingredient list, probably contain very little aloe (Tyler, 1993). One author (Swanson, 1995) found a product labeled "100% pure aloe vera," with an asterisk referring to small print reading "plus emollients, stabilizers, and preservatives to ensure potency and efficacy."

## 24.4 Pharmacologic/Toxicologic Effects

### *24.4.1 Gastrointestinal Effects*

*See also* Sections 25.4.2 and 25.4.3 for additional pertinent information.

Twelve patients with peptic ulcers treated with aloe gel emulsion and "as needed" Pro-Banthine showed a clinical recovery and no relapse 1 yr later (Blitz et al., 1963). The results of this study are controversial, as researchers did not include a control group (Anonymous, 1992). The proposed mechanism of action of aloe in treating peptic ulcer disease is that aloe may inhibit the secretion of hydrochloric acid in the stomach and prevent irritating substances from aggravating the ulcer.

One study showed aloe to be an effective treatment in patients with chronic constipation in combination with psyllium and celandine, a stimulant laxative obtained from the *Chelidonium majus* plant (Odes and Madar, 1991). An earlier study showed aloin to be effective alone, and even more effective in combination with phenolphthalein (Chapman and Pittelli, 1974). Gas and cramps were the major adverse effects with treatment.

*See also* Section 26.4.1 regarding mechanism of cathartic action.

### 24.4.2 Carcinogenicity/Genotoxicity

Melanosis coli, a harmless discoloration of the colon, may be seen on colonoscopy in those who use aloe chronically (Blumenthal, 1998). This will eventually disappear with discontinuation of the drug. A prospective study (Siegers et al., 1993b) of 1095 patients who underwent colorectal endoscopy revealed a melanosis coli incidence of 6.9% in those patients with no abnormalities in their colon, and incidences of 2.3%, 9.1%, 9.8%, and 18.6% respectively for patients with inflammatory diseases, diverticulosis, adenoma, and carcinoma. The authors calculated a relative risk of 3.04 for colorectal cancer for patients who abuse anthranoid laxatives (aloe, cascara, frangula, and rheum). This study also found that 28 of the 30 patients with adenoma or carcinoma admitted abuse of anthranoid laxatives for >10 yr. A retrospective study (Siegers et al., 1993b) of 3049 patients revealed lower incidences of melanosis coli in patients with inflammatory diseases, diverticulosis, adenoma, and carcinoma, but these results may be due to poor documentation. Data from mice fed a diet containing 0.03% aloin for 20 wk support these findings; alonin did not promote dimethylhydrazine-induced adenomas or carcinomas (Siegers et al., 1993a).

*See* Section 25.4.1 for further discussion of the mutagenicity and genotoxicity of emodin, aloe-emodin, and rhein, as well as a discussion of the association between colon cancer and laxative use. Section 26.4.3 also includes information on aloe-emodin and chrysophanol.

### 24.4.3 Hematopoietic Activity

The product CARN 750, an injectable form of acemannan derived from *Aloe barbadensis* Miller, was administered for 18 d in subcutaneous doses of 0.5 mg, 1 mg, and 2 mg to irradiated mice. Hematopoietic activity of CARN

750 at a dose of 1–2 mg/d was superior to placebo and at least comparable to that of G-CSF 3 μg/d (Egger et al., 1996).

### 24.4.4 Antimicrobial Activity

Extracts of 28 species of aloe were tested against *Mycobacterium tuberculosis*, *Staphylococcus aureus*, and *Escherichia coli* (Gottshall et al., 1949). Only *A. chinensis* Baker was effective against all three. *A. succotrina* was effective only against *M. tuberculosis*. Barbaloin, an aloe component, was found to be effective in vitro against *M. tuberculosis* (minimum inhibitory concentration [MIC] = 0.125 mg/mL) and *Bacillus subtilis* (MIC = 0.25 mg/mL) (Gottshall et al., 1950). Diluted and undiluted homogenates of the gelatinous material, the outer green vascular part of the leaves, and the entire leaf aloe did not inhibit growth of *S. aureus* or *E. coli* in another study (Fly and Kiem, 1963). It was also shown that fresh aloe juice inhibited *S. aureus* but quickly became unstable (Lorenzetti et al., 1964). Aloe juice that was heated and then freeze dried was bacteriostatic against *S. aureus*, *S. pyrogenes*, *Corynebacterium xerose*, and *S. paratyphi*. Individual components of the juice, aloe-emodin, emodin, and chrysophanic acid, did not inhibit *S. aureus* (Lorenzetti et al., 1964). A later study illustrated that Dermaide Aloe® (99.5% aloe extract) is effective at 70% concentration against *Klebesilla* sp., *P. aeruginosa*, *Enterobacter* sp., *S. aureus*, *S. agalactiae*, and *S. marcescens* (Robson et al., 1982). At concentrations exceeding 90%, Dermaide® inhibited *E. coli*, *C. albicans*, and *S. pyogenes*. It did not inhibit *B. subtilis* at any concentration. The aloe vera extract contained 3.6 mg/dL of salicylic acid. Other components, emodin, emolin, and barbaloin are converted to salicylic acid by the Kolbe reaction, perhaps explaining in part the anti-inflammatory activity of the extract (Robson et al., 1982).

Acemannan (Carrisyn®), a β-(1,4)-linked acetylated polymannan, derived from *A. barbadensis* Miller, was shown in vitro to increase the production and function of cytotoxic T cells in a dose-dependent manner, resulting in antiviral activity (Womble and Helderman, 1992). Another in vitro study showed that 15.62 μg/mL of acemannan in combination with 0.001 ng/mL of azidothymidine (AZT) inhibited HIV-1 in a synergistic manner (Kahlon et al., 1991). The combination of 15.6–125 μg/mL acemannan with 0.32 μg/mL of AZT protected the cells from rapid HIV-1 replication, which causes premature cell death. The combination of acyclovir and acemannan in respective doses of 0.025 μg/mL and 40μg/mL also inhibited HSV-1 replication. The proposed mechanism of action of acemannan's antiviral activity is inhibition of glycosylation of viral glycoproteins (Kahlon et al., 1991). A double-blind study involving 63 patients showed no significant benefit of acemannan 1600 mg vs placebo in preventing decline in CD4 count in a 48 wk study. (Montaner et al.,

1996) These results are difficult to interpret because 57 patients were taking zidovudine (AZT), and six patients were taking didanosine (ddI) along with acemannan or placebo.

### 24.4.5 Antineoplastic Activity

Aloctin A is a glycoprotein obtained from *A. aborescens* Miller. Aloctin A administered to six mice at a dose of 10 mg/kg/d intraperitoneally for 5 d inhibited growth of methylcholanthrene-induced fibrosarcoma in four of the mice vs zero of ten untreated mice. These results were attributed to aloctin A's immunomodulatory effect, not cytotoxicity (Imanishi et al., 1981).

Aloe emodin was shown to possess activity against P-388 leukemia in mice although a previous study showed that aloe emodin did not inhibit L-1210 leukemia (Kupchan and Karim, 1976). The National Cancer Institute tested aloe as an antineoplastic, with negative results (Hecht, 1981).

### 24.4.6 Anti-Inflammatory and Wound Healing Activity

In one study (Davis, 1986), subcutaneous injections of *A. barbadensis* inhibited mustard-induced rat paw edema compared to control ($p < 0.01$). The effectiveness increased with the use of RNA and vitamin C ($p < 0.001$). Another study (Vazquez et al., 1996) showed that intraperitoneally administered aloe vera extracts decreased carrageenan-induced rat paw edema and peritoneal neutrophil infiltration in response to carrageenan. It was also shown that aloe vera decreased prostaglandin $E_2$ production. Mice receiving subcutaneous injections with colorized aloe vera gel containing anthraquinones at doses of 1, 10, and 100 mg/kg for 7 d had no reduction in their wound diameter (Davis et al., 1987). However, those receiving the same doses of decolorized (i.e., without anthraquinones) aloe vera had a decrease in wound diameter. Rats injected with colorized aloe vera for 12 d also had a decrease in wound diameter. These same authors also noted that polymorphonuclear leukocyte (PMN) infiltration and inflammation are decreased by both colorized and decolorized aloe vera.

These observations might be explained by the bradykinase activity of *A. aborescens* (Fujita et al., 1976). Specifically, aloe contains a carboxypeptidase that is responsible for degrading bradykinase (Fujita et al., 1979). A later study on homogenized fetal calf skin showed that both aloe gel and aloe extract in increasing amounts inhibited the oxidation of arachidonic acid, which suggests inhibition of production of inflammatory prostaglandins (Penneys, 1982). As discussed in section 24.4.4, some aloe constituents to salicylic acid (Robson et al., 1982).

A case reported in 1935 involved a woman who developed dermatitis 14 mo after roentgen treatment for depilatory purposes (Collins and Collins 1935).

The affected area was a 4 cm by 8 cm desquamated area that oozed serous fluid. The patient reported severe itching and burning sensations in the area, and had to wear gloves to bed to prevent scratching. The dermatitis had failed treatment with boric acid, phenol in olive oil, ichthyol, a 5% mercurial ointment, and zinc oxide. She was then treated with fresh whole aloe leaf which ceased the burning and itching and resulted in complete skin healing over a period of 5 wk.

Two studies published a few years after this case report supported the observations of Collins and Collins. One investigator demonstrated that 1 g of fresh aloe gel applied for 14 d promoted complete healing in 10 of 28 rats that had received 4000 rads. of x-ray radiation in divided doses. Only 5 rats treated with saline showed marked improvement (Rowe, 1940). A later study found that fresh aloe gel applied twice a day for 3–4 wk improved healing in rats that had received 4000 rads. of x-ray radiation in a single dose. Partially decomposed gel was effective as well, but the fresh rind, aqueous extracts of the dried rind, and an ointment made of dried aloe were not effective. Fresh rind was also used to treat a patient with a chronic x-ray reaction of 7 mo duration, also with negative results (Rowe et al., 1941). Another animal study showed that acemannan wound dressing gel applied to mice that had received 30–47.5 Gy radiation produced a lower peak skin reaction to the radiation than no treatment, K-Y jelly, or Aquaphor ointment (Roberts and Travis, 1995). It was determined that the wound dressing gel was most effective if treatment began immediately after radiation and was continued for at least 2 wk. However, an ointment consisting of 2 drams of powdered aloe, mineral oil, and white petrolatum applied twice daily to irradiated rats for 3 wk did not result in increased rate of healing. In a phase III study, aloe gel from *A. barbadensis* was no more effective than placebo in preventing radiation-induced dermatitis in women receiving breast or chest wall irradiation (Williams et al., 1996). This result prompted a study of no treatment vs aloe gel, which also showed no benefit. Allergic reactions to aloe were reported in three patients. Results of animal studies might not be reproduced in humans because the experimentally produced reactions are of the acute type, rather than the chronic reactions studied in humans (Rowe et al., 1940).

A study in mice exposed to ultraviolet radiation found that aloe vera gel does not act to stimulate DNA repair after exposure nor does it act as a sunscreen; however, it was shown to prevent UV-radiation-induced suppression of immune response for 24 h after sun exposure (Strickland et al., 1994).

Aloe vera cream was shown to improve tissue survival by 24% in the experimental rabbit-ear frostbite model (Miller and Koltai, 1995). Combination with systemic pentoxifylline showed 30% improvement. Some hospitals use a protocol for frostbite developed by the University of Chicago Hospitals and Clinics that involves the use of Dermaide Aloe Cream® (70% aloe vera) on blisters every 6 h (McCauley et al., 1990).

Carrington Dermal Wound Gel®, described by the authors as "aloe vera gel extract," applied to 10 guinea pigs healed a burn covering approx 30% of the body surface area in an average of 30 d (Rodriguez-Bigas et al., 1988). This was compared to sulfadiazine cream (Silvadene®), salicylic acid, and no treatment, which effected healing in an average of 47, 45, and 50 d, respectively. Only the aloe vera gel extract was significantly ($p < 0.02$) better than no treatment. A study found concentrated aloe gel (98%) to be ineffective against experimental hydrofluoric acid burns on the hind legs of rats (Bracken et al., 1985).

Aloe vera extract 0.5% in a hydrophilic cream was shown to be more effective than placebo in treating psoriasis in a study involving 60 patients (Syed et al., 1996). Twenty-five of the thirty aloe patients compared with two of thirty placebo-treated patients were cured after 4 wk and a higher number of healed plaques were shown with aloe. No adverse effects or hypersensitivity reactions were noted.

A study found a that post-dermabrasion wounds healed 3 d faster with aloe vera gel polyethylene oxide dressing vs the same dressing without aloe vera (Fulton, 1990). Burning was reported with the aloe dressing. A later study found a delay in wound healing post-cesarean delivery or laparotomy in patients who received Carrington Dermal Wound Gel® in addition to wet-to-dry dressing using saline and Dakin's solution (0.025% sodium hypochlorite) (Schmidt and Greenspoon, 1991).

## 24.5 Case Reports of Toxicity Due to Commercially Available Products

A woman who had taken Carter's Little Pills®, which contained aloe and podophyllum, daily for 4 yr presented with unexplained hypokalemic metabolic alkalosis (Ramirez and Marieb, 1970). Carter's Little Pills® have since been reformulated and no longer contain aloe.

One retrospective study (Gold, 1980) reviewed cases of acute renal failure in 91 patients who had used herbal remedies. The majority of products used by the patients contained phenolphthalein and aloe extract or aloins. Seventy-four of the patients required peritoneal dialysis, 16 had jaundice, eight had neurologic impairment, and four died. One patient who presented with acute interstitial nephritis had ingested an aloe extract.

Dermatologic reactions to aloe have also been reported. Two weeks after a perioral chemical peel, a woman applied aloe from a houseplant to the area in an attempt to resolve some remaining pinkness. She immediately experienced a burning sensation, and the area became red, swollen, and crusted. The reaction resolved over 10 wk. (Hunter and Frumkin, 1991). Another patient who used aloe from a houseplant to treat stasis dermatitis developed dermatitis characterized by a scaly, erythematous rash on her neck, arms, and ankle (Hogan, 1988). After 3 yr of ingestion of aloe gel 1 teaspoonful three times daily, a patient developed eczema that persisted for 3 mo (Morrow et al., 1980). This patient had also been applying the gel daily, for the past year, after shaving and for the previous month had noticed urticarial lesions in his beard area that lasted 5 min after each gel application.

The FDA has received reports of four deaths as well as other adverse effects associated with the use of herbal laxative "dieters" teas (Kurtzweil, 1997). These teas contain laxatives such as senna, aloe, and buckthorn. Short-term reactions are nausea, vomiting, cramping, and diarrhea, which may last several days and usually occur in those who exceed the recommended dose. Other adverse effects include chronic diarrhea, dependence on laxatives for normal bowel function, and abdominal pain, which occur with long-term use. Severe reactions such as fainting, dehydration, and electrolyte disorders may occur in those with underlying nutritional disorders such as an eating disorder or excessive dieting.

## 24.6 Potential Drug Interactions

With long-term use hypokalemia due to intestinal potassium loss could occur (Blumenthal, 1998). Thiazide diuretics, corticosteroids, and licorice could exacerbate hypokalemia. The effects of digoxin can be potentiated by hypokalemia.

## 24.7 Pharmacokinetics/Toxicokinetics

### 24.7.1 Absorption

Aglycones (aloin, aloe-emodin, chrysophanol) in aloe preparations are thought to be absorbed in the upper small intestine, while barbaloin acts as a prodrug that is cleaved by colonic flora to yield aloe-emodin, a laxative (Anonymous, 1992; Blumenthal, 1998). Based on renal excretion data from rats fed radiolabeled aloe-emodin, at least 20–25% of a given dose is absorbed (Lang, 1993). Biliary excretion might be an important route of excretion, in which case the amount absorbed might be higher than is apparent from the urine data (i.e., drug excreted in the feces may or may not have been absorbed and excreted in the bile before being excreted in the feces) (Lang, 1993). Because aloe-emodin is metabolized quickly, its bioavailability is low — perhaps <10% (Lang, 1993).

### 24.7.2 Distribution

Aloe-emodin is 98–99% protein bound (Lang, 1993). Rhein, an active metabolite of aloe-emodin, passes into breast milk, but a laxative effect has not been noted in nursing infants (Lang, 1993; Blumenthal, 1998). Tissue concentrations of aloe-emodin and its metabolites were highest in the rat liver and kidney (Lang, 1993). Concentrations in brown fat, muscle, eyes, perirenal fat, bones, bone marrow, and gonads were low or unmeasurable.

### 24.7.3 Metabolism/Elimination

Metabolites of aloe-emodin include the active metabolite rhein, an unknown metabolite, and glucuronide, and sulfate conjugates of all three (Lang, 1993; Blumenthal, 1998). In humans, rhein was recovered in the urine after consumption of 86 mg and 200 mg of aloe powder (Blumenthal, 1998). In a study in rats (Lang, 1993) approx 20–25% of a given dose of radiolabeled aloe-emodin was excreted in the urine as rhein, aloe-emodin, an unknown metabolite, and their conjugates. The rest was excreted in the feces mainly as aloe-emodin, with small amounts of rhein and an unknown metabolite. No conjugates were found in the feces. Not all of the radioactivity in the feces was analyzed, however, owing to inability to extract all of the radioactivity with methanol. The half-life of aloe-emodin was approximately 48–50 h. Whether biliary excretion is involved, or if radioactivity found in the feces represented nonabsorbed drug is unknown.

*See also* Section 26.7 regarding biotransformation of aloe-emodin, barbaloin, and chrysophanol.

## 24.8 Analysis of Biofluids

Note that aloe use can turn the urine a harmless red color during treatment (Blumenthal, 1998). Rhein and aloin, when lightly sprayed with 3 *M* KOH on an high-performance thin-layer chromatography (HPTLC) plate and exposed to white light are yellow/red in color, and orange/red in color under UV light at 366 nm (Perkins and Livesey, 1993).

Concentrations of aloe-emodin, rhein, an unknown metabolite, and their conjugated metabolites were determined in plasma, urine, feces, liver, and kidney using TLC (Lang, 1993). Thin layer chromatograms were prepared on silica gel, and mobile phases used included an ethyl acetate–methanol–water (100/

16.5/13.5 by vol) system and a chloroform–methanol–water (59/33/8 by vol) system.

Use of HPLC to detect rhein and aloin in the urine to screen for laxative abuse has been described (Perkins and Livesey, 1993). Detection is best with three first-morning urine samples, with at least one sample collected on a Monday morning, because many laxative abusers "purge" on weekends.

## 24.9 Regulatory Status

The German Commission E does not recommend that aloe be used for more than 1–2 wk when used as a laxative in self-treatment of constipation (Blumenthal, 1998). It should be used only after failure of dietary modification or a bulk-forming laxative.

*A. perryi* Baker, *A. barbadensis* Miller, *A. ferox* Miller, and hybrids of *A. ferox* Miller with *A. africana* Miller, and *A. spicata* Baker are approved by the FDA as food flavorings (Hecht, 1981). For use as a laxative aloe is regulated as a drug by the FDA but many aloe products are classified as dietary supplements under the Dietary Supplement Health and Education Act of 1994 (Kurtzweil, 1997). The FDA has proposed to move aloe, the laxative, from Category I (generally recognized as safe and effective for the claimed therapeutic indication) to Category III (insufficient data to permit final classification) until further studies can show its benefit and safety (Anonymous, 1998). The FDA Center for Drug Evaluation and Research proposed that aloe undergo genotoxicity and carcinogenicity tests owing to its chemical similarity to phenolphthalein, which is possibly carcinogenic. They have also proposed that if these studies are not provided or if they reveal that the drug is not safe, aloe should be reclassified as a Category II (not generally recognized as safe and effective) drug. Two FDA advisory panels have shown no benefit with aloe as a treatment of minor burns and cuts and urge further studies (Anonymous, 1992). A 1995 FDA Food Advisory Committee found laxatives are not beneficial in weight loss because they do not decrease calorie absorption, and recommended labeling changes that warn consumers of the harm of laxative products used for weight loss (Kurtzweil, 1997).

## References

Anonymous. Lawrence review of natural products. St. Louis, MO: Facts and Comparisons, 1992.

Anonymous. Laxative drug products for over-the-counter human use; proposed amendment to the tentative final monograph. 21 CFR Parts 310 and 334. Fed Register 1998;63:33592–5.

Blumenthal M. The complete German Commission E monographs: therapeutic guide to herbal medicines. Austin, TX: American Botanical Council, 1998.

Blitz JJ, Smith JW, Gerard JR. Aloe vera in peptic ulcer: preliminary report. J Am Osteopath Assoc 1963;62:731–5.

Bracken WM, Cuppage F, McLaury RL, Kirwin C, Klaassen CD. Comparative effectiveness of topical treatments for hydrofluoric acid burns. J Occup Med 1985;27:733–9.

Briggs C. Herbal medicine: aloe. Can Pharmaceut J 1995;128:48–50.

Chapman DD, Pittelli JJ. Double-blind comparison of alophen with its components for cathartic effects. Curr Ther Res 1974;16:817–20.

Collins CE, Collins C. Roentgen dermatitis treated with fresh whole leaf of aloe vera. Am J Roentgenol Radium Ther 1935;33:396–7.

Cook C, Baisden D. Ancillary use of folk medicine by patients in primary care clinics in southwestern West Virginia. South Med J 1986;79:1098–101.

Davis RH, Kabbani JM, Maro NP. Aloe vera and wound healing. J Am Podiatr Med Assoc 1987;77:L165–169.

Egger SF, Brown GS, Kelsey LS, Yates KM, Rosenberg LJ, Talmadge JE. Hematopoetic augmentation by a beta-(1,4)-linked mannan. Cancer Immunol Immunother 1996;43:195–205.

Fly LB, Kiem I. Tests of aloe vera for antibiotic activity. Econ Bot 1963;14:46–9.

Fujita K, Teradaira R, Nagatsu T. Bradykinase activity of aloe extract. Biochem Pharmacol 1976;25:205.

Fujita K, Ito S, Teradaira R, Beppu H. Properties of carboxypeptidase from aloe. Biochem Pharmacol 1979;28:1261–2.

Fulton JE. The stimulation of postdermabrasion wound healing with stabilized aloe vera gel-polyethylene oxide dressing. J Dermatol Surg Oncol 1990;16:460–7.

Gold CH. Acute renal failure from herbal and patent remedies in Blacks. Clin Nephrol 1980;14:128–34.

Gottshall RY, Lucas EH, Lickfeldt A, Roberts JM. The occurrence of antibacterial substances active against *Mycobacterium tuberculosis* in seed plants. J. Clin Invest 1949;28:920–3.

Gottshall RY, Jennings JC, Weller LE, Redemann CT, Lucas EH, Sell HM. Antibacterial substances in seed plants active against tubercle bacilli. Am Rev Tuberculosis 1950;62:475–80.

Hecht A. The overselling of aloe vera. FDA Consumer 1981;15:26–9.

Hennessee OM. Some history about aloe vera. Available from: http://www.aloe-vera.com/aloe1.html. Accessed 1998 Oct 31.

Hogan DJ. Widespread dermatitis after topical treatment of chronic leg ulcers and stasis dermatitis. Can Med Assoc J 1988;138:337–8.

Hunter D, Frumkin A. Adverse reactions to vitamin E and aloe vera preparations after dermabrasion and chemical peel. Cutis 1991;47:193–6.

Imanishi K, Ishiguro T, Saito H, Suzuki I. Pharmacological studies of plant lectin, Aloctin A. I. Growth inhibition of mouse methylcholanthrene-induced fibrosarcoma (Meth A) in ascites form by Aloctin A. Experientia 1981;37:1186–7.

Kahlon JB, Kemp MC, Yawei N, Carpenter RH, Shannon WM, McAnalley BH. In vitro evaluation of the synergistic antiviral effects of acemannan in combination with azidothymidine and acyclovir. Mol Biother 1991;3:214–23.

Kupchan SM, Karim A. Tumor inhibitors in aloe emodin: antileukemic principle isolated from *Rhamnus frangula* L. Lloydia 1976;39:223–4.

Kurtzweil P. Dieter's brews make tea time a dangerous affair. FDA Consumer 1997;31:6–11.

Lang W. Pharmokinetic-metabolic studies with $^{14}$C-aloe emodin after oral adminstration to male and female rats. Pharmacology 1993;(Suppl 1):110–9.

Leung AY. Encyclopedia of common natural ingredients used in food, drugs, and cosmetics. New York: John Wiley & Sons, 1980.

Lorenzetti LJ, Salisbury R, Beal JL, Baldwin JN. Bacteriostatic property of aloe vera. J Pharmaceut Sci 1964;53:1287.

McCauley RL, Heggers JP, Robson MC. Frostbite: methods to minimize tissue loss. Postgrad Med 1990;88:67–77.

Miller MB, Koltai PJ. Treatment of experimental frostbite with pentoxifylline and aloe vera cream. Arch Otol Head Neck Surg 1995;121:678–80.

Montaner JS, Gill J, Singer J, Raboud J, Arseneau R, McLean BD, et al. Double-blind placebo-controlled pilot trial of acemannan in advanced human immunodeficiency virus disease. J Acquired Immune Def Synd Hum Retrovirol 1996;12:153–7.

Morrow DM, Rapaport MJ, Strick RA. Hypersensitivity to aloe. Arch Dermatol 1980;116:1064–5.

Morton JF. Folk uses and commercial exploitation of aloe leaf pulp. Econ Bot 1961;15:311–9.

Natow AJ. Aloe vera, fiction or fact. Cutis 1986;37:106, 108.

Odes HS, Madar Z. A double-blind trial of celanding, aloe vera, and psyllium laxative preparation in adult patients with constipation. Digestion 1991;49:65–71.

Penneys NS. Inhibition of arachidonic acid oxidation in vitro by vehicle components. Acta Dermatovener 1982;62:59–61.

Perkins SL, Livesey JF. A rapid high-performance thin-layer chromatographic urine screen for laxative abuse. Clin Biochem 1993;26:179–81.

Ramirez B, Marieb NJ. Hypokalemic metabolic alkalosis due to carter's little pills. Conn Med 1970;34:169–70.

Roberts DB, Travis EL. Acemannan-containing wound dressing gel reduces radiation-induced skin reactions in C3H mice. Int J Radiat Oncol Biol Phys 1995;32:1047–52.

Robson MC, Heggers JP, Hagstrom WJ. Myth, magic, witchcraft, or fact? Aloe vera revisited. J Burn Care Rehab 1982;3:157–63.

Rodriguez-Bigas M, Cruz NI, Suarez A. Comparative evaluation of aloe vera in the management of burn wounds in guinea pigs. Plast Reconstr Surg 1988;81:386–9.

Rowe TD. Effect of fresh aloe vera gel in the treatment of third-degree roentgen reactions in white rats. J Am Pharm Assoc 1940;29:348–50.

Rowe TD, Lovell BK, Parks LM. Further observations on the use of aloe vera leaf in the treatment of third degree x-ray reactions. J Am Pharm Assoc 1941;30:266–9.

Schmidt JM, Greenspoon JS. Aloe vera dermal wound gel is associated with a delay in wound healing. Obstet Gynecol 1991;78:115–7.

Shelton RM. Aloe vera: its chemical and therapeutic properties. Intl J Dermatol 1991;30:679–83.

Siegers CP, Siemers J, Baretton G. Sennosides and aloin do not promote dimethylhydrazine-induced colorectal tumors in mice. Pharmacology 1993a;47(Suppl 1):205–8.

Siegers CP, von Hertzberg-Lottin E, Otte M, Schneider B. Anthranoid laxative abuse—a risk for colorectal cancer? Gut 1993b;34:1099–101.

Strickland FM, Pelley RP, Kripke ML. Prevention of ultraviolet radiation-induced suppression of contact and delayed hypersensitivity by Aloe barbadensis gel extract. J Invest Dermatol 1994; 102:197–204.

Swanson, LN. Therapeutic value of aloe vera. US Pharm 1995;20:26–35

Syed TA, Ahmad SA, Holt AH, Ahmad SA, Ahmad SH, Afzal M. Management of psoriasis with aloe vera extract in a hydrophilic cream: a placebo-controlled, double-blind study. Trop Med Int Health 1996;1:505–9.

Tyler, VE, Brady, LY, Robbers JE. Pharmacognosy, 8th edit., Philadelphia: Lea and Febiger, 1981.

Tyler VE. The honest herbal, 3rd edit., Binghamton, NY: Pharmaceutical Products Press, 1993.

Vazquez, B, Avila G, Seguro, D, Escalante, B. Antiinflammatory activity of extracts from aloe vera gel. J Ethnopharmacol 1996;55:69–75.

Wichtl M. Herbal drugs and phytopharmaceuticals. Stuttgart: MedPharm, 1994.

Williams MS, Burk M, Loprinzi CL, Hill M, Schomberg PJ, Nearhood K, et al. Phase III double-blind evaluation of an aloe vera gel as a prophylactic agent for radiation-induced skin toxicity. Int J Radiat Oncol Biol Phys 1996;36:345–9.

Womble D, Helderman JH. The impact of acemannan on the generation and function of cytotoxic T-lymphocytes. Immunopharmacol Immunotoxicol 1992;14:63–77.

# Chapter 25

# Senna


## Melanie Johns Cupp


*Cassia senna* (L.) (*C. acutifolia*), known as Alexandrian senna, Aden senna, or Nubian senna; *C. angustifolia* Vahl, known as Indian senna, Tinnevelly senna, and Meca senna (Franz, 1993)

## 25.1 History and Chemistry

Senna has been used at least since the ninth century. Its medicinal use was introduced by Arabian physicians who used both the leaves and the pods. There are two species of the senna plant, one that originated in northeastern Africa, *C. senna* (L.), (Alexandrian senna) and *C. angustifolia* Vahl, from India. Indian senna is also grown in California. Both are annual shrubs that approach heights of 3 ft. Up to seven pairs of leaflets arise from each branch. The flowers are yellow and produce the fruits, or seed pods. The chemical composition of the leaves of both Alexandrian and Indian senna are similar. The anthraquinones chrysophanol, emodin, and rhein are monoanthraquinones that combine with each other and with sugar molecules to form other senna constituents. The anthraquinone glycosides (i.e., sugar-containing molecules) sennosides A and B are dimeric products (dianthrones) of rhein. This rhein dimer is called sennidin, and sennosides A and B are the two optical isomers of the β-glucosides of sennidin (De Witte, 1993). Aloe emodin and rhein are the aglycones (molecules with the sugar moieties removed) of the hetero-dianthrone sennosides C and D. Hydrocolloids found in senna are also important for its therapeutic (i.e., laxative) effect because they influence the rheology of the


From Forensic Science: *Toxicology and Clinical Pharmacology of Herbal Products*
Edited by: M. J. Cupp © Humana Press Inc., Totowa, New Jersey

intestinal contents (Franz, 1993). Other senna constituents include the monoanthrones rhein anthrone-8-monoglucoside, and rhein-8-monoglucoside (Anonymous, 1998).

## 25.2 Current Promoted Uses

Senna is used in the United States and other industrialized countries as a laxative (Nusko et al., 1993).

## 25.3 Products Available

In the United States senna is available as senna fluid extract, sennnna fruit extract, senna leaf powder, senna pod concentrate, senna syrup, and sennosides A and B (Anonymous, 1998). Sennosides A and B are available as a tablet (Ex-Lax Gentle Nature®, 20 mg). A tea (Correctol Herbal Tea®, 30 mg total sennosides per bag in lemon or cinnamon spice flavor) is also available. Senna concentrate is available as tablets (Senexon®, Senolax®, Senokot®, 187 mg [8.6 mg of sennosides]; SenokotXTRA®, 17 mg of sennosides), granules (Senokot®, 326 mg [15 mg of sennosides] per teaspoon), suppositories (Senokot® 652 mg), liquid (Dr. Caldwell Senna Laxative® or Fletcher's Castoria®, 33.3 mg/mL; X-Prep®, 49.3 mg/mL), and syrup (Senokot® and Senokot Children's®, 8.8 mg sennosides per teaspoon). Senna concentrate, 187 mg (8.6 mg of sennosides) is also available in tablet form in combination with the stool softener docusate, 50 mg (Senokot-S® and Gentlax S®), and 125 mg in combination with the laxative cascara sagrada, 20 mg (Herbal Laxative Tablets by Nature's Bounty). Herb-Lax® is a tablet containing 175 mg of senna leaf powder, and Innerclean Herbal® is a tablet containing the cut plant, psyllium seed husks, buckthorn bark, anise seed, and fennel seed. Perdiem® granules contain senna (cassia pod concentrate), 740 mg/tsp and psyllium, 3.25 g/tsp.

## 25.4 Pharmacologic/Toxicologic Effects

### 25.4.1 Carcinogenicity/Mutagenicity/Genotoxicity

Senna constituents have been tested for mutagenicity in several in vitro test systems with varying results. Emodin gave positive results with the Ames test, the hypoxanthine guanine phosphoribosyl transferase (HGPRT) test, unscheduled DNA synthesis (UDS), and cell transformation of C3H/M2 cells. Aloe-emodin was also positive in three of the four tests; with the HGPRT test, no clear reproducible results could be obtained. Rhein gave negative results with all four test systems, although a weak positive effect was found in the Ames test using *Salmonella typimurium* strains TA 1537 and an S9 mix. Senna extract gave weak to strong positive results depending on the *S. typhimurium* strain used (Heidemann et al., 1993).

An in vivo study in rats using the bromodeoxyuridine (BrdUrd) labelling technique demonstrated that sennosides administered for up to 12 wk have no effect on ileal or colonic epithelial cell proliferation, suggesting that sennosides are not tumor promoters (Geboes et al., 1993). In another rat study also designed to identify precancerous changes, the colons of rats fed sennosides for up to 12 wk were examined for acidic mucins, lectin soybean agglutinin (SBA), and cytokeratin AE1. Although acidic mucin content and cytokeratin AE1 expression were increased, these changes were not thought to be precancerous (Yang et al., 1993). A sennoside-enriched diet (0.03%) did not promote dimethylhydrazine-induced colorectal adenomas or carcinomas in mice after 20 wk (Siegers et al., 1993). A long-term study in which 5–25 mg/kg of senna extract was fed to rats for 2 yr resulted in a dose-independent mesenteric lymph node hyperplasia in preterminally killed animals (Lyden-Sokolowski et al., 1993). There were no ultrastructural alterations in the myenteric plexus, and no increased risk of gastrointestinal, liver, kidney, or adrenal neoplasms.

It has been speculated that the increase in colon cancer in Western society is associated with use of cathartics. Colorectal cancer is one of the most common malignancies in the United States, and occurs with an incidence of 25 cases per 100,000 population in Germany. This is much higher than in agricultural regions of Africa and South America. In industrialized countries, up to 20% of the population uses laxatives regularly (Nusko et al., 1993). To test the hypothesis that laxative use is associated with an increased risk of colon cancer, data from 14 case-control studies that examined risk factors for colorectal cancer were included in a meta-analysis (Sonnenberg and Muller, 1993). Eleven of these studies contained information about the use of cathartics prior to cancer diagnosis. In only one study was the use of cathartics the primary focus. Most studies found a higher incidence of colorectal cancer in patients with a history of cathartic use, but this was statistically significant in a minority of studies. The use of cathartics was associated with a pooled odds ratio of 1.46 (1.33– 1.61 for 95% CI). Because constipation was associated with an odds ratio of 1.48 (1.32–1.66 for 95% CI), the investigators hypothesized that constipation and cathartic use reflect a diet high in fat, meat, and alcohol and low in vegetables. Thus, constipation and cathartic use are not thought to be the proximate cause of colon cancer, but rather markers for dietary habits that predispose to colon cancer.

A cohort study also aimed to clarify whether laxative use and melanosis coli (a blackish-brown discoloration of the colonic mucosa caused by long-term use of anthranoid-containing laxatives) are risk factors for colorectal cancer (Nusko et al., 1993). A cohort of 2277 patients who had undergone a total of 4474 colonoscopies was identified. Diagnoses included polyps, adenoma, carcinoma, melanosis coli, inflammatory bowel disease, diverticulosis, postoperative state (e.g., resection with anastomoses), and normal mucosa. Data were analyzed in regard to family history of colorectal cancer, bowel habits, laxative use, and other medications. There was a statistically significant association between adenomas and laxative use, with a relative risk of 1.72 (1.43–2.01 for 95% CI, $p < 0.00001$) for patients exposed to laxatives. For patients who had used laxatives but had not developed melanosis coli, there was a relative risk of 1.47 (1.19–1.81 for 95% CI, $p = 0.0064$). For laxative users with melanosis coli, the relative risk was 2.19 (1.79–2.67 for 95% CI).

The results of in vitro mutagenicity studies have not been supported by rodent and human data, perhaps because of poor absorption, inability of mutagenic substances to reach DNA targets, or rapid detoxification. This is despite aloe-emodin blood levels produced in rodents that approximate the concentrations that produced genotoxicity in in vitro test systems (Heidemann et al., 1993). Aloe-emodin is not detectable in human plasma after repeated administration of commercially available senna products (Krumbiegel and Schulz, 1993). Considering that the limit of detection (0.5 ng/mL) is well below the concentrations that were mutagenic in in vitro test systems, the risk of genotoxicity would appear low (Heidemann et al., 1993).

### *25.4.2 Gastrointestinal Effects*

Chronic laxative use in general leads to a change in shape and rarefaction of the intestinal microvilli, mitochondrial damage, an increase in the number of colonocyte lysosomes, plication of the lateral cell membrane with widening of the intracellular space, and granular inclusions within the colonocytes. In the guinea pig colon, rhein damages the villi and leads to disappearance of goblet cells and superficial erosions. Sennosides also lead to colonocyte apoptosis in guinea pigs, characterized by chromatin at the periphery of the cell, and migration of cells to the intercryptal region (Muller-Lissner, 1993).

Melanosis coli is observed in 12–31% of unselected constipated patients. A causal relationship between melanosis coli and use of anthraquinone laxatives has been shown in animals and humans. Sennosides produce melanosis coli after 4–13 mo of use, which disappears 5–11 mo after cessation of sennoside use. Melanosis coli begins abruptly at the ileocolonic junction and may extend to the dentate line. The intensity is highest in the cecum and becomes less intense in the aboral direction, and may increase again in the rectum, with a prevalence of 1–8% on proctoscopy. The pigment has not been definitively identified, but it is probably lipofuscin. Even if melanosis coli cannot be seen macroscopically, pigment-filled macrophages were seen in 60% of autopsy cases in one series, and in 52% of patients taking antraquinone laxatives. The terminal ileum may contain pigmented macrophages, even if the melanosis is not visible to the naked eye. In melanosis coli, pigmented macrophages can be seen outside of the submucosa, such as in the muscularis mucosa and between crypts. Over time, the macrophages migrate to the mesenteric lymph nodes, thus dispersing the pigment. Despite the histologic abnormalities that can be seen, there is no known pathologic consequence of melanosis coli (Muller-Lissner, 1993).

"Cathartic colon" is a term used to describe certain radiologic findings in patients using laxatives chronically. Observations on barium enema include loss of haustration, dilated lumen, dilation of the terminal ileum, gaping of the ileocecal valve, and pseudostrictures (variable hourglass-shaped spasms), with a predilection for the right colon. Macroscopic and microscopic observations include muscle atrophy, superficial ulceration, submucosal infiltrates of monocytes and eosinophils, fibrosis of the muscularis mucosa and submucosa, and an increase in submucosal fat. Cathartic colon has not been associated with use of senna products and other currently available laxatives (Muller-Lissner, 1993).

Animal and human studies suggest that senna laxative use might result in damage to the colonic nerve plexus. Intraperitoneal administration of senna syrup to mice resulted in degeneration of nerve fibers seen with silver staining, but the composition of the syrup, dose, and duration of treatment were unspecified. Studies in which mice were administered 10 mg/kg/d of sennosides for 4 mo, and rats were administered 25–100 mg/kg/d of sennosides revealed no intestinal changes on electron microscopy. A similar, subsequent study also found no damage to the myenteric neurons in either rats or mice, although in mice there was an increase in the number of neurons, a finding of unclear significance. It has been hypothesized that the dissimilar results in these animal studies were due to high levels of free anthraquinones in the senna syrup administered intraperitoneally, resulting in greater systemic absorption and toxicity. Although the intestines of constipated patients who have taken laxatives for years show swollen axons with increased diameter and electron-dense inclusions, lysosomes within neurons and Schwann cells, nerve plexus abnormalities seen on silver staining, and a decrease in neurofilaments, these changes cannot definitely be attributed to senna use (Muller-Lissner, 1993).

It would be expected that pathologic findings involving the autonomic nervous system would result in functional impairment of the intestine. Spontaneous contractility of the colon in rats is not affected by chronic treatment with sennosides. "Tolerance" to laxatives has not been documented, but some patients report having to increase the dose of laxatives with long-term use (Muller-Lissner, 1993).

Other than abdominal cramps, which occur in approx 10% of patients, it does not appear that senna causes any serious adverse gastrointestinal effects (Muller-Lissner, 1993). Products containing crystalline glycosides of senna are more stable, more reliable, and cause less cramping than products made from the crude drug (Curry, 1986).

*See also* Section 26.4.1 regarding mechanism of cathartic action.

### 25.4.3 Laxative Abuse

Although when taken at recommended doses, senna laxatives do not cause changes in electrolytes, hypokalemia and resultant muscle weakness can occur when laxatives are abused for purposes of weight loss, such as in patients with anorexia nervosa or bulimia, and in Munchhausen syndrome. Hypokalemia is the most common finding in patients abusing laxatives, and is caused by fecal potassium loss as well by hyperaldosteronism caused by fecal loss of water and sodium. Hypokalemia leads to metabolic alkalosis, reduction in renal tubular concentrating ability, and reduction in creatinine clearance. The tubular epithelium also exhibits degenerative changes histologically. The dose of senna or other laxatives required to produce hypokalemia is unknown because laxative abusing patients are often unreliable historians. Other findings in laxative abusers, who are typically female, include diarrhea, weight loss, abdominal pain, and finger clubbing in anthraquinone abusers (Muller-Lissner, 1993). Use of high-performance liquid chromatography (HPLC) to detect rhein and aloin in the urine to screen for laxative abuse has been described (Perkins and Livesey, 1993).

## 25.5 Pharmacokinetics/Toxicokinetics

Additional information on rhein and aloe-emodin pharmacokinetics can be found in Section 24.7.

### 25.5.1 Absorption

Chemically, sennosides, having sugar moieties attached, are extremely hydrophilic and have a relatively high molecular weight, resulting in poor oral absorption. At low pH values, such as are found in the stomach, sennosides precipitate, further inhibiting absorption. However, rhein, a sennoside component released in the intestine, is lipophilic and has a low molecular weight, characteristics that favor absorption (De Witte, 1993).

Ten subjects were administered two different commercially available senna preparations in a crossover fashion, once daily for 4 d. After repeated administration of Agiolax® containing 378 µg of "potential" aloe-emodin (free aloe-emodin plus aloe-emodin in the form of dianthrone sennosides and monoanthrone glucosides) and Sennatin® containing 400 µg of "potential" aloe-emodin, plasma levels of aloe-emodin were below the limit of detection (0.5 ng/mL). The average rhein $C_{max}$ was 43.8 ng/mL after the first dose of Sennatin® and 49.6 ng/mL after the fourth dose, with $T_{max}$ occurring 11.3 h and 9.7 h after the first and fourth doses, respectively. This time course corresponds to the time required for the sennosides to be transported to the colon, where intestinal flora metabolize the sennosides, releasing free rhein. An additional small peak in plasma concentration was noted 1–3 h after administration, corresponding to absorption of free rhein in the formulation. For Agiolax®, the average $C_{max}$ was 65.1 ng/mL after the first dose, and 81.8 ng/mL after the fourth dose. These peak plasma concentrations occurred 3.4 h and 4.9 h after the first and fourth doses. Maximal rhein concentrations thus appear much earlier after Agiolax® administration compared to Sennatin®, reflecting a higher amount of free rhein in the former preparation (Krumbiegel and Schulz, 1993).

### *25.5.2 Distribution*

Although lactating mothers have reported milk discoloration and laxative effect in breast-fed infants while taking senna (Curry, 1986), 15 mg of sennosides administered to 20 lactating women for 3 d resulted in rhein concentrations of < 10 ng/mL in the breast milk in 94% of the women (Faber, 1988). Breast-fed infants showed no signs of laxative exposure. Data in monkeys reflect these findings (Cameron et al., 1988).

### *25.5.3 Metabolism/Elimination*

Intestinal flora metabolizes the sennosides, releasing free rhein that is subsequently absorbed. The half-life of rhein is approx 7 h (Krumbiegel and Schulz, 1993). Chrysophanic acid is excreted in urine and colors acidic urine yellowish-brown and alkaline urine reddish-violet (Curry, 1986).

## *25.6 Chemical Analysis*

Determination of sennoside content can be achieved spectrophotometrically, or via HPLC (Christ et al., 1978; Lainonen et al., 1988). There is also a USP monograph (USP, 1999) that details the chemical analysis of senna.

## *25.7 Analysis of Biofluids*

Determination of human plasma levels of aloe-emodin and rhein using HPLC with a fluorometric detector has been described (Krumbiegel and Schulz, 1993).

Additional information on rhein and aloe-emodin determination in biofluids can be found in Section 24.8.

## 25.8 Regulatory Status

Although the component or components responsible for senna's effect have not been definitively identified, most pharmacopoeias standardize senna based on its sennoside B content. Both the German and European Pharmacopoeia require 2.5% for the leaves, 3.4% in the Alexandrian pods, and 2.2% in the Indian pods (Franz, 1993).

Senna pod and senna leaf are both approved German Commission E monographs (Blumenthal, 1998).

Senna has been available in many nonprescription laxative products in the United States for many years. The FDA is proposing to reclassify senna (including sennosides A and B, senna fluid extract, senna fruit extract, senna leaf powder, senna pod concentrate, and senna syrup) from Category I (generally recognized as safe and effective for the claimed therapeutic indication) to Category III (insufficient data to permit final classification). This decision was based on the positive genotoxicity data for the senna constituents aloe-emodin, emodin, and chrysophanol, as well as the need for additional carcinogenicity information. The 2-yr carcinogenicity study reviewed by the agency was determined to lack sufficient histopathologic data. Further study should also include chemical analysis to determine quantitatively the components of the senna preparation used in the study, as well as dose-ranging studies (Anonymous, 1998).

## References

Anonymous. Laxative drug products for over-the-counter human use; proposed amendment to the tentative final monograph. 21 CFR Parts 310 and 334. Fed Register 1998;63:33592–5.

Blumenthal M. The complete German Commission E monographs. Therapeutic guide to herbal medicines. Austin, TX: American Botanical Council, 1998.

Cameron BD, Phillips MWA, Fenerty CA. Milk transfer of rhein in the rhesus monkey. Pharmacology 1988;36(Suppl 1):221–5.

Christ B, Poppinghaus T, Wirtz-Peitz H. [Isolierung und strukturaufklarung eines neuen sennosids aus *Cassi senna*]. Arzneim Forsch 1978;28:225–31.

Curry CE. Laxative products. In: Handbook of nonprescription drugs. 8th ed Washington, DC: American Pharmaceutical Association, 1986.

De Witte P. Metabolism and pharmacokinetics of anthranoids. Pharmacology 1993;47(Suppl 1):86–97.

Faber P. Relevance of rhein excretion into breast milk. Pharmacology 1988;36(Suppl 1):212–20.

Franz G. The senna drug and its chemistry. Pharmacology 1993;47(Suppl 1):2–6.

Geboes K, Nijs G, Mengs U, Geboes KPS, Van Damme A, de Witte P. Effects of "contact laxatives" on intestinal and colonic epithelia cell proliferation. Pharmacology 1993;47(Suppl 1):187–95.

Heidemann A, Miltenburger HG, Mengs U. The genotoxicity status of senna. Pharmacology 1993;47(Suppl 1):178–86.

Krumbiegel G, Schulz HU. Rhein and aloe-emodin kinetics from senna laxatives in man. Pharmacology 1993;(Suppl 1):120–4.

Lainonen H, Marvola M, Hietala P, Pariainen T. The effect of different storage conditions on the chemical stability, laxative effect and acute toxicity of sennoside solutions. Pharmacol Toxicol 1988; 63:37–41.

Lyden-Sokolowski A, Nilsson A, Sjoberg P. Two-year carcinogenicity study with sennosides in the rat: emphasis on gastro-intestinal alterations. Pharmacology 1993;(Suppl 1):209–15.

Muller-Lissner SA. Adverse effects of laxatives: fact and fiction. Pharmacology 1993;(Suppl 1):138–45.

Nusko G, Schneider B, Müller G, Kusche J, Hahn EG. Retrospective study on laxative use and melanosis coli as risk factors for colorectal neoplasma. Pharmacology 1993;47(Suppl 1):234–41.

Perkins SL, Livesey JF. A rapid high-performance thin-layer chromatographic urine screen for laxative abuse. Clin Biochem 1993;26:179081.

Siegers C-P, Siemers J, Baretton G. Sennosides and aloin do not promote dimethylhydrazine-induced colorectal tumors in mice. Pharmacology 1993;47(Suppl 1):205–8.

Sonnenberg A, Muller AD. Constipation and cathartics as risk factors of colorectal cancer: a meta-analysis. Pharamcology 1993;47(Suppl 1):224–33.

United States Pharmacopoeial Convention (USP). USP 24-NF19. Rockville, MD: United States Pharmacopeial Convention, Inc; 1999.

Yang K, Fan K, Mengs U, Lipkin M. Effects of sennosides and nonanthranoid laxative on cytochemistry of epithelial cells in rat colon. Pharmacology 1993;47(Suppl 1):196.

# Chapter 26

# Cascara Sagrada

## Amy Renner and Melanie Johns Cupp

*Rhamnus purshiana* (D.C.), synonymous with *Frangula purshiana* (D.C.) A. Gray ex J.C. Cooper; buckthorn, chittem bark, sacred bark (Anonymous, 1996)

## 26.1 History and Traditional Uses

Cascara sagrada, the dried bark of *Rhamnus purshiana*, was first used in conventional American medicine in 1877, after being introduced as a laxative by Mexican and Spanish priests in California. A European counterpart (European buckthorn; *R. frangula*) was described by the Anglo-Saxons, and the berries were included in the 1650 *London Pharmacopoeia* (Anonymous, 1996).

## 26.2 Current Promoted Uses

Cascara sagrada is a nonprescription laxative. Since the removal of phenolphthalein from the US market in 1998, it has replaced phenolphthalein in several laxative products.

## 26.3 Products Available

Cascara sagrada is available in tablets, capsules, liquids (fluid extracts), and syrups. Fluid extracts are more reliable than the solid dosage forms. Aromatic cascara fluid extract is less bitter and less active than cascara sagrada fluid extract because of the use of magnesium oxide in its preparation (Curry, 1986). Cascara tea is available, but has an extremely bitter taste (Tyler, 1994).

From Forensic Science: *Toxicology and Clinical Pharmacology of Herbal Products*
Edited by: M. J. Cupp © Humana Press Inc., Totowa, New Jersey

Specific products containing cascara sagrada include concentrated milk of magnesia-cascara (cascara sagrada equivalent to 1 mL of aromatic fluid extract per teaspoon of milk of magnesia), Kondremul® with Cascara (220 mg per teaspoon of mineral oil), Nature's Remedy® Natural Vegetable Laxative Tablets (150 mg of cascara sagrada and 100 mg of aloe in a brown, round, film-coated tablet with the logo "NR").

## 26.4 Pharmacologic/Toxicologic Effects

### 26.4.1 Gastrointestinal Effects

The primary active ingredients of cascara sagrada include cascarosides A, B, C, and D, but barbaloin, chrysaloin, chryophanol, emodin, and aloe-emodin are also present (Tyler, 1994; Anonymous, 1996). The anthrone glucofrangulin is present in the cortex of the European species *Rhamni frangula* (De Witte, 1993). As with senna and aloe constituents, these anthrones produce an active secretion of water and electrolytes within the lumen of the small intestine. In addition, the anthrones inhibit absorption of water and electrolytes from the large intestine. This causes an increase in the volume of bowel contents, and strengthens the dilatation pressure in the intestine to stimulate peristalsis (Anonymous, 1996).

The use of fresh bark, which contains free anthrones, may cause severe vomiting, intestinal cramping, and possibly spasms (Anonymous, 1996). Therefore, the bark requires either storage for at least 1 yr before use or artificial conversion by heat to allow oxidation of the harsh laxative constituents, the emodin glycosides (anthrones), to less active monomeric forms (Tyler, 1994; Anonymous, 1996).

*See also* Section 25.4.2 for information on effects of chronic laxative use.

### 26.4.2 Nutritional and Metabolic Effects

*See* Section 25.4.3.

### 26.4.3 Carcinogenicity/Mutagenicity/Genotoxicity

2-Hydroxyemodin, ω-hydroxyemodin, and aloe-emodin, metabolites of the cascara sagrada constituents emodin and chrysophanol, appear to be genotoxic (Mueller et al., 1998).

*See also* Sections 25.4.1 for additional information on emodin and aloe-emodin, and Section 24.4.2 for general information on the association between anthranoid laxative use and colorectal cancer.

## 26.5 Case Reports of Toxicity Due to Commercially Available Products

A 30-yr-old white male developed occupational respiratory allergic disease induced by cascara sagrada and passion flower (Giavina-Bianchi et al., 1997). This individual worked in a pharmacy devoted to manual preparation of products, where he prepared chemicals 8 h each day, 6 d a week, with no mask or gloves. After working in the pharmacy in this capacity for 6 mo, he began experiencing sneezing; coryza; nasal congestion, pruritus of the nose, eyes, ears, and oropharynx; and ocular tearing and pruritus. Three months later, the patient developed a dry cough, chest pain, chest tightening, dyspnea, and wheezing. Symptoms improved on Sundays and in the evenings after work, but worsened when he entered the pharmacy in the morning and when he had contact with cascara sagada and passion flower. The patient began using an inhaled β-agonist, then sought medical treatment. History revealed a smoking habit with a 16-yr pack history, but no history of allergies. Pertinent findings on physical exam included slight hypertrophy and hyperemia of the nasal turbinates, and moderate diffuse wheezing bilaterally on auscultation. Peak flow rate (PFR) was 480 L/min, compared to the predicted 622 L/min. Pulmonary function tests revealed moderate obstruction with no significant reversibility. Forced vital capacity was 71%, forced expiratory volume in one second ($FEV_1$) was 68%, FEV/FCV was 97%, $FEV_{25-75\%}$ was 47%, and PFR was 73% of predicted. Laboratory results revealed 18% eosinophils, and a total immunoglobulin E (IgE) level of 1130 IU/mL. Maxillary sinuses showed reduced transparency bilaterally on X-ray film. Prick tests were positive for cascara sagrada and passion flower at all dilutions tested (0.01–10%). Bronchial provocation challenge with passion flower and cascara sagrada were positive. Western blot revealed IgE and IgG to passion flower and cascara sagrada protein. Electrophoresis of these proteins is described in the reference. The 6-mo latent period before symptom onset supports an IgE-mediated allergy.

## 26.6 Drug Interactions

Theoretically, given that cytochrome P-450 is involved in metabolism of emodin and chrysophanol to genotoxic metabolites (Mueller et al., 1998), enzyme inducers may increase the risk of colon cancer in cascara sagrada users, assuming that such a risk exists.

## 26.7 Pharmacokinetics/Toxicokinetics

Additional information on the pharmacokinetics of barbaloin, chrysophanol, and aloe-emodin can be found in Section 24.7.

Gut flora of rats, but not guinea pigs, are able to metabolize cascarosides to aloe-emodin. *Enterococcus faecalis* and *E. faecium,* common gut flora, lack the enzymes necessary for this conversion. Human fecal flora is able to metabolize barbaloin, but the bacteria responsible have not been identified (De Witte, 1993).

In rat liver microsomes, emodin is metabolized to ω-hydroxyemodin and 2-hydroxyemodin. The metabolism of the former could not be induced, but the formation of 2-hydroxyemodin was inducible. It appears that cytochrome P-450 1A2 (CYP1A2) is involved in the formation of this metabolite, although multiple enzymes may be involved in formation of both metabolites. Chrysophanol is metabolized by CYP450 to aloe-emodin (Mueller et al., 1998).

## 26.8 Analysis of Biofluids

*See* Section 24.8 regarding aloe-emodin.

## 26.9 Chemical Analysis

The USP monograph for cascara sagrada includes chemical analysis information (Tyler, 1994).

## 26.10 Regulatory Status

Cascara sagrada is available in nonprescription form pursuant to an approved monograph. It is also sold as a dietary supplement. However, the FDA is proposing that cascara sagrada be reclassified from a category I drug (monograph; recognized as safe and effective) to category III (more data needed) based on lack of mutagenicity, genotoxicity, or carcinogenicity data (Anonymous, 1998).

There is an official USP monograph for cascara sagrada. Dried bark of USP quality contains not <7% total hydroxyanthracenes calculated as cascaroside A. The cascarosides should make up at least 60% of this total (Tyler, 1994).

Cascara sagrada bark is an approved German Commission E monograph (Blumenthal, 1998).

## References

Anonymous. The Lawrence review of natural products. St. Louis, MO: Facts and Comparisons, 1996.

Anonymous. Laxative drug products for over-the-counter human use; proposed amendment to the tentative final monograph. 21 CFR Parts 310 and 334. Fed Register 1998;63:33592–5.

Blumenthal M. The complete German Commission E monographs. Therapeutic guide to herbal medicines. Austin, TX: American Botanical Council, 1998.
Curry CE. Laxative products. In: Handbook of nonprescription drugs, 8th edit., Washington, DC: American Pharmaceutical Association, 1986.
de Witte P. Metabolism and pharmacokinetics of anthranoids. Pharmacology 1993;46(Suppl 1):86–97.
Giavina-Bianchi PF, Castro FFM, Machado MLS, Duarte AJS. Occupational respiratory allergic disease induced by *Passiflora alata* and *Rhamnus purshiana*. Ann Allergy Asthma Immunol 1997;79:449–54.
Mueller SO, Stopper H, Dekant W. Biotransformation of the anthraquinones emodin and chrysophanol by cytochrome P450 enzymes. Drug Metab Disp 1998;26:540–6.
Tyler VE. The honest herbal, Binghamton, NY: Pharmaceutical Products Press, 1994.

# Chapter 27

# Dong Quai

## Rayna DeRosa and Melanie Johns Cupp

*Angelica polymorpha* Maxim. Var. sinensis, *A. senensis*, *A. dahurica*, *A. atropurpurea*, tang-kuei, dang-gui, Chinese angelica (Anonymous, 1997)

## 27.1 History and Traditional Uses

Dong quai root has been used for centuries throughout the East (Anonymous, 1997). It is a biennial or perennial member of the carrot family that can be found in meadows and damp places in Europe, Asia, Canada, and the northern United States. It has white to greenish-white flowers that bloom from May to August (Johns, 1996). The name dong quai means "proper order" (Anonymous, 1998b). Dong quai is known historically as a female remedy and has been referred to as "empress of the herbs," "sovereign herb for women," and "the female ginseng." Historic uses include treatment of dymenorrhea, amenorrhea, metorrhagia, menopausal syndromes, anemia, abdominal pain, injuries, migraine headaches, and arthritis. It is also said to ensure healthy pregnancies and easy deliveries (Walker et al., 1998).

## 27.2 Current Promoted Uses

In the United States, dong quai is promoted primarily to alleviate problems associated with menstruation and menopause.

## 27.3 Products Available

Dong quai is available in the United States as a fluid extract, tablets, capsules, and tea. Dong quai is also available in combination with other herbs

From Forensic Science: *Toxicology and Clinical Pharmacology of Herbal Products*
Edited by: M. J. Cupp © Humana Press Inc., Totowa, New Jersey

including red raspberry leaves, ginger root, licorice root, black cohosh root, queen of the meadow herb, blessed thistle herb, and marshmallow herb.

## 27.4 Pharmacologic/Toxicologic Effects

Because dong quai is a traditional Chinese herbal medicine, studies published in English are few.

### 27.4.1 Cardiovascular Effects

Researchers have isolated seven coumarin derivatives in dong quai that may have vasodilating and antispasmodic effects that may improve circulation (Johns, 1996), lower blood pressure, and dilate coronary arteries (Walker et al., 1998) These effects may be mediated through calcium channel blockade or inhibition of phosphodiesterase activity (Walker et al., 1998). Dong quai has also been purported to have a high iron content which may prove efficacious in the treatment and prevention of iron deficiency anemia (Anonymous, 1998a). Other reported cardiovascular effects include inhibition of platelet aggregation via inhibition of platelet serotonin release; prolongation of the refractory period; and reduction of atherosclerotic plaque formation. It is claimed to stimulate hematopoiesis secondary to its vitamin $B_{12}$ (0.25–0.4 µg/100 g dried root), folinic acid, and biotin content. Cardiovascular side effects include excessive bleeding (Huang, 1993).

### 27.4.2 Neurologic Effects

The findings of an in vitro study (Hu et al., 1994) in murine neurocyte culture suggest Dong quai may accelerate the growth of neurocyte processes and prevent decline in process branch number. The authors conclude that dong quai may promote neurocyte growth and delay age-related nerve atrophy in humans.

The tranquilizing and sedative effects that have been attributed to dong quai may help alleviate of mood swings and irritability in premenstrual syndrome (Johns, 1996). Dong quai has also been recommended for the treatment of migraine headaches (Walker et al., 1998).

### 27.4.3 Musculoskeletal Effects

Components of dong quai may be capable of relaxing smooth muscle of visceral organs, including the intestines and uterus, via calcium channel blockade (Walker et al., 1998). The water-soluble, nonvolatile extract causes uterine stimulation, while the alcoholic extract (an essential oil with a high boiling point) relaxes the uterus (Huang, 1993). This relaxation may help reduce the pain associated with menstrual cramps (Johns, 1996).

Osthole, a coumarin derivative found in the root, and ferulic acid, a volatile oil component, have been shown to inhibit platelet function (Gao and Chen, 1988; Hoult and Paya, 1996). A dong quai root preparation administered intravenously was also shown to prolong prothrombin time in humans (Mei et al., 1991).

### *27.4.4 Immunologic Effects/Antineoplastic Activity/Antimicrobial Activity*

Selective inhibition of experimentally induced immunoglobulin E (IgE) production has been demonstrated with aqueous extracts of dong quai (Sung et al., 1982). Thus, the herb may prove useful in the treatment and/or the prevention of allergic symptoms. However, a polysaccharide isolated from dong quai has been demonstrated to have an immunostimulant effect, and to have an antitumor effect in murine models, (Choy et al., 1994). Thus, it may prove to have efficacy in the treatment of cancer. The coumarins found in dong quai purportedly stimulate macrophages, enhancing phagocytosis. Other immunostimulatory actions include possible B-lymphocyte mitogenic activity, complement activation, interferon production (Walker et al., 1998), and interleukin-2 production (Chen, 1994). Dong quai may have activity against both Gram-negative and Gram-positive bacteria (Walker et al., 1998).

### *27.4.5 Anti-Inflammatory Activity*

Ferulic acid, a phenolic compound of dong quai, was found to exert analgesic and anti-inflammatory activity in both the early and late phases of the inflammatory process in laboratory animals (Ozaki, 1992). The analgesic action is said to be 1.7 times greater than that of aspirin (Walker et al., 1998). Histamine-mediated inflammation is not affected by dong quai (Sung et al., 1982).

### *27.4.6 Dermatological Effects*

Dong quai has been used in the treatment of eczema, neurodermic dermatitis, and psoriasis in Chinese medicine (Huang, 1993). Psoralen and bergapten, two of the furocoumarins found in dong quai, are photoreactive and have the potential to cause severe photodermatitis. Psoralens induce skin melanization in the presence of light and have been employed in the treatment of skin depigmentation and psoriasis (Ivie, 1981). The risk of phototoxicity in humans from ingestion of dong quai has not been characterized.

### *27.4.7 Carcinogenicity*

As noted previously, the furocoumarins, psoralen and bergapten, can induce photosensitization. These agents are also photocarcinogenic, and mutagenicity persists even in the absence of light (Ivie, 1981). As with photosensitization, risks attributable to human consumption of dong quai have not been documented. Safrole, a component of the essential oil of dong quai (Anonymous, 1997), has also demonstrated carcinogenicity and its ingestion is not recommended (*see Sassafras* monograph).

### 27.4.8 Estrogenic Effect

Dong quai is purported to contain phytoestrogens and is used for treatment of conditions of both high and low estrogen levels. These phytoestrogens are reportedly lower in potency than animal estrogens. However, in conditions of low estrogen, they are said provide adequate estrogen replacement, while in conditions characterized by high estrogen levels, these lower potency phytoestrogens are thought to compete with estrogen for estrogen binding sites. Use of dong quai is also recommended for amenorrhea, dysmenorrhea, and menorrhagia (Walker et al., 1998). Dong quai has also been reported to enhance regularity of menstrual cycles, control premenstrual symptoms, and alleviate some signs and symptoms of menopause (Johns, 1996). Despite these uses, it is unclear if dong quai actually contains phytoestogens. In a 24-wk, double-blind, placebo-controlled trial (Hirata et al., 1997) involving 71 postmenopausal women, 4.5 g daily of dong quai dried aqueous extract standardized to 0.5 mg/kg ferulic acid was not found to produce estrogen-like responses or to reduce menopausal symptoms. The main outcome measures were endometrial thickness, vaginal cytology, Kupperman index, and patient diary of vasomotor symptoms. There were also no changes in serum estrone, estradiol, sex hormone-binding globulin (SHBG), blood pressure, or weight. Adverse effects included burping, gas, and headache, which occurred with similar frequencies in both the placebo and dong quai groups.

### 27.4.9 Gastrointestinal Effects

Dong quai purportedly "lubricates" the intestine, relieving constipation (Johns, 1996). It has also been used to treat dysentery (Huang, 1993).

## 27.5 Drug Interactions

A 46-yr-old black female experienced an increase in INR from 2–3 to 4.05–4.9 after taking 565 mg of dong quai once or twice daily for 4 wk. The patient's past medical history included rheumatic heart disease, stroke, and atrial fibrillation. Medications included 5 mg/d of warfarin, 0.25 mg/d of digoxin, and 20 mg/d of furosemide. Upon dechallenge from dong quai, her

INR decreased to 3.41 after 2 wk, and then to 2.48 2 wk later, with no change in warfarin dose (Page and Lawrence, 1999). Because a study in rabbits showed that 2 g/kg of dong quai increased prothrombin time (PT) but did not alter warfarin pharmacokinetics (Lo et al., 1995), the authors suspected a pharmacodynamic mechanism for the interaction. They also hypothesized that warfarin might displace a component of dong quai from protein binding sites or inhibit its metabolism, thus increasing its plasma levels and effect on PT (Page and Lawrence, 1999).

## 27.6 Chemical Analysis

Thin-layer chromatography (TLC) and gas-liquid chromatography (GLC) analysis of psoralen and bergaptan in plant material has been described (Ivie et al., 1981).

## 27.7 Regulatory Status

Dong quai is a dietary supplement in the United States. There is no German Commission E monograph for dong quai (Blumenthal, 1998).

## References

Anonymous. The review of natural products. St. Louis, MO: Facts and Comparisons, 1997.

Anonymous. Dong Quai. Available from: URL:http://www.kcweb.com/herb/dongquai.htm. Accessed 1998a Oct 28.

Anonymous. Dong-quai or Dang gui. Available from: URl:http://www.mothernature.com/articles/dongquai/article1.stm. Accessed 1998b Sept 15.

Blumenthal M. The complete German Commission E monographs. Therapeutic guide to herbal medicine. Austin, TX: American Botanical Council, 1998.

Chen YH. [Experimental studies on the effects of danggui buxue decoction on Il-2 production of blood deficient mice]. Chung Kuo Chung Yao Tsa Chih 1994;19:739–41,763.

Choy YM, Leung KN, Cho CS, Wong CK, Pang PK. Immunopharmacological studies of low molecular weight polysaccharide from *Angelica sinenses*. Am J Chin Med 1994;22:137–45.

Gao SW, Chen ZJ. [Effects of sodium ferulate on platelet aggregation and platelet thromboxane A2 in patients with coronary heart disease]. Chung Hsi I Chieh Ho Tsa Chih 1988;8:263–5, 259.

Hirata JD, Swiersz LM, Zell B, Small R, Ettinger B. Does dong quai have estrogenic effects in postmenopausal women? A double-blind placebo-controlled trial. Fertil Steril 1997;68:981–6.

Hoult JR, Paya M. Pharmacological and biochemical actions of simple coumarins: natural products with therapeutic potential. Gen Pharmacol 1996;27:713–22.

Hu G, Liu Q, Cheng J, Wang H, Ma Z, Fu D, Gao S. [Effects of Chinese herb drugs on aging-related changes in neurocyte culture]. Chung Kuo Chung Yao Tsa Chih 1994;29:336–7.

Huang KC. The pharmacology of Chinese herbs. Boca Raton, FL: CRC Press, 1993.

Ivie GW, Holt DL, Ivey MC. Natural toxicants in human foods: psoralens in raw and cooked parsnip root. Science 1981;213:909–10.

Johns J. What is dong quai and what health problems can it help relieve? Nebr Mortar Pestle 1996;59:18.

Lo ACT, Chan K, Yeung JHK, Woo KS. Danggui (Angelica sinensis) affects the pharmacodynamics but not the pharmacokinetics of warfarin in rabbits. Eur J Drug Metab Pharmacokinet 1995;20:55–60.

Mei QB, Tao JY, Cui B. Advances in the pharmacological studies of radix Angelica sinesis (Oliv) Diels (Chinese Danggui). Chin Med J 1991;104:776–81.

Ozaki Y. Antiinflammatory effect of tetramethylpyrazine and ferulic acid. Chem Pharmacol Bull 1992;40:954–6.

Page RL, Lawrence JD. Potentiation of warfarin by dong quai. Pharmacotherapy 1999;19:870–6.

Sung CP, Baker AP, Holden DA, Smith WJ, Charkin LW. Effect of Angelica polymorpha on reaginic antibody production. J Nat Prod 1982;45:398–406.

Walker C, Bigus A, Massengil D. Dong quai. Available from: URL:http://www.unc.edu/~cebradsh/main.htm. Accessed 1998 Oct 27.

# Chapter 28

# Cat's Claw

## *Melissa Dawn Bostic and Melanie Johns Cupp*

*Uncaria tomentosa*, *Uncaria guianensis*, *Uncaria gambir*, una de gato, life-giving vine of Peru, samento (Anonymous, 1996)

## 28.1 History and Traditional Uses

Cat's claw is a twining woody vine with small, sharp thorns at the base of each pair of leaves that help the vine cling to trees, allowing it to grow up to 100 ft high (Giesler and Jones, 1998). These sharp thorns resemble the claws on the paw of a cat, thus the origin of the plant's common name. The genus *Uncaria* is found throughout the tropics, mainly in Asia and South America. It has a long history of use in South America as an antiinflammatory, antirheumatic, and contraceptive. It is also traditionally used to treat gastrointestinal ulcers, tumors, gonorrhea, dysentery, various skin problems, cancers of the female genitourinary tract, and intestinal disorders. Native South Americans also use cat's claw to "cleanse the kidneys" and treat bone pain. An Asian species, *Uncaria gambir*, is used as a tanning agent, an astringent, and an antidiarrheal (Anonymous, 1996). The stem, bark, roots, and leaves are all used medicinally (Giesler and Jones, 1998).

## 28.2 Current Promoted Uses

A case report of a cancer patient in Austria who underwent a miraculous recovery helped bring attention to cat's claw in the 1970s (Giesler and Jones, 1998). Some European reports that it is useful in the treatment of AIDS when used in combination with zidovudine (AZT), as well as the purported useful-

From Forensic Science: *Toxicology and Clinical Pharmacology of Herbal Products*
Edited by: M. J. Cupp © Humana Press Inc., Totowa, New Jersey

ness of cat's claw tea in the treatment of diverticulitis, hemorrhoids, peptic ulcer disease, colitis, parasites, and "leaky bowel syndrome" have fueled demand for the bark in the United States. American sources use *Unicaria tomentosa.* Although few clinical studies support its use for the treatment or prevention of any disease, claims include benefit as an immunostimulant, antihypertensive, and hypocholesterolemic agent. Other purported benefits include the prevention of colds, influenza, heart attack, and stroke. It is also promoted in the treatment of Crohn's disease, diabetes, lupus, chronic fatigue syndrome, gastritis, and premenstrual syndrome, (Williamson and Wyandt, 1997).

## 28.3 Products Available

Cat's claw is available in 300-mg capsules to be taken three times daily; 1000-mg time-release capsules to be taken once daily; liquid concentrate (8:1 in 20% alcohol) to be diluted in water and taken one to three times daily; and bark to be used for tea.

## 28.4 Pharmacologic/Toxicologic Effects

### 28.4.1 Antiviral Effects

An in vitro study examined the ability of six components of a a cat's claw bark extract to inhibit two RNA viruses, vesicular stomatitis virus (VSV) and rhinovirus type 1B (HRV 1B) (Aquino et al., 1989). Three major glycosides and three other quinovic acid glycosides were studied. An inhibitory effect was evident for all six compounds at relatively high concentrations (i.e., the $MIC_{50}$ approached the concentration that affected host cell morphology and growth).

### 28.4.2 Antineoplastic Activity

Reportedly, scientific studies by the National Cancer Institute (NCI) verify that some constituents of cat's claw may have anticancer properties (Anonymous, 1996).

### 28.4.3 Antimutagenic Activity

Cat's claw bark extracts are not mutagenic in the Ames test, and in fact show a protective effect against mutation caused by the photosensitizer 8-methoxy-psoralen (8-MOP) and UVA radiation. In addition to testing the extracts and fractions directly, the investigators also tested urine from two volunteers (a smoker and a nonsmoker) who had ingested 6.5 g/d of cat's claw for 15 d. The decoction was prepared by boiling the dried bark in water for 3 h until the initial volume was reduced by one third. Interestingly, the smoker's urine, but not the nonsmoker's urine, was mutagenic when tested before taking the cat's claw decoction, but showed a decrease in mutagenic potential at the end of treatment. This effect persisted for 8 d following discontinuation of cat's claw (Rizzi et al., 1993).

### *28.4.4 Cytotoxicity*

Aqueous extracts of cat's claw were tested for cytotoxicity in four in vitro bioassays using Chinese hamster ovary cells and bacterial cells (Santa Maria et al., 1997). Concentrations of 10, 20, 30, 40, 50, 75, and 100 mg/mL were used. The neutral protein assay (measures inhibition of cell growth), the total protein content assay, the tetrazolium assay (measures mitochondrial succinic dehydrogenase activity), and the microtox assay (measures inhibition of light output from a luminescent bacterium) showed no evidence of cytotoxicity.

## *28.5 Case Reports of Toxicity Due to Commercially Available Products*

A 35-yr-old woman was diagnosed with systemic lupus erythematosus (SLE) in 1984 after presenting with hematuria and proteinuria in the nephrotic range. Renal biopsy revealed diffuse membranoproliferative glomerulonephritis (WHO class IV). Thereafter, she was treated periodically with immunosuppressive agents, and her serum creatinine (SCr) stabilized at 2.0 mg/dL. Hematuria and proteinuria persisted, although they were in the nonnephrotic range. In 1996, the patient presented with a SCr of 2.6 mg/dL, up from 2.0 mg/dL 1 mo earlier. Physical exam was normal, as was blood pressure. The patient had no complaints. Urinalysis revealed 2+ protein, hematuria, numerous white blood cells, and white blood cell casts. Serum complement levels were normal. Anti-double-stranded DNA titer was 1:80, compared to 1:1076 during a previous SLE exacerbation. The patient's medications included prednisone, atenolol, metolazone, furosemide, and nifedipine. The most recent addition to her medication regimen was a Peruvian cat's claw preparation that she had been taking four times daily for relief of arthritic symptoms. The diagnosis of acute allergic interstitial nephritis was made, and cat's claw was discontinued. One month later, her SCr was 2.7 mg/dL, but there was no evidence of pyuria or white blood cell casts on urinalysis (Hilepo et al., 1997).

## *28.6 Regulatory Status*

Cat's claw is considered a dietary supplement by the US Food and Drug Administration. There is no German Commission E monograph for cat's claw.

## REFERENCES

Anonymous. Cat's claw (Una de gato). The Lawrence review of natural products. St. Louis, MO: Facts and Comparisons, 1996.

Aquino R, DeSimone F, Pizza C. Plant metabolites. Structure and in vitro antiviral activity of quinovic acid glycosides from *Uncaria tomentosa* and *Guettarda platypoda*. J Nat Prod 1989;52:679–85.

Giesler M, Jones K. Cat's claw. Available from: URL: http://www.unc.edu/~cebradsh/catsclaw.html. Accessed 1998 Nov 2.

Hilepo JN, Bellucci AG, Mossey RT. Acute renal failure caused by "cat's claw" herbal remedy in a patient with systemic lupus erythematosus. Nephron 1997;77:361.

Rizzi R, Re F, Bianchi A, DeFeo V, deSimone F, Bianchi L, Stivala LA. Mutagenic and antimutagenic activities of *Uncaria tomentosa* and its extracts. J Ethnopharmacol 1993;38:63–77.

Santa Maria A, Lopez A, Diaz MM, Alban J, Galan de Mera A, Vincente Orlenna JA, Pozuelo JM. Evaluation of the toxicity of *Uncaria tomentosa* by bioassays in vitro. J Ethnopharmacol 1997;57:183–7.

Williamson JS, Wyandt CM. Herbal therapies: the facts and the fiction. Drug Topics 1997;(Aug 4):7885.

# Part III

# Summary of Toxicities and Drug Interactions

# Chapter 1

# *Summary of Toxicities and Drug Interactions*

Types of data supporting toxicity or drug interaction:

C = case report
E = epidemiologic data
A = animal data
V = in vitro data
T = theoretical concern

Allergic
- *Aloe* — C
- Cascara sagrada — C
- Cat's Claw — C
- Chamomile — C
- *Echinacea* — C
- Garlic — C

Carcinogenicity
- *Aloe* — E, V
- Cascara sagrada –E
- Chaparral — C
- Colt's foot — A
- Comfrey — A
- *Sassafras* — A
- Senna — E, V

Cardiovascular
- *Ephedra* — C

Dermatologic
- Garlic — C
- Kava — C
- St. John's wort — C

Hematologic
- Feverfew — V
- Garlic — V, C
- *Ginkgo* — C

Hepatic
- Chaparral — C, A
- Colt's foot — C, A
- Comfrey — C, A
- *Sassafras* — A
- Scullcap — C (coingestants involved)
- Valerian — C (coingestants involved)

Neurologic
- *Ephedra* — C
- *Ginkgo* — C
- Kava — C
- St. John's Wort — C
- Valerian — C

From Forensic Science: *Toxicology and Clinical Pharmacology of Herbal Products*
Edited by: M. J. Cupp © Humana Press Inc., Totowa, New Jersey

Reproduction
- Colt's foot — C
- Valerian — T

Renal
- Cat's claw — C
- Chaparral — C, A
- *Ephedra* — C
- Licorice — C

Drug interactions
- *Aloe* — T
- Cascara sagrada — V
- Chaparral — V
- Comfrey — V
- Dong quai — A, C
- *Ephedra* — T
- Feverfew — T
- Garlic — T
- Ginger — T
- *Ginkgo* — C
- Ginseng — C
- Hawthorn — T, V
- Kava — C
- St. John's wort — C, V
- Valerian — A

# Index

## B



## C

**L**

**M**

## N



## O



## P

**W**



**X**



**Y**

**Z**